Seminars
in Child and Adolescent

8.9289

College Seminars Series

Series Editors

Professor Anne Farmer Professor of Psychiatric Nosology, Institute of Psychiatry and Honorary Consultant Psychiatrist, South London and Maudsley NHS Trust, London

Dr Louise Howard Research Fellow, Institute of Psychiatry, London

Dr Elizabeth Walsh Clinical Senior Lecturer, Institute of Psychiatry, London

Professor Greg Wilkinson Professor of Liaison Psychiatry, University of Liverpool and Honorary Consultant Psychiatrist, Royal Liverpool University Hospital

---

Praise for the first editions of books in the series

This very reasonably priced textbook should improve knowledge and stimulate interest in a common and challenging topic.

BMJ

The editors state that this book is not intended to be a substitute for supervised clinical practice. It is, however, the next best thing.

Psychological Medicine

...this book joins others in the series in being both readily understandable and accessible.. should be on every psychiatrist's bookshelf...

Journal of Psychopharmacology

... an excellent, up-to-date introductory text. It can be strongly recommended for residents, clinicians, and researchers.

American Journal of Psychiatry

Every chapter informs, but also pleases. This is expert teaching by skilled and committed teachers.

Journal of the Royal Society of Medicine

Congratulations are due to the editors for the breadth of their vision and to the authors for the thoroughness and liveliness of their contributions.

Psychological Medicine

...an excellent teaching and revision aid for psychiatric trainees...

Criminal Behaviour and Mental Health

Seminars in Child and Adolescent Psychiatry

Second edition

Edited by Simon G. Gowers

Gaskell

Gaskell is an imprint of the Royal College of Psychiatrists, 17 Belgrave Square, London SW1X 8PG
http://www.rcpsych.ac.uk

British Library Cataloguing-in-Publication Data.
A catalogue record for this book is available from the British Library.
ISBN 1-904671-13-6

Distributed in North America by Balogh International Inc.

The views presented in this book do not necessarily reflect those of the Royal College
of Psychiatrists, and the publishers are not responsible for any error of omission or fact.

The Royal College of Psychiatrists is a registered charity (no. 228636).
Printed by Bell & Bain Limited, Glasgow, UK.

Contents

Tables, boxes and figures

Figures

Contributors

Sue Bailey, Adolescent Forensic Services, Salford and Trafford Mental Health NHS Trust, Bury New Road, Prestwich, Manchester M25 3BL

Dora Black, Honorary Consultant, Department of Child and Adolescent Mental Health, Great Ormond Street Hospital, London WC1N 3JH

Andrew J. Cotgrove, Young People's Centre, Pine Lodge, 79 Liverpool Road, Chester CH2 1AW

Stephen Earnshaw, Dewi Jones Unit, Mulberry House, Alder Hey, Eaton Road, Liverpool L12 2AP

Mary Eminson, Child and Adolescent Mental Health Services, Royal Bolton Hospital, Minerva Road, Bolton BL4 0JR

David M. Foreman, Child and Adolescent Mental Health Services, Skimped Hill Health Centre, Market Square, Bracknell, Berkshire RG12 1LH

Robin Glaze, St Edwards Hospital, 7 Garden View Court, Leeds LS8 1EA

Ian M. Goodyer, Developmental Psychiatry Section, University of Cambridge, Douglas House, 18B Trumpington Road, Cambridge CB2 2AH

Simon G. Gowers, Professor of Adolescent Psychiatry, University of Liverpool, Child and Adolescent Psychiatry and Psychology, Pine Lodge Academic Unit, 79 Liverpool Road, Chester CH2 1AW

Latha Hackett, The Winnicott Centre, 195–197 Hathersage Road, Manchester M13 0JE

Steve Hughes, Birch Hill Hospital, Union Road, Rochdale OL12 9QB

Lindsey Kent, Developmental Psychiatry Section, University of Cambridge, Douglas House, 18 Trumpington Road, Cambridge CB2 2AH

David M. Kingsley, Orchard Young People's Unit, Cheadle Royal Hospital, 100 Wilmslow Road, Cheadle, Cheshire SK8 3DG

Clare Lamb, North Wales Adolescent Service, Cedar Court, 65 Victoria Park, Colwyn Bay, Conwy LL29 7AJ

Ann Le Couteur, Fleming Nuffield Unit, Burdon Terrace, Newcastle upon Tyne NE2 3AE

Sean Maskey, Michael Rutter Centre, Maudsley Hospital, De Crespigny Park, London SE5 8AF

Paul McArdle, Fleming Nuffield Unit, Burdon Terrace, Newcastle upon Tyne NE2 3AE

Tim Morris, Mary Burbury Unit, East Lancashire CAMHS, Casterton Avenue, Burnley BB10 2PQ

Bobby Smyth, Bridge House Addiction Service, Cherry Orchard Hospital, Ballyfermot, Dublin 10, Ireland

Paul Tiffin, Newberry Centre, Westlane Hospital, Acklam Road, Middlesborough TS5 4EE

Judith Trowell, Tavistock and Portman NHS Trust, 120 Belsize Lane, London NW3 5BA

Andrew Weaver, Child and Adolescent Mental Health Services, Alderley Building, Macclesfield District General Hospital, Victoria Road, Macclesfield SK10 3BL

Alison Wood, Adolescent Psychiatry Service, Bolton, Salford and Trafford Mental Health NHS Trust, Bury New Road, Prestwich, Manchester M25 3BL

Foreword

Series Editors

We are very pleased to introduce the second editions of *College Seminars*, now updated to reflect changes in the understanding, treatment and management of psychiatric illness and mental health, as well as changes in the MRCPsych examination and the need for continuing professional development. These titles represent a distillation of the collective wisdom of hundreds of individuals, written in approachable, tutorial-style prose.

As the body responsible for maintaining professional standards and developing the MRCPsych curriculum, the Royal College of Psychiatrists has a duty to assist trainees in psychiatry as well as all practising psychiatrists throughout their careers. The first of the *College Seminars*, a series of textbooks covering the breadth of psychiatry, were published by the College in 1993. Widely acclaimed as essential and approachable texts, they were each written and edited to the brief of 'all the College requires the trainee to know about a sub-specialty, and a little bit more'.

Anne Farmer
Louise Howard
Elizabeth Walsh
Greg Wilkinson

Preface

In the 12 years since the publication of the first edition of *Seminars in Child and Adolescent Psychiatry*, considerable changes have taken place in the provision of UK child and adolescent mental health services and in postgraduate medical education. In many respects these developments have been very positive; government expenditure on child psychiatry has grown considerably in recent years with expansion of multidisciplinary teams throughout much of the country. Research has grown and we have an increasing evidence base for our interventions, some backed by guidance from the National Institute for Clinical Excellence.

The Royal College of Psychiatrists has recognised the importance of our sub-specialty, and experience in child and adolescent psychiatry or learning disabilities has become mandatory in basic training schemes. As postgraduate education undergoes its latest reorganisation, the opportunity for 'taster' experience of child psychiatry in foundation programmes for non-career psychiatrists is evolving, providing the opportunity for a broader range of doctors to gain familiarity with a sometimes bewildering branch of medicine.

The second edition of this book has been extensively updated and extended, with a number of new chapters covering the major disorders and the range of service provision. It is aimed at juniors requiring a basic introduction to the field, while at the same time providing enough depth to satisfy the requirements of trainees taking postgraduate examinations and those wanting greater levels of knowledge, evidence and understanding.

Simon G. Gowers

Acknowledgements

The first edition of this book, edited by Dora Black and David Cottrell, became essential reading for trainees in psychiatry and attracted many into our sub-specialty. Thanks are due to them for preparing the groundwork on which this new edition is based.

Grateful thanks also to Linda Rhodes for liaising with the authors and preparing the first draft of the manuscript. We are grateful to Lauren Thomas (illustrations below and overleaf) and to the five anonymous contributors of the artwork used on pp. 19–20.

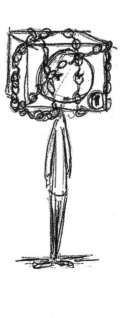

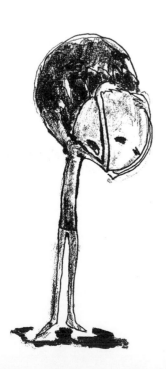

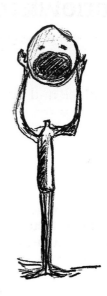

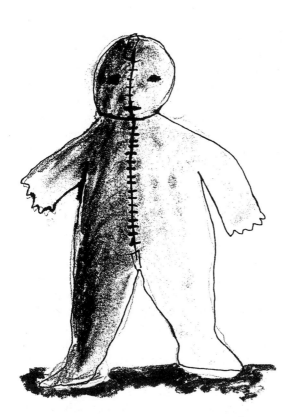

CHAPTER 1

A brief history of child and adolescent psychiatry

Dora Black and Simon G. Gowers

The history of the treatment of children's deviant behaviour goes back centuries (Wardle, 1991), but the first child guidance clinic, established in Boston in the early 1920s, continued the focus on delinquent children and marked the beginning of the child guidance movement. This launched the application of 'scientific' methods to the study and treatment of deviant children, and quickly extended to the UK and Europe.

The first child guidance clinic in the UK was founded by the Jewish Health Organisation in the East End of London in 1927. Emanuel Miller, a psychiatrist, was appointed as honorary director together with a psychiatric social worker who had trained in the Boston Clinic, and a psychologist. A year later, the London Child Guidance Centre opened under the direction of Dr William Moody, who had trained at the Maudsley Hospital where children and adolescents had been treated for some years. When Miller moved to the Tavistock Clinic in 1933, a new department for children was established, pioneering the recognition of family influences on child psychopathology, and a focus on the assessment and treatment of the whole family (Hersov, 1986).

Although general psychiatrists had sometimes treated children and adolescents, and some paediatricians had considered the psychological as well as physical aspects of paediatric disorder, it was only after the Second World War that child psychiatry separated as a specialty from general psychiatry. By the late 1940s, child guidance clinics were spreading rapidly and by the time of the establishment of the National Health Service (NHS) in 1948, many local authority districts provided a rudimentary service. By the end of the 1960s, most child psychiatrists in the UK were employed by the NHS and were working in child guidance clinics with social workers, educational psychologists and sometimes child psychotherapists and teachers. The services were usually housed in accommodation owned by the local education authority, which provided administrative services. Occasionally there was joint provision with the NHS, but hospital-based child psychiatric clinics were still relatively rare. The geographical isolation of the clinics from other health facilities led to the alienation of some child psychiatrists from their roots in medicine and general psychiatry, while educational psychologists were divorced from colleagues in academic and clinical psychology. As social workers were equally separated from their colleagues in local authority departments, there was little cross-fertilisation of ideas and few opportunities for teaching, research or the development of the political expertise to enable effective expansion of services to take place. A shortage of trainees in child psychiatry to challenge established dogma contributed to the entrenchment of outdated and ineffective practices in some clinics. Classification was rudimentary, the aetiology and treatment of most disorders was poorly understood and there had been almost no research on the therapies being used (Black, 1987).

By the 1970s services were developing rapidly, but were rarely based on any assessment of the needs of the community. Kolvin (1973) found that less than 1% of the child population were receiving help from child guidance clinics, yet 7–20% of children were identified as suffering from a definite and functionally disabling psychiatric disorder (Rutter *et al*, 1970). The lack of available therapeutic resources was sometimes exacerbated by a focus on psychoanalytic training, and consequent intensive and lengthy treatment.

Academic departments of child and adolescent psychiatry were established earlier in the USA than in Europe. The first academic department of child psychiatry to open in England in 1972 was led by Professor Michael Rutter at the Maudsley Hospital. However, the growth of academic departments was slow. Kanner's delineation of the new syndrome of infantile autism (Kanner, 1943), Robertson's films on children in hospital (Robertson, 1952, 1958), Bowlby's seminal ideas on attachment and loss (Bowlby, 1969, 1973, 1980), Winnicott's concept of 'good-enough' mothering and his attention to mother–child relationships (Winnicott, 1965), Robin's long-term follow-up of child guidance patients (Robin,1966), Rutter's work on epidemiology (Rutter *et al*, 1970) and Kolvin's careful assessment of treatment strategies (Kolvin *et al*, 1981) are landmarks in the history of child psychiatry.

By the end of the 20th century, most UK medical schools employed academic child and adolescent psychiatrists, while most postgraduate higher training schemes had links to a university department.

The late 20th century also saw a number of developments in therapeutics. Early treatments had been based on psychoanalytic theory and technique, as applied to children by Anna Freud (1928) and Melanie Klein (1932), and play therapy, as described by Lowenfeld (1935), with concurrent guidance for the mother (but rarely the father) by psychiatric social workers. Other treatment approaches such as behaviour therapy (developed mainly by clinical psychologists), family therapy in its various schools, group therapies and occasionally drug therapies were integrated into eclectic practice in the 1970s and 1980s. Although some services might have specialised in a form of therapy or a type of disorder until the mid 1980s, more comprehensive services subsequently developed. Pharmacotherapy became more widespread as the practice of child and adolescent psychiatry became eclectic and more evidence-based. More recently, cognitive–behavioural therapy, cognitive–analytic therapy, dialectical behaviour therapy and other approaches have been developed, often with a focus on particular patient groups. Many parts of the UK have seen a great expansion of child psychiatric services into the 21st century, and although most of these services have become multidisciplinary, many have seen a withdrawal of social work input. This is despite the establishment in the 1990s of child protection teams and moves towards the joint commissioning of child and adolescent mental health services (CAMHS) by health, education and social services.

The advent of clinical audit in the NHS required all services to measure performance against standards, following the 'purchaser/ provider split', to report on these to service commissioners. The establishment of the UK National Institute for Clinical Excellence at the turn of the 21st century heralded the introduction of national treatment guidelines, the first on the use of methylphenidate (National Institute for Clinical Excellence, 2000), to be followed by guidelines on the treatment on childhood eating disorders and depression, in order to standardise clinical practice.

Training for child psychiatry

A famous debate on training took place in the 1960s between Dr Donald Winnicott of Paddington Green Hospital and Professor Aubrey Lewis of the Maudsley Hospital (Lewis, 1963; Winnicott, 1963), with Winnicott advocating the route for training child psychiatrists through paediatrics and Lewis through general psychiatry. Although there is much to be said for child and adolescent psychiatrists having a sound basic training in both disciplines before starting higher training, many now have little or no experience of paediatrics. The Royal College of Psychiatrists requires all higher trainees in child and adolescent psychiatry to have passed the membership examination after training in general psychiatry. By the turn of the 21st century, it was mandatory for all those completing basic training to have had 6 months' experience of either child and adolescent psychiatry or services for children with learning disabilities. Higher training had by this time, however, been reduced from 4 years to 3 years in order to bring postgraduate training into line with the rest of Europe. During higher training, the Royal College of

Psychiatrists has become increasingly prescriptive about training requirements; balancing clinical training with research and the development of a wide range of therapeutic skills. Management experience is also required in a very full training programme, which is formally reviewed at annual intervals to ensure attainment of a Certificate of Completion of Satisfactory Training after 3 years. As the evidence base for the practice of child psychiatry is growing rapidly, clinicians have appreciated the necessity to update skills and knowledge on a regular basis. The necessity for 'life-long learning' is now established, and 21st-century practitioners are required to regularly update personal development plans and submit to annual appraisal within the NHS.

Organisation of services

A series of studies and reports in the 1970s and 1980s (Brunel Institute of Organisation and Social Studies, 1976; Royal College of Psychiatrists, 1978, 1986; Interdisciplinary Standing Committee, 1981) exposed difficulties in the traditional way of organising child guidance services. A perceived lack of clearly defined leadership and a muddled management structure led to intractable problems in some clinics. Some (Graham, 1976; Rutter, 1986) saw positive trends in the practice of child psychiatry – a reflection of the efforts that had been made over the years to maintain good relationships in the multidisciplinary team, although this was often at the expense of efficiency and good practice. By the early 1980s, child psychiatric practice had moved on little from the historical child guidance model based on the disciplines of psychiatry, social work and educational psychology, in a style of practice unsuited to the developing NHS. Modern practice needed to be more flexible, with contributions from the disciplines of clinical psychology, psychiatric nursing, child psychotherapy, teaching, dietetics, occupational therapy, art and music therapies, physiotherapy, paediatrics, general psychiatry, radiology, neurology and others as needed. By the early 1990s, reviews of child and adolescent mental health services consistently reported that services were incomplete and uncoordinated, as well as being patchy across the country (Kurtz et al, 1994). Services were criticised on the basis of their failure to meet local need and their exclusion of those who did not meet criteria for the particular treatments offered by the local service. There was often a lack of planning, particularly where liaison between the three statutory agencies (education, health and social services) was required. There was also poor communication with the voluntary sector.

In 1995 the Health Advisory Service proposed a strategic approach to commissioning and delivering a comprehensive CAMHS (Health Advisory Service, 1995). This emphasised a continuum of care, a range of treatments in a variety of settings (community, day care and residential) and a seamless transition from one level of care to the next. In the UK the Department of Health recommended the adoption of a tiered model of service, in which Tier 1 comprises services delivered in primary care, Tier 2 CAMHS professionals working singly, Tier 3 the multidisciplinary specialist CAMHS, and Tier 4 very specialised out-patient services for children and young people with complex disorders and in-patient care. With the development of NHS trusts, child and adolescent mental health services found themselves in a range of acute, community and mental health organisations. In the early 21st century, a number of these reorganised into specialist mental health or 'partnership' trusts. The private sector became a significant provider of CAMH services for the first time (particularly Tier 4), with NHS commissioners purchasing private services for NHS patients where there were gaps – particularly in the field of eating disorders. The implementation of the Children's National Service Framework (Department of Health, 2004) will see a blueprint for services that can begin to even out inequalities. The Commission for Health Improvement and later the Commission of Health Audit and Inspection were also designed to improve and monitor the quality of services. Although the demands on child psychiatrists are constantly growing, with a greater expectation of their having a role in youth offending teams and the treatment of those with early-onset psychosis, funding for CAMHS has grown and services are now able to provide a more comprehensive range of interventions than ever before in their history.

References

Black, D. (1987) The future of child guidance. In *Progress in Child Health:* vol. 3 (ed. J. A. Macfarlane), pp. 155–163. Edinburgh: Churchill Livingstone.

Bowlby, J. (1969) *Attachment and Loss, vol. 1.* London: Hogarth Press.

Bowlby, J. (1973) *Attachment and Loss, vol. 2. Separation.* London: Hogarth Press.

Bowlby, J. (1980) *Attachment and Loss, vol. 3. Loss.* London: Hogarth Press.

Brunel Institute of Organisation and Social Studies (1976) *Future Organisation in Child Guidance and Allied Work* (Working Paper HS1). Uxbridge: Brunel University.

Department of Health (2004) National Service Framework for Children Young People and Maternity Services (http://www.dh.gov.uk/PolicyAndGuidance/ HealthAndSocialCareTopics/ChildrenServices/ChildrenServicesInformation/fs/en).

Freud, A. (1928) *Introduction to the Technique of Child Analysis.* New York: Nervous and Mental Disease Publishing.

Graham P. (1976) Management in child psychiatry: recent trends. *British Journal of Psychiatry,* **129**, 97–108.

Health Advisory Service (1995) *Child and Adolescent Mental Health Services. Together We Stand.* London: HMSO.

Hersov, L. (1986) Child psychiatry in Britain – the last 30 years. *Journal of Child Psychology and Psychiatry,* **27**, 781–802.

Interdisciplinary Standing Committee (1981) *Interdisciplinary Work in Child Guidance*. London: Child Guidance Trust.

Kanner, L. (1943) Autistic disturbance of affective contact. *Nervous Child*, **2**, 217–250.

Klein, M. (1932) *The Psychoanalysis of Children*. London: Hogarth Press.

Kolvin, I. (1973) Evaluation of psychiatric services for children in England and Wales. In *Roots of Evaluation* (eds J. K. Wing & J. Hafner), pp. 131–173. Oxford: Oxford University Press.

Kolvin, I., Garside, R. F., Nicol, A. R., *et al* (1981) *Help Starts Here: The Maladjusted Child in the Ordinary School*. London: Tavistock.

Kurtz, Z., Thornes, R. & Wolkind, S. (1994) *Services for the Mental Health of Children and Young People in England, A National Review* (report to the Department of Health South West Thames Regional Health Authority). London: HMSO.

Lewis, A. (1963) Symposium: Training for child psychiatry. *Journal of Child Psychology and Psychiatry*, **4**, 75–84.

Lowenfeld, M. (1935) *Play in Childhood*. London: Gollancz.

National Institute for Clinical Excellence (2000) *Guidance on the Use of Methylphenidate for Attention Deficit Hyperactivity Disorder (ADHD)*. Technology Appraisal Guidance No.13. London: National Institute for Clinical Excellence.

Robertson, J. (1952) *A Two Year Old Goes to Hospital* (film). Ipswich: Concord Films Council.

Robertson, J. (1958) *Going to Hospital with Mother* (film). Ipswich: Concord Films Council.

Robins, L. (1966) *Deviant Children Grown Up*. Baltimore, MD: Williams & Wilkins.

Royal College of Psychiatrists (1978) The role, responsibilities and work of the child and adolescent psychiatrist. *Bulletin of the Royal College of Psychiatrists*, **2**, 127–131.

Royal College of Psychiatrists (1986) The role, responsibilities and work of the child and adolescent psychiatrist. *Bulletin of the Royal College of Psychiatrists*, **10**, 202–206.

Rutter, M. (1986) Child psychiatry: looking 30 years ahead. *Journal of Child Psychology and Psychiatry*, **27**, 803–841.

Rutter, M., Tizard, J. & Whitmore, K. (1970) *Education, Health and Behaviour*. London: Longman.

Wardle, C. (1991) Historical influences on services for children and adolescents before 1900. In *150 Years of British Psychiatry, 1841–1991* (eds G. E. Berrios & H. Freeman), pp. 279–293. London: Gaskell.

Winnicott, D. (1963) Symposium: training for child psychiatry. *Journal of Child Psychology and Psychiatry*, **4**, 85–91.

Winnicott, D. (1965) *The Family and Individual Development*. London: Tavistock.

Normal development and developmental theories

Latha Hackett

Development, or the expectation of orderly change, is the backdrop against which all child psychiatry is practised. It is arguable that all psychiatric disorders in children represent deviations or delays of development. An understanding of development, and the theories and evidence for what carries it forward, holds it up or deviates it from the expected path, is important because it affects our judgement of what is normal. It also informs our clinical method, and governs the framework in which we formulate cases and plan treatment.

Development is a lifelong process. It involves a continuous interaction between heredity and environment. Genetic determinants express themselves through the process of maturation. Motor development is largely a maturational process, as normal children acquire skills such as crawling, standing and walking in the same orderly sequence at roughly the same age. Development in other areas such as language, academic ability and personality may be permanently affected by early experiences.

This chapter briefly describes normal development and theories of development. Global developmental delay is described in Chapter 8.

The range of normal development is wide and merges with the abnormal. Table 2.1 describes the main features of development at different ages. For a detailed description, see Illingworth (1990).

Normal child development

Motor development

Of all mammals, human infants are the most immature at birth and require the longest period of development before they are capable of all the skills characteristic of their species. The sequence of development is the same in all healthy children, although some infants reach each stage ahead of others. Motor development is in the cephalocaudal direction, head control preceding hand control, which precedes walking.

Table 2.1 Developmental milestones

Age	Motor	Speech	Vision and hearing	Social development
4–6 weeks				Smiles at mother
6–8 weeks		Vocalises		
3 months	Prone: head held up for prolonged periods. No grasp reflex	Talks a great deal	Follows dangling toy from side to side. Turns head to sound	Squeals with pleasure appropriately Discriminates smile
5 months	Holds head steady. Goes for objects and gets them. Objects taken to mouth	Enjoys vocal play		Smiles at mirror image
6 months	Transfers objects from one hand to the other. Pulls self up to sit and sits erect with supports. Rolls over prone to supine. Palmar grasp of cube	Double syllable sounds such as 'mumum' and 'dada'	Localises sound 45 cm lateral to either ear	May show 'stranger shyness'
9–10 months	Wriggles and crawls. Sits unsupported. Picks up objects with pincer grasp	Babbles tunefully	Looks for toys dropped	Apprehensive of strangers
1 year	Stands holding furniture. Stands alone for a second or two, then collapses with a bump	Babbles 2 or 3 words repeatedly	Drops toys, and watches where they go	Cooperates with dressing, waves goodbye, understands simple commands
18 months	Can walk alone. Picks up toy without falling over. Gets up/ down stairs holding onto rail. Begins to jump with both feet. Can build a tower of 3 or 4 cubes and throw a ball	'Jargon'. Many intelligible words		Demands constant mothering. Drinks from a cup with both hands. Feeds self with a spoon
2 years	Able to run. Walks up and down stairs 2 feet per step. Builds tower of 6 cubes	Joins 2–3 words in sentences		Parallel play Dry by day
3 years	Goes up stairs 1 foot per step and downstairs 2 feet per step. Copies circle, imitates cross and draws man on request. Builds tower of 9 cubes	Constantly asks questions. Speaks in sentences		Cooperative play Undresses with assistance Imaginary companions
4 years	Goes down stairs 1 foot per step, skips on 1 foot. Imitates gate with cubes, copies a cross	Questioning at its height. Many infantile substitutions in speech		Dresses and undresses with assistance Attends to own toilet needs
5 years	Skips on both feet and hops. Draws a man and copies a triangle. Gives age	Fluent speech with few infantile substitutions		Dresses and undresses alone
6 years	Copies a diamond. Knows right from left and number of fingers	Fluent speech		

Normal feeding

The feeding relationship between the newborn infant and mother in the first few days of life is largely dependent on instinctively determined behaviour based on physiological mechanisms. It also depends on whether it is mutually enjoyable or not. The secretion of breast milk is a neurohumoral response; the infant's suckling triggers the milk letdown reflex. After a few days, a rhythm is usually established between the baby's need and milk production. Similarly, in bottle-fed babies a pattern of feeding is established with gradual lengthening of the period between late-night and morning feeds.

Newborn infants usually cannot place their lips tightly around the areola of the breast or the teat of the bottle, so milk leaks out at the corner of the mouth. As they mature, they are able to do so. They are able to drink out of a cup at 4–5 months, to chew at 6 months, and like to hold a bottle. At 15 months, they are able to manage a cup without dropping it. They can manage a knife and fork by the age of 2–3 years.

Both the child and the mother influence early feeding. The child should have an intact gastrointestinal system and a normal mouth. Premature infants, those who experienced perinatal trauma, or have cerebral palsy and other forms of brain damage, and infants with a cleft palate or lip could have difficulty in feeding. Medication used in the intrapartum period might impair the baby's ability to suck. Some babies can be difficult temperamentally, and this will affect their feeding (Thomas & Chess, 1977).

Early feeding is commonly affected by the emotional state of the mother, especially depression or anxiety. Mothers may be generally anxious or anxious specifically about feeding. A young and inexperienced mother with little social and family support may have particular difficulties. The supply of breast milk may be affected by local problems affecting the nipple or breast, or impairment of general physical health.

There is no evidence that whether a child is breast-fed or bottle-fed influences the later development of behavioural or emotional problems in the child (Orlansky, 1949; Sewell & Mussen, 1952).

Sleep

Newborn babies tend to alternate frequently between waking and sleeping. The total sleeping time drops from 16–17 hours per day to 13 hours per day within the first 6 months of the infant's life. A rhythm of two shorter naps during the day and a longer sleep at night is usually established. By the age of 6 months, over 80% of babies sleep through the night and only 10% at the age of 12 months are still waking every night (Graham, 1994).

Environmental influences also affect the sleep patterns of infants during the first year of life. A change in the sleeping arrangements, an alteration in the bedtime ritual, or anxiety or depression in the mother may disturb the infant's sleep pattern. Difficulties in getting to sleep are common in 2-year-olds and 3-year-olds, and may be related to children's limited capacity at this age to retain an image in their mind of their parents. Inappropriate parental responses to the waking child may also reinforce night-time waking. 'Transitional objects' (Winnicott, 1958) such as a teddy bear or a 'security blanket' may help some children to settle at night. Temperamentally difficult children commonly experience sleep problems.

Dreams

By the time children are 3–4 years old, they are able to recognise dreams as such and to speak of them, although only one-fifth of children under 5 are able to describe traumatic dreams (Terr, 1987). Adults may infer that younger children dream as they vocalise or make movements in their sleep. Nightmares, troubled and frightening dreams associated with actual fears and traumas, may occur at any age and must be distinguished from night terrors (pavor nocturnus). Nightmares occur in rapid eye movement sleep; children are asleep during the episode but fully awake afterwards, have vivid recall and usually there is no family history of nightmares.

Night terrors are thought to be prevalent in about 3% of children, mainly in later childhood. The episodes start before the age of 7 years and continue on an average for about 4 years. The episode usually lasts for a few minutes, ends abruptly and the child has no memory of the event. This occurs in deep non-rapid eye movement sleep; the child is unaware during the episode, confused if awakened or following episodes, and a family history is common. Occasionally, night terrors indicate an underlying psychological disturbance that may precipitate and maintain their occurrence and predict severity.

High rates of serious sleep problems are reported in adolescence. This is thought to be due to the marked psychological and social changes that are present during this stage of development. The disorders could be due to an erratic sleep–wake schedule, worries and anxiety, excessive caffeine intake, alcohol and tobacco, illegal substances or psychiatric disorders.

Normal sleep in childhood and adolescence reflects the serenity and stability, or the reverse, of the life led by the sleeper. The content of dreams may be associated with the waking world through play, art, visualised memories and speech, which may allow access to traumatic memories. Sleep disturbances form one route to the knowledge of the child's life events (Terr, 1991).

Bowel and bladder control

In the newborn period, micturition is a reflex. Babies usually empty the bladder or bowels immediately after a meal; they can be conditioned at any age to pass urine when placed on a pot. Voluntary control does not begin until the age of 15–18 months, depending on maturation of the nervous system, which is influenced by genetic factors. Most children are reasonably dry by day at 18 months. By two years, 50% are dry at night; by three, 75%; and by five some 90% are dry.

For children to be continent, they need an intact nervous system supplying the bladder, no congenital malformation of the urinary system, physiological maturity, an understanding of what is required of them and the motivation to achieve this. In a child with generalised learning difficulties, a delay in bowel and bladder control could be one aspect of general immaturity. If the family is under stress when the child is between the ages of 18 months and 3 years, he or she will achieve dryness more slowly. Parents who take a relaxed view of toilet training and start when the child is sufficiently mature, between the ages of 18 months and 2 years, and praise successful efforts, are likely to see their children gain control of their bowel and bladder with less effort. If bedwetting (enuresis) persists beyond the age of 5 years, it is considered abnormal.

Bowel control is usually acquired before control of the bladder. Children generally would have achieved normal control by the age of 3–4 years, although they might have accidents.

Sexual development

The process of sexual development enables the individual to conform to the gender-specific modes of behaviour and appearance expected by society, form stable relationships with members of the opposite sex, and produce and rear children. Many areas of our lives are affected by our gender, from our choice of shoes to our choice of partner, from our chances of developing rheumatoid arthritis to our chances of ending up in prison.

It is clear that sexual development covers an enormous area of change, ranging from universal aspects of physical development to relatively culture-specific aspects of social behaviour. It is conventional to divide this sweep of human development into its physiological aspects (which will be described first), gender identity, gender role and, finally, sexual orientation. For a review, please refer to Zucker & Bradley (1995).

Physical development

A happy sexual adjustment in adult life requires the necessary anatomical and physiological changes to have taken place. At about 2 months' gestation, the sex chromosomes cause the primitive, undifferentiated gonad to develop into either ovaries or testes. The ensuing phenotype depends on the secretion of foetal androgens, as without their masculinising influence female genitalia will result regardless of genotype.

The next decisive move towards a sexually adult body occurs some years before puberty. The maturing hypothalamus activates the pituitary gland, leading to increased release of luteinising hormone and follicle-stimulating hormone. These in turn encourage the ovaries to secrete oestrogen (from the age of about 7 years) and the testes androgens, although the adrenals contribute to androgen output from the ninth year (adrenal puberty). Early on in puberty, before the final balance between oestrogen and androgens is established, temporary anomalies such as transient gynaecomastia in boys can commonly be observed.

The development of genitalia and secondary sexual characteristics starts earlier and proceeds faster in girls than boys, menarche occurring between the ages of 10 and 16, and the equivalent event – the capacity to ejaculate semen – happening between the ages of 13 and 17 years. The neural substrate of sexual activity responsible for erection, pelvic movements and ejaculation is present from an early age in the spinal cord, although pathways mediating the latter two functions require an appropriate hormonal input.

Human sexual behaviour and its development are influenced strongly by culture. Every society places some restrictions on sexual behaviour, and incest is prohibited by almost all cultures. By about 3–4 years of age, most children can identify correctly their own sex as well as that of other children.

Gender identity

This is the degree to which children regard themselves as male or female, and is usually well established by the age of 4 years. Transsexualism, which usually starts with cross-dressing and feminine behaviour (in the case of boys) in early or middle childhood, represents an extreme aberration of gender identity. Studies have suggested that an indulgent maternal attitude to the child's preference for behaving and dressing like a member of the opposite sex, and lack of interest and failure to act as a role model on the part of the father, may contribute to gender identity problems (Green, 1985). Although less extreme than the complete reversal of gender identity described above, insecurity of sexual identity can complicate late physical maturation, especially in boys. Such boys have been shown to feel dominated by their better-developed peers and have a poorer self-concept as males.

Gender role

This refers to the ability of an individual to carry out the repertoire of behaviours considered socially appropriate for his or her sex. By 3 years, children show a preference for particular activities (e.g. boys for rough and tumble play) and gender-stereotyped toys. Throughout childhood and adolescence, many of these differences become accentuated. Processes by which the arrays of behaviour that constitute sex role are acquired include selective reinforcement by parents and identification.

Sexual orientation

This refers to an individual's choice of sexual stimulus and outlet. There is evidence of a genetic contribution to sexual orientation, particularly in homosexuality (Heston & Shields, 1968). The prenatal hormonal environment also plays a part (Money & Ehrhardt, 1972). Sexual orientation represents a continuum from exclusive hetero-sexuality to exclusive homosexuality; only about 4% of men and 1–2% of women become exclusively homosexual (Kinsey et al, 1948, 1953).

The wish to achieve sexual pleasure by stimulation of the genitalia is present from birth. This sexual drive persists throughout childhood and increases in early adolescence, to peak in late adolescence and early adulthood. Masturbation is common in both boys and girls between the ages of 2 years and 5 years; sex play involving undressing and sexual exploration and interest in the genitalia of siblings and playmates is common and normal during this period. It is only around puberty that the three components of sexuality – gender identity, gender role and sexual orientation – become incorporated into the formation and maintenance of emotional dyadic relationships, and our sexual orient-ation becomes organised and relatively fixed.

Infants develop their first feelings of affection and trust through a warm, loving, nurturing relationship with the mother. This is a prerequisite for a satisfactory interaction and affectionate relationships with youngsters of both sexes, and for intimacy of later sexual relationship among young adults.

Language development

There are many ways to describe normal language development, but the two major ones are the age-related method and the skills-related model. The age-related method (Lees & Urwin, 1997) suggests that a child should have mastered skills by a certain age. The first 5 years is seen as the important period for language development and is divided into age bands. In the skills-related model (Lees & Urwin, 1997), a child's development is considered as the acquisition of certain skills that run alongside each other and overlap. There are two important points that need to be borne in mind about normal child development in relation to understanding language impairment in childhood. The first is the growing understanding of the importance of the pre-lingual period, and the second is that most children develop language without too many difficulties.

There is considerable research about the paralinguistic period that shows that the infant has communication skills well before the appearance of his or her first words. In children with deviant language development, these very early communication skills are missing.

Communication needs the parent or carer and the child to alternate the role of initiator and receiver. It starts off with innate signals at birth and develops through interaction into an increasingly elaborate and complex pre-verbal exchange.

The pre-verbal communications include eye gaze, gesture and early vocalisation. Infants are born with affective behaviours that allow them to express their basic needs. These innate behaviours bring about appropriate nurturing responses; for example, a parent delighted by the infant's social smile at 2 months will go to any length to encourage it. This innate behaviour could have developed historically and evolved precisely for strengthening the parent–child relationship. Hence, an infant is not a passive partner but is involved actively in influencing his or her own parenting. Another aspect of early communication is the pattern of turn-taking sequences, and this is seen as the precursor of turn-taking in conversations.

Infants are also able to see and aim their gaze. Gaze and basic orientating movements are the initial things that can be used to measure the attention of an infant. It is joint attention that is the basic necessity for successful communication. By 3–6 months, infants achieve head and neck control, and orientation of head and gaze are signs that the infant is ready to communicate. When visual contact ends, this is seen by the infant or parent as withdrawal from communication.

Pointing is one of the most important pre-verbal gestures and is observed as exploratory, in the first few months. By about 9 months, this is used along with eye gaze to draw the carer into a communication. In 9–18 month-old children, pointing was found by Bates *et al* (1979) to be the strongest predictor of language development.

Between the stages of babbling and conventional words, the vocal phenomenon of protowords occurs. They are used to express approval, disapproval, wanting and rejecting. Protowords are accompanied by gestures from 14 months to 19 months, followed by single-word utterances also accompanied by gestures. By 20 months, children develop a considerable communicative repertoire and this includes vocal, verbal and non-verbal acts.

Most children develop language without any major difficulties and by the age of 5 years have mastered the basic building blocks. From then on, the rest of childhood is spent in focusing on refining language so that it can be used in increasingly complex tasks such as reading, writing, debating and hypothesising. The development of speech depends on the interaction of genetic, auditory, environmental and intellectual factors. There are wide variations in the development of speech in normal children, and girls tend to speak earlier than boys.

Play

Play is the work through which children learn about themselves, others, and the world in which they live. The earliest play, from a few weeks old, is social; smiling and moving the head to catch the eye of another soon leads to peep-boo, then the copying of other movements and attempts to copy sounds and rhythms (see also the account of attachment theory below; Bowlby, 1977).

By the end of the first year, children are learning to clap, smile, hide and seek, and to look for approval of shared jokes, tasks and movements. Rhythm, rhymes, stories, songs, dancing, imitation of adults at work, for the development of cooperative play with other children, solving puzzles, building, drawing (Figs 2.1 to 2.5) and modelling all become available as activities for the maturing child. However, play should not be an end in itself; children require opportunities to contribute to the life around them by succeeding at household tasks, helping to care for siblings, preparing food, running errands and so on. For children, there is no clear line between work and play; the need is for a valued role in family and community life.

The provision of such rich experience is as important for the psychosocial well-being of the child, the adolescent in transition and the adult he or she will become, as is the care of bodily needs and acquisition of language. Indeed, language, play and social learning are intertwined and are all essential for the development of autonomy, reciprocity, ethical awareness, creativity and resilience in adult life, and for the availability of adults to each new generation of children.

Some theories of development

Theories of development are summarised in Table 2.2. except for that of Bowlby (1951, 1973, 1977, 1982), which does not lend itself to tabular presentation.

Psychoanalytic theory

The psychoanalytic theory of Sigmund Freud (1856–1939) described a predictable sequence of qualitatively distinct stages (Table 2.2) through

Table 2.2 Stages in psychosocial development

	Freud	Erikson	Piaget	Kohlberg
1st year	Oral stage	Trust v. mistrust	Sensorimotor (0–2 years)	Pre-conventional morality: level I
2nd year	Anal stage	Autonomy v. shame and doubt		
3rd to 5th year	Phallic stage	Initiative v. guilt	Preoperational (2–7 years)	
6th year to puberty	Latency period	Industry v. inferiority	Concrete operational (7–12 years)	Conventional morality: level II
Adolescence	Genital stage	Identity v. confusion	Formal operational (over 12 years)	
Early adulthood		Intimacy v. isolation		Post-conventional morality: level III
Middle adulthood		Generativity v. self-absorption		
Ageing years		Integrity v. despair		

which children pass, each differing as to the physical function that is invested with pleasure (Freud, 1905).

Freud stated that the personality is composed of three major structures – the id, the ego and the superego – each having its own function but interacting to govern behaviour. The id, being the most primitive part of the personality, is present in the newborn infant, operates on the pleasure principle and from it, the ego and the superego later develop. The ego obeys the reality principle. The superego is the internalised representation of the values of society as taught to the child by the parents and others. The superego develops in response to parental rewards and punishment. It strives for perfection. Freud's theory of personality dynamics explains that there is a constant amount of psychic energy (libido) for every individual. When an impulse or forbidden act is suppressed, this energy has to seek an outlet in some other form and this is expressed in dreams or neurotic symptoms. The theory assumes that impulses that are unacceptable cause anxiety and defence mechanisms can reduce them.

Psychoanalytic theory has always been controversial. Critics have pointed out that it has no empirical evidence to support the conclusion that identifying with the same-sex parent or discovering genital sex differences determines sex typing and gender identity. Over the years, Freud's structural theory (id, ego and superego), the psychosexual theory and the energy concept have not fared well, whereas his dynamic theories of anxiety and defence mechanisms have withstood the test of time, observation and research much better.

Cognitive development

Jean Piaget (1896–1980) was a Swiss psychologist who derived his theory of cognitive development from the observation of children: his own, those attending a nursery and, subsequently, school children (Piaget, 1932, 1951, 1952; Piaget & Inhelder, 1969). As well as describing a stage theory of development, he identified four necessary factors that brought this development about:

1. maturation – physical development of the nervous system governed by inherent factors;
2. interactions with inanimate objects – learning as an ongoing experiment in the world of objects and physical forces;
3. opportunities for social interactions – learning derived from contact with other people, including imitation as well as formal teaching;
4. the ability to construct an internal representation of the world.

He described four stages through which children's cognitive development passes:

1. **Sensorimotor stage (0–2 years)** By encountering objects and people around them, infants acquire the ability to distinguish between self and other.
2. **Pre-operational stage (2–7 years)** Having acquired familiarity with the properties of objects and the ability to retain a stable, internalised representation of them, the child learns that they can be represented by symbols, particularly words. This stage has four characteristics: egocentrism, animism, pre-causal logic and an authoritarian morality.
3. **Stage of concrete operations (7–12 years)** Children lose their egocentrism, animism and authoritarian morality during this stage. They start to use categories; they are able to abstract from a number of objects a common property that allows them to be classified together. In a similar way, a child of 9 years is able to ignore superficial differences such as the height of a column of water, while attending to its more essential characteristic, its volume. Conservation of number occurs at the age of 6 years, followed by conservation of weight at 7 years on average. Children are now able to engage in cooperative activities with others. Justice is more a central concept than obedience.

4.   **Formal operations (12 years onwards)** By this stage, children can entertain novel constructions and possibilities, completely divorced from objects around them. In addition they can anticipate consequences by manipulating mental constructions. Essentially, they can now hypothesise. This ability allows them to imagine the world from the point of view of others, an essential, albeit not always achieved, task of adolescence.

New methods of testing reveal that Piaget's theory underestimated children's abilities. Several alternative approaches to the assessment of cognitive abilities have been proposed, such as the information-processing approach. This approach views cognitive development as a reflection of the gradual development of attention and memory processes. The knowledge acquisition approach proposes that after infancy children and adults have the same cognitive processes and capacities, but the essential difference between them is that the adults have a more extensive knowledge base.

Moral development

Kohlberg (1969, 1973) used Piaget's approach to account for the development of conscience and proposed the following three stages.

1.   **Pre-conventional morality (level 1)** This applies to children up to about 7 years. Behaviour is guided entirely by external contingencies. Socially acceptable behaviour is exhibited purely to avoid punishment. Later on in this stage, adherence to social rules also becomes driven by reward for conformity.

2.   **Conventional morality (level II)** At first, the child conforms to avoid the disapproval of others. This develops into a sense of an externally imposed obligation so that children will feel bad if they do not 'do their duty' (authority orientation).

3.   **Post-conventional morality (level III)** Actions are guided by the principle of a social contract where one behaves towards others as one would wish them to behave to oneself. This finally evolves into 'ethical principle orientation', in which actions are determined according to abstract values such as justice and dignity, and are driven by the urge to avoid self-condemnation. According to Kohlberg, many individuals never progress beyond level II. He sees the stages of moral development as parallel to Piaget's stages of cognitive development. By the age of 13 14 years, only those who have developed the capacity of abstract thought are able to function at this level. He also reports that only 10% of his subjects over the age of 16 years were at the highest stage of moral development, the stage of 'ethical principle orientation.'

Fig. 2.1 A painting by a 15-month-old child. Only one or two colours are used, layered on thickly. The painting did not use the whole sheet of paper.

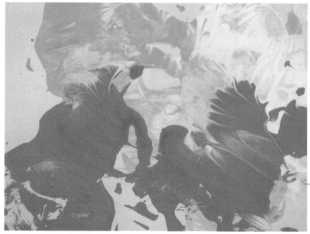

Fig. 2.2 A painting by a 1-year-old child. Lots of colours are used, filling the whole sheet of paper.

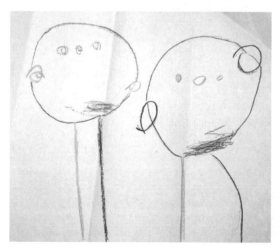

Fig. 2.3 A painting by a 4-year-old child. Note the large head and relative lack of detail, typical at this age.

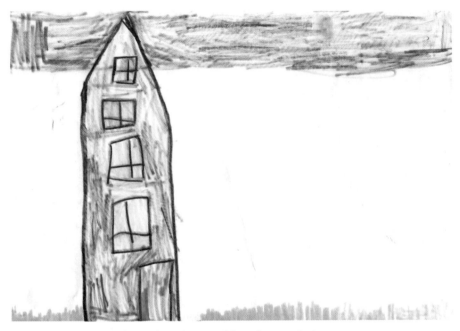

Fig. 2.4 A typical painting by a 6-year-old; a picture of a house.

Fig. 2.5 A painting by an 8-year-old. Shows greater sense of proportion, more detail and use of appropriate colours.

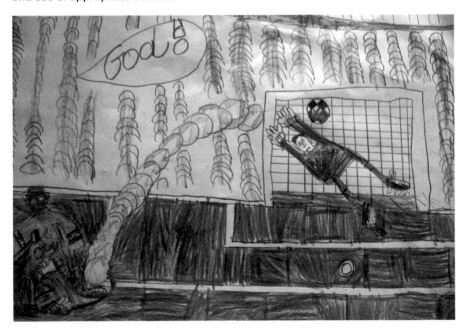

Erikson (1968) proposed a series of eight psychosocial stages to describe development from cradle to grave, based on the individual's ability to resolve a series of psychosocial crises and to establish appropriate social relations at each of these life stages (see Table 2.2).

Personality and temperament

Temperament refers to mood-related personality characteristics and is thought of as composed of enduring traits that have a biological basis and are relatively stable over time. These are assumed to be pure at birth but modified by environmental, social and cultural factors. Personality has been described as the characteristic manner in which the person, thinks, feels, behaves and relates to others (Widiger et al, 1999).

Studies have approached the concept of personality and temperament from many different theoretical perspectives (Bates & Wachs, 1994). The two main approaches are homothetic and idiographic. In the homothetic approach, study focuses on the differences between individuals; the idiographic approach suggests that every individual is unique and has an integrated whole (Deary & Power, 1998).

Recent studies have focused on identifying dimensions of personal characteristics on which individuals differ. One of the pioneering studies in the field of temperament has been the New York Longitudinal Study (Thomas et al, 1963; Thomas & Chess, 1986). This study described a nine-trait classifi-cation of infant temperament. The authors described the following categories: activity level, regularity of biological functions, approach to or withdrawal from new stimuli, adaptability to new stimuli or altered situations, the intensity of reaction, the threshold of responsiveness, the quality of mood, distractibility and persistence/attention span. Further analysis of this led to three clinically useful temperamental categories: 'easy', 'difficult' and 'slow to warm up'. Children with an 'easy' temperament were characterised by biological regularity, an adaptable approach to a new stimulus and altered situations, and a positive mood. These children accounted for 40% of the sample. 'Difficult' children accounted for 10% of the sample and they were characterised by the reverse of these behaviours. On the other hand, 'slow to warm up' children, who accounted for 15% of the sample, were characterised by withdrawal tendencies to new situations, slow adaptability and frequent negative outbursts of low intensity. A number could not be classified.

Buss & Plomin (1975) have put forward four temperamental factors that are described as EASI: emotionality, activity, sociability and impulsivity. They suggested that these characteristics were inherited, observed in the first year and remained stable over time to form the foundation of personality traits later.

Kagan and colleagues (Kagan *et al*, 1988; Kagan & Snidman, 1991; Kagan, 1994) described temperamental traits in children as 'inhibited' and 'uninhibited'. 'Inhibited' children are characterised by timidity in response to unfamiliar situations, whereas 'uninhibited' children are described as sociable, talkative and less fearful when faced with new, unfamiliar situations. The 'inhibited' group also differed from the 'uninhibited' group by having a relatively high but stable heart rate, higher salivary cortisol levels and larger eye pupils. Kagan's hypothesis was that this was because 'inhibited' children were born with a lower threshold of arousal to unexpected changes in the environment. The stability of this classification has been supported by longitudinal studies of children aged from 14 months to 7 years.

Other theories of adult personality structure include Eysenck's neuroticism (N), extraversion–introversion (E) and psychoticism (P) model, largely consigned to history (Eysenck & Eysenck, 1969).

A more recent theory of personality is the Big Five theory, the five factors being openness, conscientiousness, agreeableness and emotional stability (acronym OCEAN). This was proposed by Costa & McCrae (1992) and is not rooted in any particular theoretical approach (John & Srivastava, 1999).

The five-factor model of personality seems more appropriate to adult study. Some studies have suggested that seven factors, the Big Five factors plus an additional two, are more appropriate for childhood personality structure. The two additional factors of irritability and activity become more integrated into the big five over the adolescent period.

Many studies in children have shown evidence of three personality types that are referred to as 'resilients,' 'overcontrollers' and 'undercontrollers' (Van Leishout & Haselager, 1994; Caspi & Silva, 1995; Robins *et al*, 1996; Hart *et al*, 1997). The resilient personality type functions effectively on all the Big Five factors. The 'overcontrollers' score highly on agreeableness and conscientiousness, and low on extraversion. The undercontrollers score low on agreeableness and conscientiousness and low on emotional stability. These personality categories have been shown to be predictive of psychological adjustment, resilient children generally showing a high level of psychological adjustment.

In general temperament and personality are largely stable throughout life, but individuals can change their patterns of behaviour, thoughts and ways of relating as a result of learning, experience and illness.

Attachment

Attachment is described as the infant's tendency to seek proximity to particular people and to feel more secure in their presence. Initially, this was thought to be due to the mother being the source of food, food being one of the basic needs of the infant. This was not observed to be the case in species that can feed themselves from birth, like ducklings, who still followed their mothers. A series of well-known animal experiments were conducted to study this phenomenon and found that there is more to mother–infant relationships than satisfying feeding needs (Harlow & Harlow, 1969). These researchers conducted their experiments on infant monkeys separated from their mothers shortly after birth and placed with two artificial mothers; one had a body of bare wire and the other was covered in terry cloth. Both were equipped to provide milk. In these experiments, no matter which mother provided the food for the monkey, the infant clung on to the one that provided it with comfort rather than just the food (Harlow & Harlow, 1969).

These monkeys, who were separated from their mothers and deprived of all social contacts with other monkeys during their first 6 months, were later found to have bizarre behaviours in adulthood. They did not engage normally with other monkeys, and if female monkeys were mated they neglected their infants. However, these female monkeys became better mothers with their subsequent infants. If monkeys with artificial mothers were allowed to interact with their peers in their first 6 months, they did not have significant problems as adults.

In humans, most of the original work on attachment in infants was developed by John Bowlby in the 1950s and 1960s. Bowlby's research suggested that if a child fails to develop a secure attachment with one or two caregivers in his early years, he would be unable to develop close personal relationships in adulthood (Bowlby, 1951, 1973, 1982).

Mary Ainsworth, who was an associate of Bowlby, studied children in Uganda and the USA extensively and developed the 'strange situation procedure', a laboratory procedure to assess infant attachment style (Ainsworth *et al*, 1978). In this procedure, the baby is observed when his or her main caregiver leaves and later returns to the room. The baby is watched through a one-way screen and several observations are made, such as the child's activity level and play involvement, crying and other distress signs, proximity to and attempts to gain the attention of the mother, and proximity to and willingness to interact with a stranger.

Episodes in the 'strange situation' procedure

1. A mother and her baby enter the room. The mother places the baby on the floor, surrounded by toys. She goes to sit at the opposite end of the room.
2. A female stranger enters the room. She at first sits quietly in the room for a minute, then converses with the mother for a minute and then attempts to engage the baby in play with the toys.

3.   The mother leaves the room unobtrusively. The stranger sits quietly if the baby is not upset. If the baby is upset the stranger tries to soothe him or her.
4.   The mother returns to the room and engages the baby in play. The stranger leaves the room.
5.   The baby is left alone in the room as mother leaves again.
6.   The stranger returns. If the baby is upset the stranger soothes the baby.
7.   The mother returns and the stranger leaves the room.

On the basis of these observed behaviours in the strange situation procedure babies were classified into three groups: securely attached; insecurely attached: avoidant; and insecurely attached: ambivalent. A fourth category, disorganised, was later added (Main & Solomon, 1986).

Securely attached

Babies classified as securely attached seek to interact with their mother when she returns, regardless of whether they were upset when she left the room. Such children could behave in different ways: some are happy to acknowledge her return and carry on playing, others seek physical contact, and some are preoccupied by her throughout the session and are distressed intensely when she leaves the room. Around 60–65% of American children are classified in this group.

Insecurely attached: avoidant

About 20% of American children fall into this group. These babies avoid interacting with their mother on her return. Some choose to ignore her entirely, and some show mixed attempts to interact and to avoid any interactions. These babies show little interest while the mother is in the room and do not seem distressed when she leaves the room. They can be equally well comforted by the stranger as by the mother.

Insecurely attached: ambivalent

These babies show resistance to the mother when she returns to the room. They seek and resist physical contact simultaneously. They may cry, wanting to be picked up, but squirm angrily when they are picked up and quickly want to get down. Some are passive, crying for their mother but not making any approaches towards her such as crawling to her on her return. When she approaches they show resistance. Ten per cent of American children are classified in this group.

Disorganised

About 10–15% of American children are classified as disorganised. These children show contradictory behaviours. They may approach their mother without looking at her. They may approach her and then show avoidance or cry suddenly after having settled down. Some look depressed, emotionless or disoriented. There are high rates of maltreated children or children of parents with mental illness in this group.

A baby's attachment classification has been found to be stable when tested many years later, if there is no major change of life circumstances in the child's life. Stressful life events can affect caregiving skills in mothers and these may in turn affect the child's feeling of security.

Studies have shown that children who are securely attached by their second year are better equipped to manage new experiences. It is difficult to assume that the child's early attachment is directly linked with their later competency as this may depend on the current parent–child relationship. Children's temperament can also affect their behaviour in the 'strange situation' procedure, and this can influence their competency later.

Conclusion

A number of factors within the child, the child's family and the external world influence development. A number of theories to explain aspects of development have been proposed, with a growing tendency for these to be based on observation rather than theory alone. Although some theories are now of mainly historical interest, the concepts of attachment and temperament have stood the test of time and are helpful in contributing to clinical understanding.

References

Ainsworth, M. D. S., Blehar, M. C., Walters, E., *et al* (1978) *Patterns of Attachment: A Psychological Study of the Strange Situation*. Hillsdale, NJ: Erlbaum.

Bates, E., Benigni, L., Bretherton, I., *et al* (1979) *The Emergence of Symbols: Communication and Cognition in Infancy*. New York: Academic Press.

Bates, J. E. & Wachs, T. D. (1994) *Temperament: Individual Difference at the Interface of Biology and Behaviour*. Washington, DC: American Psychological Association.

Blehar Ainsworth, M. D. & Waters, E. (1978) *Patterns of Attachment: A Psychological Study of the Strange Situation*. Hillsdale, NJ: Erlbaum.

Bowlby, J. (1951) *Maternal Care and Mental Health*. Geneva: World Health Organization.

Bowlby, J. (1973) *Attachment and Loss: vol. 2.Separation: Anxiety and Anger*. London: Hogarth Press.

Bowlby, J. (1977) The making and breaking of affectional bonds. *British Journal of Psychiatry*, **130**, 201–210.

Bowlby, J. (1982) *Attachment and Loss: Attachment* (2nd edn). New York: Basic Books.

Buss, A. H. & Plomin, R. (1975) *Temperamental Theory of Personality Development*. New York: Wiley.

Caspi, A. & Silva, P. A. (1995) Temperamental qualities at age three predict personality traits in young adulthood: longitudinal evidence from a birth cohort. *Child Development*, **66**, 486–498.

Costa, P. T. & McCrae, R. R. (1992) *Revised NEO Personality Inventory (NEO–PI–R) and NEO Five Factor Inventory (NEO–FFI): Professional Manual*. Odessa, FL: Psychological Assessment Resources.

Deary, I. & Power, M. J. (1998) Normal and abnormal personality. In *Companion to Psychiatric Studies* (eds E. C. Johnstone, C. P. L. Freeman & A. K. Zealley), pp. 565–596. Edinburgh: Churchill Livingstone.

Erikson, E. (1968) *Identity, Youth and Crisis*. London: Faber.

Eysenck, H. J. & Eysenck, S. B. G. (1969) *Personality Structure and Measurement*. London: Routledge.

Freud, S. (1905) *Three Essays on the Theory of Sexuality*. Reprinted in the *Standard Edition of the Complete Works of Sigmund Freud* (trans. and ed. J. Strachey), vol. 7. London: Hogarth Press.

Graham, P. (1994) *Child Psychiatry: A Developmental Approach*. Oxford: Oxford University Press.

Green, R. (1985) Atypical sexual development. In *Child and Adolescent Psychiatry: Modern Approaches* (2nd edn) (eds M. Rutter & L. Hersov). Oxford: Blackwell Scientific.

Harlow, H. F. & Harlow, M. K. (1969) Effects of various mother–infant relationships on rhesus monkey behaviours. In *Determinants of Infant Behaviour*, vol. 4 (ed B. M. Foss).

Hart, D., Hoffman, V., Edelstein, W., *et al* (1997) The relationship of childhood personality types to adolescent behaviour and development: a longitudinal study of Icelandic children. *Developmental Psychology*, **33**, 195–205.

Heston, L. L. & Shields, J. (1968) Homosexuality in twins: a family study and a Register study. *Archives of General Psychiatry*, **18**, 149–160.

Illingworth, R. S. (1990) *The Development of the Infant and Young Child, Normal and Abnormal*. Edinburgh: Churchill Livingstone.

John, O. P. & Srivastava, S. (1999) The Big Five Trait Taxonomy: history, measurement and theoretical perspective. *Handbook of Personality*, **55**, 359–375.

Kagan, J. (1994) *Galen's Prophecies*. New York: Basic Books.

Kagan, J. & Snidman, N. (1991) Temperamental factors in human development. *American Psychologist*, **46**, 856–862.

Kagan, J., Reznick, J. & Snidman, N. (1988) Biological basis of childhood shyness. *Science*, **240**, 167–171.

Kinsey, A. C., Pomeroy, W. B., Martin, C. E., *et al* (1948) *Sexual Behaviour in the Human Male*. Philadelphia: Saunders.

Kinsey, A. C., Pomeroy, W. B., Martin, C. E., *et al* (1953) *Sexual Behaviour in the Human Female*. Philadelphia: Saunders.

Kohlberg, L. (1969) Stage and sequence: the cognitive developmental approach to socialisation. In *Handbook of Socialisation Theory and Research* (ed. D. A. Goslin), pp. 81–83. Chicago, IL: Rand McNally.

Kohlberg, L. (1973) Implications of developmental psychology for education: examples from moral development. *Educational Psychologist*, **10**, 2–14.

Lees, J. & Urwin, S. (1997) *Children with Language Disorders* (2nd edn). London: Whurr.

Main, M. & Solomon, J. (1986) Discovery of an insecure-disorganised/disoriented attachment pattern: procedures, findings and implication for the classification of behaviours. In *Affective Development in Infancy* (eds T. B. Brazelton & M. Yogman), pp. 95–124. Norwood, NJ: Ablex.

Money, J. & Ehrhardt, A. A. (1972) *Man and Woman, Boy and Girl: Differentiation and Dimorphism of Gender Identity from Conception to Maturity.* Baltimore: Johns Hopkins University Press.

Orlansky, H. (1949) Infant care and personality. *Psychological Bulletin,* **46**, 1–48.

Piaget, J. (1932) *The Moral Judgement of a Child.* London: Routledge & Kegan Paul.

Piaget, J. (1951) *The Child's Conception of the World.* London: Routledge & Kegan Paul.

Piaget, J. (1952) *The Language and Thought of the Child.* London: Routledge & Kegan Paul.

Piaget, J. & Inhelder, B. (1969) *The Psychology of the Child.* London: Routledge & Kegan Paul.

Robins, R. W., John, O. P., Caspi, A., *et al* (1996) Resilient, overcontrolled and undercontrolled boys: three replicable personality types? *Journal of Personality and Social Psychology,* **70**, 157–171.

Sewell, W. H. & Mussen, P. H. (1952) The effect of feeding, weaning and scheduling procedures on childhood adjustment and the formation of oral symptoms. *Child Development,* **23**, 185–191.

Terr, L. C. (1987) Children's nightmares. In *Sleep and its Disorders in Children* (ed. C. Guilleminault). New York: Raven Press.

Terr, L. C. (1991) Childhood traumas: an outline and overview. *American Journal of Psychiatry,* **148**, 10–20.

Thomas, A. & Chess, S. (1977) *Temperament and Development.* New York: Brunner/Mazel.

Thomas, A. & Chess, S. (1986) The New York Longitudinal Study: from infancy to adult life. In *The Study of Temperament: Changes, Continuities and Challenges* (eds R. Plomin & J. Dunn), pp. 39–52. Hillsdale, NJ: Erlbaum.

Thomas, A., Chess, S., Birch, H. G., *et al* (1963) *Behavioral Individuality in Early Childhood.* New York: New York University Press.

Van Leishout, C. F. M. & Haselager, G. J. T (1994) The Big Five Personality factors in Q-sort description of children and adolescent. In *The Developing Structure of Temperament and Personality from Infancy to Adulthood* (eds C. F. Halverston, G. A. Kohnstamm & R. P. Martin), pp. 293–318. Hillsdale, NJ: Erlbaum.

Widiger, T. A., Verheul, R. & Van Den Brink, W. (1999) Personality and psycho-pathology. In *Handbook of Personality: Theory and Research* (eds L. A. Pervin & O. P. John), pp. 3–27. New York: Guilford.

Winnicott, D. W. (1958) Transitional objects and transitional phenomena. In *Collected Papers: Through Paediatrics to Psychoanalysis.* London: Tavistock (reprinted 1975 as *Through Paediatrics to Psychoanalysis.* London: Hogarth Press).

Zucker, K. J., & Bradley, J. S. (1995) *Gender Identity Disorder and Psychosocial Problems in Children and Adolescents.* London: Guilford.

Further reading

Atkinson, R. L., Atkinson, R. C., Smith, E. E., *et al* (2000) *Hilgard's Introduction to Psychology* (13th edn). London: Harcourt College Publishers.

Illingworth, R. S. (1990) *The Development of the Infant and Young Child, Normal and Abnormal.* Edinburgh: Churchill Livingstone.

Lees, J. & Urwin, S. (1997) *Children with Language Disorders* (2nd edn). London: Whurr Publishers.

Rutter, M. & Taylor, E. (2003) *Child and Adolescent Psychiatry: Modern Approaches* (4th edn). Oxford: Blackwell Scientific.

CHAPTER 3

Influences on development

David M. Kingsley and Simon G. Gowers

Although normal development might simply seem to be a sequence of stages that occur in an invariant and predetermined order and reach an end-point when the process is complete, the reality is often more complex. Development encompasses physical, cognitive, social, moral, emotional and spiritual domains. All have differing patterns of progression, ranges of normality and variations from the norm. Many influences, internal and external, positive and negative, affect outcomes in each developmental domain. Moreover, the attainment of a developmental 'milestone' is not usually an all or nothing phenomenon, achieved on a single day. For example, in the acquisition of urinary continence there is usually a transitional phase in which wetting is more or less likely and may be situational. Particular stresses or changes may lead to the re-emergence of wetting well after continence has been achieved. So the normal developmental process may be less a case of a smooth continual process than a case of two steps forward and one step back.

It is important to always bear in mind the extent of normality that exists. One child aged 3 years may speak in long sentences, whereas a peer may utter only a few words. Although they might be at opposite ends of the spectrum, both children's language would be considered developmentally 'normal'. So it is important to be familiar with normal ranges in order to be competent to identify abnormality. Generally, children develop across developmental domains at a broadly even pace. One pattern that may suggest a problem is where a child's ability in a particular area lags significantly behind his or her general level of functioning. In such cases, further assessment may be needed.

Development is the backdrop against which child psychiatry is practised and it may be argued that all mental health problems in children represent, or are associated with, developmental delays or deviations in one or more domains. This chapter reviews some key influences on development that are of particular relevance to child psychiatric practice.

Genes and environment

For many years, a somewhat naïve debate has taken place as to whether genetic or environmental influences make the prime contribution to developmental outcomes. However, recent studies suggest that the reality is more complex and interactive. Although our genes play a significant part in predisposing us to a whole range of traits and competencies, they also influence the environment into which we place ourselves, consequently predisposing us to differing life experiences. Furthermore, our genes then mediate the way in which we respond to our circumstances. The following scenario illustrates this gene–environment interaction.

Mark is an 8-year-old boy with mild learning disability and a sensitive temperament. He attends a learning support unit within a mainstream primary school. He is prone to being teased by other children, who say he is an 'idiot'. His emotional sensitivity makes it particularly hard to shake off these comments and he becomes increasingly sad, withdrawn and socially isolated.

This case shows how a significantly genetic trait (low intellect) predisposes this boy to the experience of being teased. Furthermore, his sensitive temperament (also genetically influenced) moderates the way in which he copes with the taunting, leading him to become withdrawn, unhappy and socially isolated. So genes and environment are involved in a complex interplay in all areas of human experience and behaviour. It is helpful to keep this in mind as we go on to discuss some specific influences on child development; meanwhile, the genetics of psychiatric disorder are discussed more fully in Chapter 15.

Influences on development

Cognitive development

Intelligence

Although we tend to think of intelligence as a single cognitive ability, it actually comprises a number of competencies that together determine our capacity to learn from, make sense of and adapt to the environment around us. Our tendency to see intelligence as a single entity has been, somewhat unhelpfully, encouraged by the development of intelligence tests and the concept of the intelligence quotient, or IQ. Although the IQ score may be useful in giving a broad idea of the general level of intellectual functioning, it remains important to understand that it only gives an average score of tests measuring differing skills. So a child may have a normal global IQ score, but still show a significant specific intellectual deficit. For example, a child with a high IQ, but who has a reading ability of two standard deviations below this (which may still fall within the normal range), will meet criteria for a diagnosis of specific reading disorder. Conversely, a child with a learning disability, often autism, may be gifted with particular ability in a subject such as art or mathematics.

It is generally accepted from genetic studies that the heritability of intelligence is about 50–60%, which leaves a significant role for environmental factors. Parents are perhaps the most important such influence. It has been shown that encouragement and assistance with learning by parents who themselves value education and have a good intellectual capacity significantly contributes to the achievement of a child. In addition, Tomlinson-Keasey & Little (1990) showed that the strongest predictor of occupational achievement in mid-life is educational attainment, which in turn is best explained by parents' level of education, reflecting their intellectual skills as well their attitude to educational attainment. A child's intellectual ability potentially acts as a protective factor against the risks associated with socio-economic adversity, opening up as it does the possibility of academic achievement and occupational success. Such achievement may boost self-esteem, and hence also protect against child mental health problems. However, factors such as attention, confidence, commitment and social skill are also important mediators to achievement – not all intelligent people attain occupational success.

It is sometimes hard to distinguish between quantitative and qualitative deficits in intellectual development. Most intellectual competencies form a normal distribution within populations. So a small proportion of people will always fall at the low end of the normal range of intelligence without a 'disease process' to explain this. In others, conditions such as birth anoxia, chromosomal anomalies, brain trauma or infection may cause similar or more serious levels of mental retardation.

Children with learning disabilities (those with a general IQ of less than 70) are particularly prone to psychiatric difficulties for a variety of reasons. First, a common neurological abnormality may lead to poor intellectual function as well as psychiatric syndromes such as autism or psychosis. Second, the frustration and distress caused by a lack of ability to cope with ordinary situations, or to think or express oneself clearly, may predispose to emotional and behavioural disorders. In addition, many children with learning disabilities, particularly in the 'severe' range (IQ<35), may also have physical health problems, such as epilepsy. Emotional and behavioural symptoms may be caused by partial complex seizures, or indirectly due to post-ictal states, epilepsy-related syndromes, side-effects of anticonvulsant medication or a combination of these. Families may struggle to cope with the demands of a child with a learning disability. Parents may overprotect and overcompensate for such children, or may resent their additional needs. Siblings may tease a disabled brother or sister, perhaps begrudging the extra time and attention that parents have to give to caring for their sibling. It should also be said that many families feel that the individual qualities and love that they experience from a relative with a learning disability outweigh the struggles they face.

Language

Language may well be the most highly developed of all human skills and has an impact on all aspects of our lives. The effortless way that children seem to learn language during their early years belies the monumental nature of the task. As well as developing phonetic abilities, children need to understand both the explicit meaning of words and phrases (semantics) and the appropriate use of language in a social context (pragmatics). Given this complexity, it is perhaps unsurprising that language problems are common, broadly defined difficulties being present in 15–25% of children. Tomblin *et al* (1997) reported a prevalence of developmental language disorders in 7.4% of pre-school children, only a third of which had been previously identified. There may be various reasons for this underdiagnosis. Standard language tests tend to focus on the word level and may not adequately assess understanding of whole phrases or social conversation. Expectations are often based on the average skills of children of a similar age, thereby missing children of above-average general ability who have specific language deficits. Also, as children with language problems are more likely to have comorbid emotional and behavioural problems, their language difficulties may thus remain hidden behind other, more prominent, presentations.

Children with language problems have been shown in several studies to be at increased risk of psychiatric difficulties (Rapin, 1996). Rates of anxiety disorders, social difficulties and attention problems are all increased – although interestingly, conduct problems have not been shown to be more prevalent. Such comorbid psychopathology is more common in those with low IQ and is particularly associated with mixed expressive and receptive language difficulties. In addition, language delays may in themselves be secondary to autistic spectrum disorders or learning disabilities. Children with predominantly receptive language difficulties tend to have persistent social impairments, which may lead to significant social disabilities in adult life. These children also have an increased risk of developing psychotic disorders in adolescence, which may point to common neurobiological precursors to these disorders.

Social development

Attachment

John Bowlby (1971) suggested that the relationships that a young child forms with its parents, particularly its mother, act as an internal template for future relating with others. He felt that it was therefore of key importance that a child should experience unconditional love, through sensitive and responsive parenting. Although there may be intrinsic factors in both parents and children that influence the nature of the relationship that develops between them, it remains clear that attachment is very much influenced by the behaviour of the parent. Styles of attachment have been classified and were described in Chapter 2. Children with insecure styles of attachment appear to be at greater risk of later emotional and behavioural problems, although by no means all develop such difficulties. More common presentations may include separation anxiety and school refusal. In cases of severe early emotional deprivation or abuse, children may show significant deficits in physical and emotional development. Children may fall behind their expected developmental milestones, and may fail to grow and gain weight as expected (non-organic failure to thrive). The later emotional effects of such early trauma, particularly where there has been a series of caregivers, include attachment disorders. In the 'reactive' type, children may appear afraid and 'watchful'. They may be emotionally unresponsive or ambivalent with others or aggressive towards either themselves or others. In 'disinhibited' attachment disorder, children show little interest in who is caring for them and may show indiscriminately friendly behaviour to unknown adults or children. In both variants, children may also present with hyperactivity, poor attention and aggression. They may struggle to make successful relationships with peers and adults.

Temperament

Temperament has been defined as those 'biologically rooted individual differences in behaviour tendencies that are present early in life and are relatively stable across various kinds of situation and over the course of time' (Bates, 1989). Such tendencies constitute behavioural qualities of emotion, attention and activity that have particular relevance in the context of interactions with others. Frequently cited examples include positivity versus negativity of emotional responses to varying stimuli, soothability when distressed, distractibility of attention, levels of motor activity and self-modulation of such activity. The presence of certain temperamental characteristics may have significance either as pre-disposing factors for developmental difficulties or as protective factors against them. Although temperament may of itself be largely genetically determined, it would appear that there is a need for a 'goodness of fit' between temperament and environment for a child to thrive (Chess & Thomas, 1990). For instance, Kochanska (1995) reported that for infants who demonstrated a pattern of negative emotionality (increased intensity of distress and demands for attention) at 6 months of age, the quality of their parenting appeared to predict the level of subsequent behaviour problems at age 3 years. However, this mediating effect of parenting quality on later behaviour was not present for infants who demonstrated positive emotionality at 6 months. Again, it is the interplay between genes and environment that determines develop-mental outcome.

Family

Clearly the most important context for children is their family, and it is therefore a central influence towards the achievement of healthy development across all domains. See Chapter 16 for a full discussion of family issues.

Education

After the family, school is the place where children and young people spend the most time. The school experience offers children many challenges in various developmental domains. There are academic demands, behavioural expectations and relationships to be negotiated with teachers as well as with large numbers of peers. For some children, this new world is exciting and empowering. For others it may compound existing difficulties or introduce new ones. As is often the case, difficulties in one domain tend to influence development in others. For instance, children with specific reading disorder have an increased incidence of anxiety and depression as well as conduct disorder and delinquency. Such comorbidity may lead to missed cases of specific reading disorder, as teachers may notice an obvious behavioural problem but overlook the underlying reading difficulty. One might expect this to be more likely to happen if an overworked teacher is trying to manage a large class of children in a deprived area where other classmates may also have similar difficulties; so school context may also be an important factor in the development and maintenance of problems. Interestingly, the research seems to suggest that the contextual factors that contribute to the greatest variance in both academic and social outcomes for pupils are those that relate to school ethos and organisation rather than practical considerations such as the physical environment, teacher:pupil ratio or firm discipline strategies (Rutter, 1980). The things that seem most important are high academic expectations, teachers setting good models of behaviour, pupils being praised and given responsibilities, and well-conducted lessons.

An important time during school life is the transition between primary and secondary school, and this may also be accompanied by difficulties. Studies have shown that pupils' academic achievements, self-esteem and enjoyment of school may all decline during the early stages of this transition. The comforting structure of a single classroom and class teacher as well as a relatively small school environment, in which a child is well established, is suddenly exchanged for a massive complex of buildings full of threatening older children and numerous teachers, classrooms and new challenges. It is perhaps unsurprising that some children do not immediately thrive in this hostile territory.

Another important consideration in the modern school system is the increasing emphasis on testing and examinations. Children in the UK are now subject to formal assessments from the beginning of primary school and will be subject to numerous such tests during their school career. Such scrutiny can only lead to children feeling increasingly pressured to perform academically. One study showed that the level of anxiety symptoms in Year 7 predicted both anxiety and achievement scores in Year 11 (Ialongo *et al*, 1995). Children in the top third for anxiety were ten times more likely to be in the bottom third for achievement in Year 11, irrespective of their academic attainment in Year 7. So it is important for schools and authorities to be aware that children who experience excessive stress will actually perform less well. Those pupils who do not achieve to expectations may lose self-esteem and disengage from the educational process, thereby missing out on the possibility of reaching their academic potential and, in some cases, even dropping out of the school system. Such children are at increased risk of emotional problems, delinquency and depression (Dryfoos, 1991). It is therefore important to support pupil inclusion programmes that make adequate educational provision for children who either drop out of school or are excluded.

Peers

During childhood and adolescence there is a steady social progression from total dependence on parents to independent adult lives. This process involves a gradual increase in the quantity and quality of relationships with peers. Pre-school children begin to initiate verbal interchanges and coordinated play with others, seeing peers as playmates and companions. In middle childhood, friendships begin to form that are more based on helping and sharing. Adolescents seek more intimate friendships based on mutual social support. This being said, even young children clearly attach an affective component to friendships. Audiotapes of children aged 3–5 years in conversation with their best friends have revealed numerous instances of intimacy, shared confidences and emotional support (Gottman & Parkhurst, 1980). Children may have difficulties in forming social relationships for a variety of reasons. Success in a peer group may be influenced by a child's physical appearance, ethnicity, academic competence, athletic ability, disability or socio-economic status. This being said, the most prominent influence seems to be the pattern of their social behaviour. Children appear to be better accepted if they are more pro-social, more cooperative in play, participate in social conversations and share more often (Dodge, 1983). Such children have longer and more affectively positive encounters with others and are less likely to terminate social interaction. In contrast, poorly accepted children tend to be more disruptive, aggressive and uncooperative, and to engage in solitary play that excludes others. Their interactions tend to be shorter and may be with smaller groups, younger children or other marginalised children. Poorly accepted aggressive boys may demonstrate faulty social attributions, interpreting others' ambiguous behaviour in a hostile way (Dodge, 1980), leading to inappropriately aggressive responses. A lack of peer acceptance may lead children to experience overt rejection, or even victimisation or bullying. Moreover, there is evidence that peer rejection is linked to feelings of depression in children (Vosk et al, 1982) and to other 'internalising' emotional disorders, such as somatisation. Conversely, other rejected children may express their distress more externally through conduct disorder and later delinquency (Rubin et al, 1990).

In adolescence, young people are in the process of separating from their parents, and are searching for their own identity and values. Peers are influential during this time, as young people experiment with new experiences. Some such experiences may put young people at both physical and emotional risk (for example, drug use, crime or premature sexual activity). It is important to be aware, however, that parents still play the major part in influencing a young person's values and behaviour. When peer groups assume an unusually dominant role in the life of an adolescent, this may be due to inadequate parental attention rather than the attractiveness of the peer group (Galambos & Silbereisen, 1987).

Physical development

Somatic illness

Around 5–10% of children suffer from a chronic physical condition, the most common being asthma, followed by eczema. Other relatively common disorders include diabetes mellitus, epilepsy and cerebral palsy. Many children with such illnesses (especially if mild and/or well treated) live relatively normal lives. However, any physical illness or disability will have an impact on children's views of themselves, as well as affecting the expectations that others place upon them. Such pressures may contribute to the finding that twice as many children with such physical conditions suffer psychiatric disorder as their peers (Rutter et al, 1970b). Those with more severe difficulties may, as well as dealing with the everyday demands of their disability, have to cope with the stress of hospitalisation. Children vary in their response to such stress, but Quinton & Rutter (1976) found that children admitted to hospital in early and mid-childhood had a mildly increased incidence of emotional and behavioural problems in adolescence. Important factors to minimise the stress of a hospital stay for a child are the presence and involvement of parents during admission, adequate preparation of the child beforehand, and child-friendly staff and surroundings on the ward (Graham, 1991). Physical disorders may also necessitate extended periods of absence from school, leading to educational failure. Rutter *et al* (1970*a*) found that children with physical disabilities had 2–3 times the rates of reading difficulties of children in the general population.

Puberty

Pubertal changes and associated physical growth form a significant phase in physical development, and have emotional consequences as young people come to terms with the transition from childhood to adulthood. Divergence from the normal range of pubertal development can accentuate the emotional angst of the process and cause young people to struggle in their development of social relationships and sexual identity. Teenagers often feel a keen need to conform to their peer group and an enforced physical difference may make them stand out in an unwelcome way. In particular, short stature and late puberty (which are associated) tend to have a negative effect on the self-esteem of boys. In turn, late-developing boys are less popular with peers and adults, although these difficulties may be overcome in later adolescence as they catch up with their peers (Davis, 2001). As completion of puberty puts a brake on growth, those undergoing late puberty may in the end overtake their earlier developing peers in physical stature. Early male puberty is associated with popularity and greater self-esteem, but also with an increase in risk-taking behaviours, particularly smoking and drug use (Coleman & Hendry, 1998). Girls, meanwhile, are less adversely affected by short stature, and later puberty may indeed be protective. Tall stature is often perceived negatively by girls and has been reported as a risk factor for eating disorders (Joughin *et al*, 1992). Early female puberty is associated with body dissatisfaction, depression and eating disorders. The menarche is often experienced negatively by such girls, who are unprepared for this life change at a young age, an example of the risks inherent in uneven development. Early-developing girls may be burdened by the expectation that they should be more emotionally mature than their years. They may also be increasingly pressured to engage in premature sexual activity.

Sphincter control

Children vary widely in the ages at which they attain sphincter control. This may reflect parents' own experiences, as age of bladder control has high heritability. The syndromes of enuresis and encopresis may indicate quantitative or qualitative abnormalities of development, or indeed may simply reflect normality. For instance, parents who have high expectations of their children to toilet-train early will be more likely to complain than those parents who are willing to wait until the child is ready. Fergusson *et al* (1986) found primary nocturnal enuresis in 93% of 2-year-olds, 16% of 5-year-olds and 10% of 7-year-olds. Anxious parents of bedwetting 4- and 5-year-olds can be reassured that about half of these children will improve spontaneously by the age of 8 years. It is important to distinguish between *primary* and *secondary* enuresis (those with secondary enuresis having previously achieved continence that they subsequently lose), as secondary enuresis may be more related to recent psychological trauma, including sexual abuse. Children with day- and night-time wetting as well as voiding difficulties are more apt to have urinary tract abnormalities. In all cases of enuresis, urinary infection and diabetes mellitus should also be excluded. By age 7–8 years, both children and parents may become anxious about persistent wetting. A child's social life may be limited by embarrassment about sleeping away from home. Parents may become frustrated with a child who wets the bed, and enuresis may lead to disrupted sleep and turmoil for the whole family. Studies suggest that 20–35% of parents will punish their children for bedwetting, leading to feelings of distress and low self-esteem in these children, who may feel that they have little control over their wetting. It is important to emphasise that the child is not at fault in enuresis. Coexistence of enuresis with attention-deficit hyperactivity disorder (ADHD) is 30% greater than would be expected by chance, although it is unclear why this should be.

Encopresis is defined in ICD–10 as 'the repeated passing of faeces in places that are inappropriate for the purpose' (e.g. clothing, floor) in a child over the age of 4 years with no organic condition to explain this behaviour (World Health Organization, 1992). A primary and secondary distinction is made, as in enuresis. Foreman & Thambirajah (1996) found that boys with primary encopresis tended to have other developmental delays and enuresis, whereas those with secondary encopresis had experienced more psychosocial adversity and had more comorbid conduct problems. A minority of cases may be associated with severe emotional difficulties, often resulting from serious abuse or neglect. In these cases, carers may be understandably distressed by behaviours such as smearing and defecation in socially inappropriate places. Such 'acting out' may be understood as an outward expression of deep inner distress and a challenge towards a care figure as to how much they care and are therefore prepared to tolerate from the child.

Conclusion

Development is not always a smooth process, and delays and regressions may occur along the way. This chapter has explored the complex interaction between genes and environment across many developmental domains. In addition, we have examined some key influences that can help or hinder development during the hazardous journey from infancy to adulthood. We have found that particular skills and abilities can be protective, but also that difficulties in a wide range of developmental situations may be associated with behavioural and emotional problems in children, some of which may extend into their adult lives. Children inhabit a developmental context. It follows that if we wish to understand the nature of psychiatric disorders in children and adolescents, we need to incorporate a developmental perspective into our framework for assessing and working with young people and their families.

References

Bates, J. E. (1989) Concepts and measures of temperament. In *Temperament in Childhood* (eds G. A. Kohnstamm, J. E. Bates & M. K. Rothbart), pp. 3–26. London: John Wiley.

Bowlby, J. (1971) *Attachment and Loss, vol. 1: Attachment.* London: Penguin.

Chess, S. & Thomas, A. (1990) Continuities and discontinuities in temperament. In *Straight and Devious Pathways from Childhood to Adulthood* (eds L. Robins & M. Rutter), pp. 205–220. Cambridge: Cambridge University Press.

Coleman, J. C. & Hendry, L. (1998) *The Nature of Adolescence* (3rd edn). London: Routledge.

Davis, R. (2001) Influences on the development of psychopathology in adolescence. In *Adolescent Psychiatry in Clinical Practice* (ed. S. G. Gowers), pp. 30–59. London: Arnold.

Dodge, K. A. (1980) Social cognition and children's aggressive behaviour. *Child Development*, **51**, 162–170.

Dodge, K. A. (1983) Behavioral antecedents of peer social status. *Child Development*, **54**, 1386–1399.

Dryfoos, J. G. (1991) Adolescents at risk: a summation of work in the field: programs and policies. *Journal of Adolescent Health*, **12**, 620–637.

Fergusson, D. M., Horwood, L. J. & Shannon, F. T. (1986) Factors related to the age of attainment of nocturnal bladder control: an 8-year longitudinal study. *Pediatrics*, **78**, 884–890.

Foreman, D. M. & Thambirajah, M. S. (1996) Conduct disorder, enuresis and specific developmental delays in two types of encopresis: a case-note study of 63 boys. *European Child and Adolescent Psychiatry*, **5**, 33–37.

Galambos, N. L. & Silbereisen, R. K. (1987) Influence of income change and parental acceptance on adolescent transgression proneness and peer relations. *European Journal of Psychology of Education*, **1**, 17–28.

Gottman, J. M. & Parkhurst, J. T. (1980) A developmental theory of friendship and acquaintanceship processes. In *Minnesota Symposia on Child Psychology* (ed. W. A. Collins), vol. 13, pp. 197–253. Hillsdale, NJ: Erlbaum.

Graham, P. (1991) *Child Psychiatry: A Developmental Approach.* Oxford: Oxford University Press.

Ialongo, N., Edelsohn, G., Werthamer-Larsson, L., *et al* (1995) The significance of self-reported anxious symptoms in first grade children: prediction to anxious symptoms and adaptive functioning in fifth grade. *Journal of Child Psychology and Psychiatry*, **36**, 427–437.

Joughin, N., Varsou, E., Gowers, S. G., *et al* (1992) Relative tallness in anorexia nervosa. *International Journal of Eating Disorders*, **12**, 195–207.

Kochanska, G. (1995) Children's temperament, mothers' discipline, and security of attachment: multiple pathways to emerging internalization. *Child Development*, **66**, 597–615.

Quinton, D. & Rutter, M. (1976) Early hospital admission and later disturbances of behaviour: an attempted replication of Douglas' findings. *Developmental Medicine and Child Neurology*, **18**, 447–459.

Rapin, I. (1996) Developmental language disorders: a clinical update. *Journal of Child Psychology and Psychiatry*, **37**, 643–655.

Rubin, K. H., LeMare, L. J. & Lollis, S. (1990) Social withdrawal in childhood: developmental pathways to peer rejection. In *Peer Rejection in Childhood* (eds S. R. Asher & J. D. Coie), pp. 217–249. New York: Cambridge University Press.

Rutter, M. (1980) School influences on children's behaviour and development. *Pediatrics*, **65**, 208–220.

Rutter, M., Tizard, J. & Whitmore, K. (1970a) *Education, health and behaviour*. London: Longman.

Rutter, M., Graham, P. & Yule, W. (1970b) *A Neuropsychiatric Study in Childhood*. London: Heinemann.

Tomblin, J. B., Records, N. L., Buckwalter, P., *et al* (1997) Prevalence of specific language impairment in kindergarten children. *Journal of Speech, Language and Hearing Research*, **40**, 1245–1260.

Tomlinson-Keasey, C. & Little, T. D. (1990) Predicting educational attainment, occupational achievement, intellectual skill and personal adjustment among gifted men and women. *Journal of Educational Psychology*, **82**, 442–455.

Vosk, B., Forehand, R., Parker, J. B., *et al* (1982) A multimethod comparison of popular and unpopular children. *Developmental Psychology*, **18**, 571–575.

CHAPTER 4

Continuities and discontinuities from childhood to adult life

Ian M. Goodyer

Since the 1990s there has been a significant increase in our understanding of the links between development in early childhood and adolescence and well-being in early adult life. Longitudinal studies of large unselected populations of children repeatedly assessed through the formative school-age years into young adult life have begun to illustrate the pathways and trajectories that result in differential levels of risk and resilience, and the subsequent onset of psychiatric disorder.

This chapter provides a selected overview of three domains where child–adult links for psychopathology have been sought: first, the notion of the child at risk; second, childhood antecedents of adult psychiatric disorders; and third, continuities between child and adult psychiatric disorder.

The nature of risk for psychopathology

Risk can be defined as the degree to which the likelihood of a given adverse outcome will occur following exposure to a defined toxic agent. The relative importance of exposure is estimated by the probability of the outcome occurring in a given population compared with the level of occurrence in a non-exposed population. Risks are suspected causes and outcomes are undesirable. A detailed discussion of the quantitative analysis of risk is beyond the scope of this chapter. The magnitude of the risk is the degree to which the likelihood of outcome is increased as a consequence of exposure to the agent. A critical issue in risk evaluation is the importance of defining and characterising the risk factor. Risks for psychopathology occur from a variety of sources, both within and external to the subject. They may be defined at the level of the individual, the family or the community at large. For example, individuals may be born with genes that render them susceptible to psychiatric illness, acquire lesions such as head injury that alter their capacity for learning, or become exposed to negative social environments that diminish emotional and cognitive development. Familial environmental risks might include a neglectful or hostile parenting environment, or an environment that is physically inadequate (such as in failure to ensure food and shelter) without being overtly emotionally negative. In addition, physical neighbourhood risks might occur (such as poor housing) or functional risks (such as living in a violent or dangerous society).

Invariably, risks of these types are not independent of each other and determining their degree of association prior to the occurrence of the undesirable outcome is essential. This is because it is increasingly apparent that most risk profiles for psychopathology involve multiple adverse events from different levels of biology (genetic, physiological, social, and so on).

The general approach to determining the importance of a set of risk characteristics is probabilistic. This approach involves comparing two populations, one exposed and the other not, and determining a meaningful level above chance that outcome occurs in association with exposure. Demonstrating a statistical association between the putative agent and undesirable outcome is, in itself, insufficient. The size of this assoc-iation provides an important indication of the likelihood of an effect. This has been termed the 'potency' of a risk factor, and is the maximal discrepancy achievable between exposed and unexposed groups (often referred to as high and low risk, indicating exposed and not exposed). Many quantitative statistics are used to denote the size of the effect (potency).

The precise statistic used depends on the population being studied. Thus, relative risk has been used to calculate the magnitude of association between acute recent negative life events and psychiatric disorder in case–control studies. For example, in both child and adult studies of this type, events occurring in the months prior to onset are estimated to increase the risk of psychiatric disorder between 2 and 7 times (Paykel, 1978; Goodyer *et al*, 1985). This estimate is not appropriate for population-based studies, where a relatively precise enumeration of the incidence of the disease in the exposed and non-exposed population is required. For example, the proportion of participants subsequently exposed and not exposed to personally disappointing life events was determined in 171 adolescents at high risk of psychopathological disorder followed over a 12-month period. Among these individuals, 30 developed a first-episode major depressive disorder over the study period compared with 141 who did not (Goodyer *et al*, 2000*a*). The number of events per month over the follow-up year was computed. Among the 30 who became ill, 18 (60%) had experienced such an event in the month before onset, compared with 31 of the 141 (22%) who did not develop the disorder – a highly significant difference (Goodyer *et al*, 2000*b*). From these proportions, it can be seen that highly proximal negative life events are neither necessary nor sufficient to 'explain' the onset of major depression in this age range. Indeed, calculating the attributable risk suggests that only some 27% of all cases of major depression in this cohort can be attributed to exposure to highly proximal acute life events. This is because there are multiple potential risk pathways involved in the emergence of depression, in which acute life events have only a modest role (Kendler *et al*, 2002). Of course, such events are going to be important in those cases that have experienced them, but it would not be possible to construct a psychological theory of the depressions on the knowledge of recent life events alone. Neither would it be advisable to develop a social policy of prevention focusing on acute event reduction, as no more than a third of such cases at best could be reduced, even if such a strategy was 100% successful. Including other potential risk processes considerably increases the opportunity for 'capturing' those adolescents most likely to become depressed in the above population. Analysis of the five psychosocial risks measured in the adolescent study described above showed that the median number of risks was three and that 91% of the participants at high risk for psychopathology were exposed to two, three or four psychosocial risks in the 12 months before follow-up (Goodyer *et al*, 2000*b*). Furthermore, 30 (97%) out of 31 of the participants who developed major depression came from this multiple high-risk group. Note, however, that even among those at very high risk, 141 did not become depressed over the follow-up period. The attributable risk of becoming depressed among those exposed to multiple psychosocial risks compared with those exposed to no such risks is now 88%. Thus, we might be on better ground for social policy-making by targeting very high-risk populations, because we can say with some confidence that they have a very high attributable risk for subsequent onset of depression. Nevertheless, it is not immediately clear how we would construct our interventions, knowing that, in the short term, no more than around 1 in 5 of even this population will develop major depression over the ensuing 12 months. This analysis also indicates that we are unlikely to devise a psychosocial theory alone that will 'explain' the onsets of all cases. Other non-social factors need to be taken into account. These examples illustrate the importance of understanding the complexities of risk analysis from different perspectives from a relatively straightforward prospective cohort study. There are, however, further important issues to consider regarding the effects of risk factors for psychopathology.

For example, it is difficult to find two risk factors that are truly independent of each other and therefore each is likely to carry a moderate effect at most even in the best-designed studies and using the most sensitive of measures. Statistical procedures must be able to cope with a risk profile that is more often than not going to determine the relative contribution of two or more risk factors in the onset of a given disorder. Risk can be best expressed as more than a threefold increase in the liability to psychiatric disorder following exposure, or stating that more than 50% of the onsets of a symptom or syndrome are attributable to the measured risk. Such statements are a necessary but insufficient first step in interpreting with confidence a causal association (through exposure) between risk and outcome. Returning to the adolescent study described briefly above, multivariate analyses of psychoendocrine risk processes measured at the beginning of the study showed that the patterning of all measured risks most likely to correlate with the subsequent onset of major depression involved social adversity, changes in hormones and the level of depressive features at onset of the study. Under these conditions, the true role of highly proximal life events in those becomes apparent for a small but significant group of adolescents. Thus, in those participants with high levels of cortisol and dehydro epiandrosterone (DHEA), personally disappointing events occurring in the month before onset increased the risk of onset by no less than 7 times and on average by around 50 times, compared with those at high psychosocial risk but with no hormonal changes. The risk statistic derived from this multivariate analysis is the odds ratio, which reflects the liability of each variable to be associated with the outcome of interest for each unit change of its measurement, having taken into account any correlated liabilities between the risk variables themselves.

At the level of measurement, risk factors must precede and be independent from the outcome variable of interest. For example, high scores on a self-report behaviour scale often precede the onset or emergence of a clinically significant disorder, with the latter invariably being detected because of an increase in symptoms, greater symptom severity and personal and/or social impairment. The preceding self-report scores cannot denote a pure risk factor, as they might also contain features of the disorder itself, albeit in a low-level or non-impairing form. In contrast, adverse social circumstances, temperamental style and physical and psychosexual growth represent features that are independent of mental states and may be viewed as potential candidate risk markers for different forms of emotional and behavioural difficulty or disorder.

Many of the psychiatric disorders of interest (depression, schizophrenia, disruptive behaviour disorders) are episodic in nature, occurring in their first episode during a fairly wide developmental period (e.g. 8–20 years of age), within which changes in physical and psychological characteristics are prominent and interplay closely with alterations in social experience. The risk profile most associated with onset of these conditions is likely to be drawn from more than one level of this complex biology. For example, we have just described how both severe personal disappointments in combination with cortisol and DHEA hypersecretion are significantly associated with the onset of first-episode major depression in adolescents. This indicates that different levels of physiological and social risk additively contribute to these forms of psychopathology (Goodyer *et al*, 2000*a*,*b*). The candidate risks for affective disorders are not, however, confined to these domains alone, as being at least Tanner stage three with high testosterone and/or oestrogen levels are also associated with a marked increase in a range of depressive conditions (Angold *et al*, 1999). In other words, the population specificity of candidate risks may involve considerably more processing levels than the social or the physiological environment. Recent findings have also implicated the potential importance of genetic risks probably operating through gene–environment interactions. Thus, possession of the short allele of the serotonin transporter gene increases the occurrence of negative life events and together this results in increasing the risk of depression (Caspi *et al*, 2003). Whether differentiated risk patterns involving social, psychological, physiological and genetic components are sufficient to distinguish between clear-cut forms of psychopathology is not yet clear.

From the developmental perspective, it is critical to consider the issue of timing of risk exposure and to be able to determine the effects (potency) of risk profiles over time. From the temporal perspective, the potency of risk may vary. The association between increasing levels of sex hormones, Tanner stage three and increased incidence of affective disorder, or the onset of disruptive behaviour disorders in adolescents exposed to a deviant peer group but with no prior history of behavioural disorder (Moffitt & Caspi, 2001), are examples of developmental timing effects.

Determining the effects of risks over time requires longitudinal designs and repeated measurement of the candidate risk profile determined prior to the study. Such cohort studies are uncommon, particularly developmentally sensitive studies. One example is that of Rueter *et al* (1999), who demonstrated that among adolescents, persistent or escalating stressful events, such as disagreements with parents, indirectly increase the risk for the onset of internalising disorders through their direct association with high or increasing symptom levels. These findings suggest that for many adolescents, first-episode major depression is a rather slow-growing affair, arising through the persisting interplay of family difficulties and rising levels of depressive symptoms over a period of years. No other candidate risks, social or physiological, were measured, therefore it is not easy to determine what the risk processes were that led to eventual disorder. The study is virtually unique in this age range for demonstrating quite clearly the interplay between social family adversity and rising self-reported depressive symptoms, and how there is not a clear direct impact of family disagreements in young teenagers for the onset of major depression in late adolescence. These findings demonstrate that a longitudinal perspective on candidate risks provides a more succinct analysis of the processes involved in the formation of psychopathology.

The effects of potency may also vary with time. Thus, what may be an important risk candidate at one time may be less so at another. There are few invariate psychosocial risk models that continue to exert effects of the same potency for psychopathology throughout the lifespan (severe learning disability may be one of a few exceptions). When considering risks for disorder, it is critical to take into account the potential variation in potency effect on the emergence of the same condition at different ages. Equally it may be that the characteristics of the disorder will vary with time because of developmental influences on the emergent phenotype. For example, child maltreatment is strongly associated with general emotional and behavioural problems in 3-year-olds, but somewhat more specifically with major depression in adolescence and again more generally with psychopathology and poor social adjustment in young adult life. These differences in phenotype probably reflect developmental differences in the formation of psychopathology during the first three decades within individuals exposed to severe child abuse in the first decade.

Finally, determining risk factors is only the first step in elucidating risk processes (Kraemer *et al*, 1997). For example, if cortisol hypersecretion had true direct risk effect of significant potency acting as a causal agent, then lowering cortisol levels in high-risk adolescents might diminish the subsequent population incidence of first-episode major depression in this age range. Demonstrating that the risk factor can be altered and that this leads to a diminution in psychopathology would definitively demonstrate the causal nature of an antecedent risk factor.

Child and adolescent risks for adult-onset disorders

Schizophrenia

Schizophrenia has a prevalence of around 1% in adults, with first episodes generally occurring between the ages of 16 years and 25 years (Andreasen, 1999). The symptoms manifest in multiple domains of behaviour, language, thought and affect, but their origins, sequential emergence and precise relationship have yet to be adequately documented. A neurodevelopmental aetiology has been influential in an attempt to explain the emergence of this complex disorder in late adolescence and early adult life (Kemppainen *et al*, 2001). There have been two important birth cohort studies whose design has allowed correlates to be determined between early developmental events, mental symptoms in childhood, and the onset of schizophrenia and related mental disorders in young adult life (Isohanni *et al*, 2000; Cannon *et al*, 2002). There is a converging body of findings that significant impairments in neuromotor, language and cognitive development, including being late in walking and delayed toilet training (bowel and bladder), are associated with the onset of first-episode schizophrenia by the person's mid-twenties (Isohanni *et al*, 2001). Overall, early milestones may reduce and later milestones increase the risk in a linear manner. These developmental correlates are not associated with non-psychotic psychiatric outcomes, suggesting a relatively specific effect on the adult form of the disorder. Interestingly, these neurodevelopmental delays, while in themselves rather non-specific, also predict the development of psychotic symptoms in both childhood and adulthood. Self-reported psychotic symptoms at age 11 years predicted a very high risk of a schizophreniform diagnosis at age 26. In 42% of schizophreniform cases in the cohort one or more psychotic symptoms were reported at age 11 years (Cannon *et al*, 2002). This finding was not mediated through non-psychotic child psychiatric difficulties in these patients, suggesting a relatively specific association between child psychotic symptoms and later schizophrenia, with the former themselves arising in populations with neurodevelopmental delay. These findings confirm the long-standing observations that some, perhaps many, forms of schizophrenia have developmental origins (Isohanni *et al*, 2001; Silverstein *et al*, 2002). Moreover, the recent findings take us further, showing that the rather non-specific and somewhat generalised delays in early motor and language development are associated with more particular and subsequent abnormalities in language and thought associated with psychotic symptoms. This implicates the emergence in childhood of cortical systems dysfunction related to receptive language development. Quite how this leads to a widening of the symptoms and subsequent first-rank symptoms and social impairment remains to be clarified. In a longitudinal study of a group of people at genetically high risk of schizophrenia, compared with controls the presence of psychotic symptoms was preceded by a decline in memory and general IQ, suggesting a decline in performance skills occurring in individuals already neurodevelopmentally at risk. The implication is that there may be a second neurodevelopmentally sensitive set of events occurring in late childhood or early adolescence that promotes the onset of psychotic symptoms through a further decline in language and executive processing abilities.

Major depression

Childhood antecedents of major depression in adult life have received less scientific attention than might be expected, given the strong theoretical emphasis on early parental loss, subsequent negative self-perception and the onset of affective disorder. Recent findings from national and birth cohort studies have confirmed that compared with people with no early difficulties, adults exposed to childhood adversities occurring from birth through the school-age years do indeed report a higher prevalence of adult affective disorder (Kessler & Magee, 1993). There are some important principles arising from these general findings. First, there is no evidence that any single early adversity has sufficient potency in itself to cause adult depression (Kessler *et al*, 1997). Overall, it is the multiplicity of adversities that is associated with subsequent major depression in adult life. Second, this multiple adverse risk pattern is not confined to social adversities alone, but also includes perinatal insults and motor skills deficits. A significant confounding factor for direct links between child adversities and adult depression is the potential effects of child psychopathology occurring as a con-sequence of these childhood adversities. This is not only possible but highly likely, given the clear-cut associations between such adversities and common emotional and behavioural psychopathologies in the school-age years. The most common effect is likely to be that both adversity and childhood psychiatric disorder contribute to adult disorder. For example, a retrospective study of depressed women has demonstrated that teenage depression is an important contributory factor to the onset of adult depression in addition to prior child sexual abuse (Bifulco *et al*, 1998).

A more recent birth cohort study (Jaffee *et al*, 2002) has extended these findings by examining the links between a wide range of childhood adversities (social, family, perinatal, temperamental) and the onset of depression in juveniles. Four groups of adults were studied: those who either recover or develop recurrent depression into adult life; adults with first onset after 17 years of age; and well adults with no lifetime psychiatric history who none the less experienced childhood adversities. A comparison of these four groups revealed that the two juvenile-onset groups (recovered and recurrent) had similar high-risk profiles on a range of childhood adversity measures. Compared with the adult-onset depression group, the juvenile-onset groups experienced more perinatal insults and motor skill deficits, caretaker instability, criminality and psychopathology in their family of origin, and behavioural and socio-emotional problems. The adult-onset group's risk profile was similar to that of the never-depressed group, with the exception of elevated childhood sexual abuse. The findings confirm and substantially extend the previous retrospective reports that generalised child adversities are associated with early-onset depression (<17 years of age), of which cases around 60% might have at least one further episode into adult life. Importantly, however, adults who have depression but no juvenile history of depression show a significantly greater exposure to unwanted childhood sexual contact than lifetime well controls, but not other depressions. This supports a potentially direct effect over time for child sexual abuse into adulthood for those 'escaped' adolescent onset.

The one finding to show significant association with all depressive types in this study was unwanted sexual contact. The implication is that rather than loss events (i.e. the permanent exit of a parent), abuse and maltreatment appear to be the most potentially risky childhood experience for depressive disorders in the first three decades of life. The psychiatric outcome from child sexual abuse is not, however, specific to affective disorders. Individuals of both sexes who reported a history of unwanted sexual contact as a child are more likely to come from difficult adverse circumstances, including alcohol-related parent difficulties. Multiple family adversities result in a series of correlated early psychosocial adversities with a range of psychiatric outcomes, including different forms of affective disorders, anxiety states, conduct difficulties and substance misuse-related conditions (Molnar *et al*, 2001; Nelson *et al*, 2002). The evidence from both cohort and twin studies is that child sexual abuse exerts an independent and particular effect of some importance for adult psychopathology in general. This appears to be most likely for those with severe abusive histories, including rape and intercourse, and multiple abusive experiences in childhood. There is also some evidence to suggest that among depressive conditions, such a history is somewhat more associated with severe rather than milder depressions in adult life (Harkness & Monroe, 2002). In addition, it seems that the pathway through which abusive experiences exert these effects is different from the pathway through which poor parental care is associated with subsequent adult affective (and other) disorders (Sadowski *et al*, 1999; Hill *et al*, 2001).

Adult deviant behaviour

Much adult psychopathology has some of its roots in childhood difficulties, and nowhere is this more apparent than in the tendency for continuities between child and adult antisocial behaviour (Farrington, 1995; Robins, 1996). The core childhood predictor for adult antisocial behaviour is the pattern of severe behavioural difficulties evident across different social domains and leading to the Axis II diagnosis of antisocial personality disorder. Looking back, one sees that the great majority of adults with severe antisocial personality disorder had severe conduct disorder as children. New-onset antisocial conduct disorder in adulthood is rare, occurring in around 10% of cases at the most. Looking forward from childhood, however, around 60% of children showing antisocial behaviour do not develop antisocial personality disorder in adulthood (Robins & Price, 1991). Rates of antisocial personality disorder appear to rise with the number of childhood problems, and it is the number rather than the specific type of early childhood behaviour that is the better predictor of later poor adult outcome. The same pattern of child-to-adult problems holds for both men and women, despite marked secular change in overall rates of childhood difficulties. Finally, earlier-onset conduct problems, with onsets before the age of 13 years, appear to be especially ominous in terms of long-term persistence (Loeber & Farrington, 2000). Childhood conduct problems also show robust links with later offending (Farrington, 1995). Modest associations have been reported between childhood aggression in those as young as 3 and adult offending, but the majority of findings pertain to aggression in boys in middle childhood and girls in early adolescence, associated with later young adult offending. Looking back, chronic adult offenders show an early onset of offending and engage in a diverse range of offences, both violent and non-violent. In addition to specific continuities for antisocial behaviour, childhood conduct disorders are associated with a broader set of later deviancies, including alcohol and substance misuse and a wide range of subsequent affective and psychotic psychopathologies (Zoccolillo, 1992; Robins, 1998). The poor outcome for those with persisting conduct disorder includes considerable social and personal morbidity, with increased risks for school drop-out, poor work record, teenage pregnancy and marital instability. It appears that a large number of violent adults with childhood histories of antisocial behaviour have other psychiatric disorders that increase the liability to aggressive behaviour (Arseneault *et al*, 2000).

Adult outcomes of child and adolescent psychopathology

Anxiety disorders

Anxiety disorders are one of the least well understood groups of conditions in child and adolescent psychopathology. Accordingly, there are few data on their natural history, course and outcome (Ost & Treffers, 2001), although there is growing evidence to suggest that these disorders are not uncommon in childhood and adolescence (Silverman & Treffers, 2001). The form of anxiety appears somewhat developmentally sensitive, with younger populations having a higher prevalence of separation anxiety, and simple phobias with social phobias, generalised anxiety disorder and panic disorders being more apparent in adolescents. Post-traumatic stress disorder does not appear to vary in prevalence with age. Overall, the history of any anxiety disorder in childhood or adolescence is associated with a large increase in the risk of anxiety disorder in adult life (Newman *et al*, 1996). The level of specificity for the same anxious condition recurring over time appears to be low (Ferdinand & Verhulst, 1995; Pine *et al*, 1998). The most specific continuity reported is that of social phobia being present with much the same characteristics in adolescence and early adult life (Pine *et al*, 1998). Generalised anxiety disorder in adolescence appears to precede the onset of major depression in adults, but the exact relationship remains unclear (Last *et al*, 1997; Pine *et al*, 1998). It may be that in some cases of anxiety, major depression or dysthymia was already present. This is possible because there is considerable symptom overlap between anxious and depressive diagnoses. What little evidence there is suggests that anxiety–depression has a worse early adult outcome than pure anxiety disorders (Last *et al*, 1997). Indeed, many people with anxiety disorders have a good prognosis, being indis-tinguishable from well controls at follow-up, apart from being somewhat less sociable and showing reluctance to leave the parental home. Continuity for adult anxiety disorders in general is positively correlated with the number of anxiety disorders experienced during adolescence, even after controlling for the confounding effects of socio-familial and individual factors (Woodward & Fergusson, 2001). Adolescents with three or more episodes of anxious conditions are 3.5 times more likely to have anxious disorders in adult life. Equally, however, a history of child and adolescent anxiety disorder carries a more generalised risk of illicit drug use, poor socialisation, depression and educational underachievement by early adult life (Pine *et al*, 1998; Woodward & Fergusson, 2001). The precise relations between anxiety in the school years, adult psycho-pathological disorder and poor social and educational adjustment remain unknown. The possibility that some childhood anxiety disorders may be early-forming major depressive states deserves more extensive longitudinal study. Determining what variables distinguish single-episode from recurrent anxious disorders at first presentation would help to delineate those at risk of future mental health and social adjustment difficulties. What little infor-mation we have suggests that neither social environmental difficulties nor family factors (such as anxious, over-involved parenting) are strong predictors of recurrence (Last *et al*, 1997). A more recent observation is that childhood motor impairment is strongly associated with persistent anxiety among male, but not among female, adolescents (Sigurdsson *et al*, 2002). This suggests a putative neurodevelopmental aetiology for persistent anxiety states in males and a gender-differentiated set of causal processes for chronic anxiety states in the first 20 years of life.

Depression

Considerable advances have been made since the 1990s in our under-standing of the natural history and outcome of major depression (Harrington & Dubicka, 2001). There is now good evidence that both depressive symptoms and disorder show continuities over time. Clinical follow-up studies into adult life have shown that adolescent depression is associated with a high risk of depressive relapse, extending well into the third decade (Fombonne *et al*, 2001*a*). Contrary to expectations, this risk of recurrence was unaffected by non-depressive comorbid diagnoses. Thus, depressive conduct disorder is associated with equally severe affective and more severe non-affective adverse outcomes. Among the depressive conduct subgroup, the undesirable long-term effects of adolescent depression may be worse for women than for men. The reasons for this gender difference in outcome is unclear, but may be related to narrowing social opportunities for women, with increased rates of teenage pregnancy, social isolation and poverty. Depressive conduct disorder during adolescence also shows outcomes consistent with those for antisocial behaviour without overt depressive disorder. Thus in this depressive subgroup there are increased rates of suicide, alcoholism, substance misuse and antisocial personality disorders (Fombonne *et al*, 2001b). Indeed there is evidence that a history of major depressive disorder in childhood or adolescence may be associated with an increased likelihood of an Axis II personality disorder in adult life (Kasen *et al*, 2001). This increased risk is not confined to depressive conduct disorders, suggesting that the nature of major depression itself has long-term effects on those social, cognitive and neuro-psychological processes that are involved in the formation of behavioural traits and style over time. The notion that depression is bad for you in general, independent of non-depressive comorbid disorders, appears to be particularly true for those with recurrent rather than single-episode disorders. Recurrent depressions in adolescents do appear to be more closely associated with the emergence of depressogenic thinking styles than single-episode disorders, suggesting deleterious effects of the disorder on cognitive development (Lewinsohn *et al*, 1999). These negative effects on social cognition do not appear to be gender-related, suggesting that once established through adolescence, recurrent depression is psychologically bad for both men and women. In addition, poor social adjustment in adults that is associated with recurrent child and adolescent depressions may be a direct function of the adverse social circumstances of the adolescent at that time and not a direct effect of their mental state *per se* (Fergusson & Woodward, 2002). Thus, there are direct and specific effects of affective psychopathology in adolescence for the same form of disorder in adult life, but equally there are continuities for social adversity effects independent of the risks exerted by the presence of recurrent depression.

Obsessive–compulsive disorder

Unlike anxiety disorders, it appears that as far as clinically presenting obsessive–compulsive disorder (OCD) in childhood is concerned, there is no developmental effect on the form of disorder over time, but the prognosis is moderate to poor, with as many as 50% of cases showing recurrent episodes into adult life (March & Leonard, 1996). In addition, other psychiatric diagnoses, including depression and personality disorders, may arise over time (Thomsen, 1995; Wewetzer *et al*, 2001).

An interesting finding from a recent epidemiological study of the outcome of child-onset OCD is a potentially aetiologically important three-way relationship between tics, attention-deficit hyperactivity disorder (ADHD) and OCD (Peterson, 2001). In this study, childhood OCD symptoms (diagnosis before 11 years of age) were associated with tic symptoms in childhood and an increased risk of ADHD symptoms in adult life as well as OCD, even if ADHD had not been diagnosed in childhood. In childhood, tics and ADHD symptoms were positively associated with an increase in OCD symptoms in adulthood. This suggests that OCD developing before age 11 years and OCD developing in late adolescence have different aetiologies, phenotypes and potentially different outcomes. The childhood form may be more associated with other neurodevelopmental symptoms and syndromes such as hyperkinesis and Tourette syndrome, whereas the adolescent-onset form is associated with emotional symptoms and affective disorders. The childhood form appears more obsessional and less responsive to treatment, but there appear to be individual differences in this general finding (Rosario-Campos *et al*, 2001). Since these disorders are uncommon and most studies are on small samples or quantitative symptom data from questionnaires, further longitudinal studies are much needed to determine if the natural history and outcome of these two subtypes are as markedly different as currently suggested.

Attention-deficit hyperactivity disorders

The attention-deficit hyperactivity syndromes represent a heterogeneous set of disorders whose natural history, course, treatment and outcome into adult life have been the subject of numerous studies (Sandberg, 1996). The disorders are often highly comorbid with other neurodevelopmental problems, such as tics and motor coordination difficulties. These children often show high levels of general worry and social anxiety as well as behavioural difficulties, evolving in many cases into comorbid conduct disorder by middle childhood. By early and middle adolescence, relative deficits are commonly seen in academic and social functioning, ADHD symptoms remain problematic in two-thirds to three-quarters of cases, and antisocial behaviours, in some cases amounting to conduct disorder, are common (Mannuzza & Klein, 2000). When patients are evaluated in their mid-twenties, dysfunctions are apparent in these same areas. Compared with controls, adults with a history of ADHD in childhood complete less schooling, hold lower-ranking occupations, and continue to suffer from poor self-esteem and social skills deficits. Antisocial personality and perhaps substance misuse in adulthood may also be more common, but it is unclear if this is directly associated with ADHD or with correlated risks such as conduct disorder, social adversity and exposure to risky environments

(Gillberg & Hellgren, 1996). The effectiveness of treatment has been cited as an important variable in diminishing the poor outcome for these disorders. It has been suggested that intervention in childhood diminishes the risk of conduct disorder and educational impairment in adolescence, reducing the risks of poor adult outcome through lowering the rate of secondary psychiatric and psychosocial handicap in the group as a whole (Silver, 2000). This is an important and encouraging suggestion for child psychiatry, indicating a potential improvement in the developmental trajectory of children with a condition with known effective pharmacological and psychosocial treatments.

Recent observations have noted that children with ADHD are at risk of other psychiatric disorders in adult life, including bipolar disorder (Geller et al, 2002) and OCD (Peterson et al, 2001). This raises important questions about a potential change in the form of disorder in some cases. The suggestion that a small group of patients with ADHD may develop bipolar disorder in late adolescent or adult life requires considerable verification, but if true may be more likely in those with a high familial loading in first-degree relatives for mood disorders in general, and perhaps bipolar disorders in particular. The suggested emergence of obsessional symptoms by adult life in other children with ADHD also requires more systematic inquiry before a direct correlation between the two groups of symptoms and/or disorders can be established. It does, however, appear from these studies that ADHD may have a significant and differential effect on emotional and cognitive development and contain perhaps two or more subtypes whose adult trajectories and psychopathologies may be different. Currently, there appears to be no clear-cut set of childhood predictors to help determine the likely form of psychiatric disorder in adult life.

It is important to also note that for many children with ADHD, outcomes can be good. A review of long-term studies noted that by their mid-twenties, nearly all such people were gainfully employed (Mannuzza & Klein, 2000). Furthermore, some had achieved a higher-level education (e.g. completed a master's degree, enrolled in medical school) and occupation (e.g. accountant, stockbroker). In addition, two-thirds of these children showed no evidence of any mental disorder in adulthood. In conclusion, although children with ADHD as a group fare poorly compared with their non-ADHD counterparts, the childhood syndrome does not preclude attaining high educational and vocational goals, and most children no longer exhibit clinically significant emotional or behavioural problems once they reach their mid-twenties.

Conduct disorders

Prospective studies of epidemiological samples have noted that there is considerable validity for childhood-onset conduct disorders to show

53

persistence across the life course and for adolescent-onset cases to remit within early adulthood in the majority of cases (Moffitt & Caspi, 2001). New-onset conduct disorder or antisocial personality disorder arising in adolescence seems relatively rare, occurring in only about 10% of cases (Newman *et al*, 1996). The observation that age of onset has a significant predictive effect has resulted in a developmental taxonomy dividing the antisocial population of young people into two distinct groups: a small early-onset group who show a life-course persistence of deviant and antisocial behaviours, and an adolescent-limited group with little or no long-term difficulty into adult life (Moffitt & Caspi, 2001). In the Dunedin Multidisciplinary Health and Development Study, individuals with childhood-onset delinquency had childhoods of inadequate parenting, and neurocognitive, temperament and behaviour problems, whereas individuals with adolescent-onset delinquency did not have these pathological backgrounds. Gender comparisons showed a male-to-female ratio of 10:1 for childhood-onset delinquency, but a ratio of only 1.5:1 for adolescent-onset delinquency. Showing the same pattern as males, females with childhood-onset delinquency had high-risk backgrounds, but those with adolescent-onset delinquency did not. The implications of these findings are that the aetiology of conduct disorder is distinctly different, with childhood-onset processes arising from neurocognitive deficits, emotional dys-functions and language problems (particularly pragmatics or social discourse). Adolescent-onset delinquency, meanwhile, arises from social psychological difficulties involving peer-group deviancy and cultural values incorporating high levels of group aggression. In some cases, children with child-onset conduct disorders recover, indicating a 'childhood limited' subgroup whose nature and characteristics remain unclear. Whether these arise from social factors alone, in the absence of neurocognitive and emotional dysfunction within the child, is not clear. In addition, not all adolescent conduct disorders show a time-limited course, suggesting that some such adolescents may either possess some other set of risks, or their adolescent social developmental trajectory does not ameliorate. In these, social adversities persist and lead to greater adult deviancy than would otherwise be expected (Moffitt *et al*, 2002). Social cognitions remain open to considerable influence in the adolescent years and it may be that for some cases social information processing becomes disorganised and dysfunctional as a consequence of adolescent peer-group experiences such as rejection (Laird *et al*, 2001). In addition, some adolescents interpret interpersonal cues as personally threatening when others do not (hostile attributional bias); this may come about in part as a consequence of exposure to high levels of threat in the adolescent peer environment (Lochman & Dodge, 1994). Interest-ingly, deviant peer relations are among the most powerful correlates of adolescent delinquency and, for males, such relationships appear very 'sticky', persisting over time and being highly correlated for some individuals with male offending (Vitaro et al, 2001). This raises the intriguing and important issue that proximal social environments can shape behaviours that may persist. Thus, interventions to diminish the risk of persistence for adolescent conduct disorder are likely to involve a focus on peer group deviancy and preventing their secondary behavioural effects (drug/alcohol misuse, stealing, violence to others) on developmental aspects of social information processing in the adolescent years. In contrast, the interventions in childhood-onset disorders may require more individual approaches, for example to aid parents in minimising the effects of neurocognitive and emotional deficits, and improving tolerance to frustration in their child, developing new ways of appreciating the needs of others in challenging interpersonal circumstances.

Longitudinal studies will continue to inform us about the nature and characteristics of this heterogeneous and important group of behavioural syndromes, whose variations in nature, characteristics and outcome are much more variable than considered hitherto (Maughan & Rutter, 2001).

References

Andreasen, N. (1999) Understanding the causes of schizophrenia. *New England Journal of Medicine*, **340**, 645–647.

Angold, A., Costello, E. J., Erkanl, A., et al (1999) Pubertal changes in hormone levels and depression in girls. *Psychological Medicine*, **29**, 1043–1053.

Arseneault, L., Moffitt, T. E., Caspi, A., et al (2000) Mental disorders and violence in a total birth cohort: results from the Dunedin Study. *Archives of General Psychiatry*, **57**, 979–986.

Bifulco, A., Brown, G. W., Moran, P., et al (1998) Predicting depression in women: the role of past and present vulnerability. *Psychological Medicine*, **28**, 39–50.

Cannon, M., Caspi, A., Moffitt, T. E., et al (2002) Evidence for early-childhood, pan-developmental impairment specific to schizophreniform disorder: results from a longitudinal birth cohort. *Archives of General Psychiatry*, **59**, 449–456.

Caspi, A., Sugden, K., Moffitt, T. E., et al (2003) Influence of life stress on depression: moderation by a polymorphism in the 5-HTT gene. *Science*, **301**, 386–389.

Farrington, D. P. (1995) The Twelfth Jack Tizard Memorial Lecture. The development of offending and antisocial behaviour from childhood: key findings from the Cambridge Study in Delinquent Development. *Journal of Child Psychology and Psychiatry*, **36**, 929–964.

Ferdinand, R. F. & Verhulst, F. C. (1995) Psychopathology from adolescence into young adulthood: an 8-year follow-up study. *American Journal of Psychiatry*, **152**, 1586–1594.

Fergusson, D. M. & Woodward, L. J. (2002) Mental health, educational, and social role outcomes of adolescents with depression. *Archives of General Psychiatry*, **59**, 225–231.

Fombonne, E., Wostear, G., Cooper, V., et al (2001a) The Maudsley long-term follow-up of child and adolescent depression: 1. Psychiatric outcomes in adulthood. *British Journal of Psychiatry*, **179**, 210–217.

Fombonne, E., Wostear, G., Cooper, V., et al (2001b) The Maudsley long-term follow-up of child and adolescent depression: 2. Suicidality, criminality and social dysfunction in adulthood. *British Journal of Psychiatry*, **179**, 218–223.

Geller, B., Craney, J. L., Bolhofner, K., *et al* (2002) Two-year prospective follow-up of children with a prepubertal and early adolescent bipolar disorder phenotype. *American Journal of Psychiatry*, **159**, 927–933.

Gillberg, C. & Hellgren, L. (1996) Outcome. In *Hyperactivity Disorders of Childhood* (ed. S. Sandberg), pp. 477–503. Cambridge: Cambridge University Press.

Goodyer, I. M., Kolvin, I. & Gatzanis, S. (1985) Recent undesirable life events and psychiatric disorder in childhood and adolescence. *British Journal of Psychiatry*, **147**, 517–523.

Goodyer, I. M., Herbert, J., Tamplin, A., *et al* (2000*a*) First-episode major depression in adolescents. Affective, cognitive and endocrine characteristics of risk status and predictors of onset. *British Journal of Psychiatry*, **176**, 142–149.

Goodyer, I., Herbert, J., Tamplin, A., *et al* (2000*b*) Recent life events, cortisol DHEA in the onset of major depression amongst 'high risk' adolescents. *British Journal of Psychiatry*, **177**, 499–504.

Harkness, K. L. & Monroe, S. M. (2002) Childhood adversity and the endogenous versus nonendogenous distinction in women with major depression. *American Journal of Psychiatry*, **159**, 387–393.

Harrington, R. C. & Dubicka, B. (2001) Natural history of mood disorders in children and adolescents. In *The Depressed Child and Adolescent* (ed. I. Goodyer), pp. 311–343. Cambridge: Cambridge University Press.

Hill, J., Pickles, A., Burnside, E., *et al* (2001) Child sexual abuse, poor parental care and adult depression: evidence for different mechanisms. *British Journal of Psychiatry*, **179**, 104–109.

Isohanni, M., Jones, P., Kemppainen, L., *et al* (2000) Childhood and adolescent predictors of schizophrenia in the Northern Finland 1966 birth cohort – a descriptive life-span model. *European Archives of Psychiatry, Clinical Neuroscience*, **250**, 311–319.

Isohanni, M., Jones, P. B., Moilanen, K., *et al* (2001) Early developmental milestones in adult schizophrenia and other psychoses. A 31-year follow-up of the Northern Finland 1966 Birth Cohort. *Schizophrenia Research*, **52**, 1–19.

Jaffee, S. R., Moffitt, T. E., Caspi, A., *et al* (2002) Differences in early childhood risk factors for juvenile-onset and adult-onset depression. *Archives of General Psychiatry*, **59**, 215–222.

Kasen, S., Cohen, P., Skodol, A. E., *et al* (2001) Childhood depression and adult personality disorder: alternative pathways of continuity. *Archives of General Psychiatry*, **58**, 231–236.

Kemppainen, L., Veijola, J., Jokelainen, J., *et al* (2001) Birth order and risk for schizophrenia: a 31-year follow-up of the Northern Finland 1966 Birth Cohort. *Acta Psychiatrica Scandinavica*, **104**, 148–152.

Kendler, K. S., Gardner, C. O. & Prescott, C. A. (2002) Toward a comprehensive developmental model for major depression in women. *American Journal of Psychiatry*, **159**, 1133–1145.

Kessler, R. C. & Magee, W. J. (1993) Childhood adversities and adult depression: basic patterns of association in a US national survey. *Psychological Medicine*, **23**, 679–690.

Kessler, R. C., Davis, C. G. & Kendler, K. S. (1997) Childhood adversity and adult psychiatric disorder in the US National Comorbidity Survey. *Psychological Medicine*, **27**, 1101–1119.

Kraemer, H. C., Kazdin, A., Offord, D., *et al* (1997) Coming to terms with the terms of risk. *Archives of General Psychiatry*, **54**, 337–343.

Laird, R. D., Jordan, K. Y., Dodge, K. A., *et al* (2001) Peer rejection in childhood, involvement with antisocial peers in early adolescence, and the development of externalizing behavior problems. *Developmental Psychopathology*, **13**, 337–354.

Last, C. G., Hansen, C. & Franco, N. (1997) Anxious children in adulthood: a prospective study of adjustment. *Journal of the American Academy of Child and Adolescent Psychiatry*, **36**, 645–652.

Lewinsohn, P. M., Allen, N. B., Seeley, J. R., *et al* (1999) First onset versus recurrence of depression: differential processes of psychosocial risk. *Journal of Abnormal Psychology*, **108**, 483–489.

Lochman, J. E. & Dodge, K. A. (1994) Social-cognitive processes of severely violent, moderately aggressive, and nonaggressive boys. *Journal of Consulting and Clinical Psychology*, **62**, 366–374.

Loeber, R. & Farrington, D. P. (2000) Young children who commit crime: epidemiology, developmental origins, risk factors, early interventions, and policy implications. *Developmental Psychopathology*, **12**, 737–762.

Mannuzza, S. & Klein, R. G. (2000) Long-term prognosis in attention-deficit/hyperactivity disorder. *Child and Adolescent Psychiatric Clinics of North America*, **9**, 711–726.

March, J. S. & Leonard, H. L. (1996) Obsessive-compulsive disorder in children and adolescents: a review of the past 10 years. *Journal of the American Academy of Child and Adolescent Psychiatry*, **35**, 1265–1273.

Maughan, B. & Rutter, M. (2001) Antisocial children grown up. In *Conduct Disorders in Childhood and Adolescence* (ed. B. Maughan), pp. 507–552. Cambridge: Cambridge University Press.

Moffitt, T. E. & Caspi, A. (2001) Childhood predictors differentiate life-course persistent and adolescence-limited antisocial pathways among males and females. *Developmental Psychopathology*, **13**, 355–375.

Moffitt, T. E., Caspi, A., Harrington, H., *et al* (2002) Males on the life-course-persistent and adolescence-limited antisocial pathways: follow-up at age 26 years. *Developmental Psychopathology*, **14**, 179–207.

Molnar, B. E., Buka, S. L. & Kessler, R. C. (2001) Child sexual abuse and subsequent psychopathology: results from the National Comorbidity Survey. *American Journal of Public Health*, **91**, 753–760.

Nelson, E. C., Heath, A. C., Madden, P. A., *et al* (2002) Association between self-reported childhood sexual abuse and adverse psychosocial outcomes: results from a twin study. *Archives of General Psychiatry*, **59**, 139–145.

Newman, D. L., Moffitt, T. E., Caspi, A., *et al* (1996) Psychiatric disorder in a birth cohort of young adults: prevalence, comorbidity, clinical significance, and new case incidence from ages 11 to 21. *Journal of Consulting and Clinical Psychology*, **64**, 552–562.

Ost, L.-G. & Treffers, P. (2001) Onset, course and outcome for anxiety disorders in children. In *Anxiety Disorders in Children and Adolescents* (ed. P. Treffers). Cambridge: Cambridge University Press.

Paykel, E. S. (1978) The contribution of life events to the causation of psychiatric illness. *Psychological Medicine*, **8**, 245–253.

Peterson, B. S. (2001) Neuroimaging studies of Tourette syndrome: a decade of progress. *Advances in Neurology*, **85**, 179–196.

Peterson, B. S., Pine, D. S., Cohen, P., *et al* (2001) Prospective, longitudinal study of tic, obsessive-compulsive, and attention-deficit/hyperactivity disorders in an epidemiological sample. *Journal of the American Academy of Child and Adolescent Psychiatry*, **40**, 685–695.

Pine, D. S., Cohen, P., Gurley, D., *et al* (1998) The risk for early-adulthood anxiety and depressive disorders in adolescents with anxiety and depressive disorders. *Archives of General Psychiatry*, **55**, 56–64.

Robins, L. N. (1996) Deviant children grown up. *European Child and Adolescent Psychiatry*, **5**, 44–46.

Robins, L. N. (1998) The intimate connection between antisocial personality and substance abuse. *Social Psychiatry and Psychiatric Epidemiology*, **33**, 393–399.

Robins, L. N. & Price, R. K. (1991) Adult disorders predicted by childhood conduct problems: results from the NIMH Epidemiologic Catchment Area project. *Psychiatry*, **54**, 116–132.

Rosario-Campos, M. C., Leckman, J. F., Mercadante, M. T., *et al* (2001) Adults with early-onset obsessive–compulsive disorder. *American Journal of Psychiatry*, **158**, 1899–1903.

Rueter, M. A., Scaramella, L., Wallace, L. E., *et al* (1999) First onset of depressive or anxiety disorders predicted by the longitudinal course of internalizing symptoms and parent–adolescent disagreements. *Archives of General Psychiatry*, **56**, 726–732.

Sadowski, H., Ugarte, B., Kolvin, I., *et al* (1999) Early life family disadvantages and major depression in adulthood. *British Journal of Psychiatry*, **174**, 112–120.

Sandberg, S. (ed.) (1996) *Hyperactivity Disorders of Childhood*. Cambridge: Cambridge University Press.

Sigurdsson, E., Van Os, J. & Fombonne, E. (2002) Are impaired childhood motor skills a risk factor for adolescent anxiety? Results from the 1958 UK birth cohort and the National Child Development Study. *American Journal of Psychiatry*, **159**, 1044–1046.

Silver, L. B. (2000) Attention-deficit/hyperactivity disorder in adult life. *Child and Adolescent Psychiatric Clinics of North America*, **9**, 511–523.

Silverman, W. & Treffers, P. (2001) *Anxiety Disorders in Childhood and Adolescence*. Cambridge: Cambridge University Press.

Silverstein, M. L., Mavrolefteros, G. & Close, D. (2002) Premorbid adjustment and neuropsychological performance in schizophrenia. *Schizophrenia Bulletin*, **28**, 157–165.

Thomsen, P. H. (1995) Obsessive–compulsive disorder in children and adolescents. A 6–22 year follow-up study of social outcome. *European Child and Adolescent Psychiatry*, **4**, 112–122.

Vitaro, F., Tremblay, R. & Bukowski, W. M. (2001) Friends, friendships and conduct disorders. In *Conduct Disorders in Childhood and Adolescence* (ed. B. Maughan), pp. 346–378. Cambridge: Cambridge University Press.

Wewetzer, C., Jans, T., Muller, B., *et al* (2001) Long-term outcome and prognosis of obsessive-compulsive disorder with onset in childhood or adolescence. *European Child and Adolescent Psychiatry*, **10**, 37–46.

Woodward, L. J. & Fergusson, D. M. (2001) Life course outcomes of young people with anxiety disorders in adolescence. *Journal of the American Academy of Child and Adolescent Psychiatry*, **40**, 1086–1093.

Zoccolillo, M. (1992) Co-occurrence of conduct disorder and its adult outcomes with depressive and anxiety disorders: a review. *Journal of the American Academy of Child and Adolescent Psychiatry*, **31**, 547–556.

CHAPTER 5

Classification and epidemiology

Simon G. Gowers and Robin Glaze

Classification is concerned with the naming, categorisation and ordering of diseases. Categorising information and setting it in the context of what is known about normal development is central to the practice of child and adolescent psychiatry. Classification also provides a language for communication between professionals in writing clinical reports, disseminating research findings and in mapping the epidemiology of child mental health problems. Diagnosis involves selecting key symptoms, behaviours or abnormalities in social functioning, which an individual shares with others bearing the same condition. Rather than specifying unique features about the child, classification involves grouping shared characteristics.

If a classification system is to be useful, it must satisfy the needs of professionals who might have different theoretical views, and its diagnoses must be reliable (between clinicians and over time). In addition, the diagnoses must have validity, enabling predictions about course, prognosis and response to treatment, as well as, sometimes, aetiology.

A classification system should be practical, set out in a clear, unambiguous, convenient form and show adequate differentiation between disorders, with minimal overlap. The system should encompass all the important conditions known to professionals and be clinically relevant, identifying conditions that warrant attention and aid in decision-making. Ideally, the system should have conceptual coherence and logical consistency, although the present state of knowledge best suits a descriptive approach without undue inference about aetiology.

The diagnosis of a mental disorder does not imply the presence of an organic disease state. Cantwell (1988) described nine important questions in the diagnostic process:

- Does the child have a psychiatric disorder (a problem in behaviour, emotions, relationships or cognition of sufficient severity and duration to cause distress, disability or disadvantage)?
- Does the disorder meet criteria for a clinical syndrome?

- What are the intra-psychic, family, sociocultural and biological roots of the disorder, and what are their relative strengths?
- What forces maintain the problem?
- What forces facilitate the child's normal development?
- What are the strengths and competencies of the child and the family?
- What is the likely outcome without treatment?
- Is intervention necessary in this case?
- What types of intervention are most likely to be effective?

Disadvantages of diagnosis

If diagnosis is to be justified, its clinical value must be demonstrated. It should help clarify thinking about the nature of a child's disturbance. By improving therapeutic responses and the delivery of services, it should serve to help the child. However, objections are sometimes raised against the labelling involved in the diagnostic process. It has been claimed that the process obscures individual differences, hinders a detailed understanding of disordered mental functioning and highlights difficulties rather than strengths. Diagnosis has been held responsible for producing social stigma and negative impact on the child. The implication of deviance can lead to an altered view of one's self and hence to a self-fulfilling prophecy. It may lead to a change in the way others act towards the individual, even to the extent of justifying inappropriate social control. It is argued that the expectations of others can be altered by the labelling process, with increased likelihood of a poor outcome for the child, for example with regard to teacher expectations of low achievers (Rutter, 1978).

The diagnosis should reflect problems of adjustment, rather than qualities of individuals. A classification of people is not only morally offensive, but can convey an assumption of persistence that is often incorrect. Furthermore, diagnosis does not necessarily imply the need for psychiatric treatment or other forms of administrative action. The harmful effects of labelling are therefore to be found in the misuse of the diagnostic label, rather than in the process of diagnosis itself. Importantly, informal – and sometimes much more harmful – labelling has often already taken place in the network of the child long before mental health professionals become involved. Correcting mis-conceptions is often an important part of the assessment.

Categorical v. dimensional systems

Approaches to modern classificatory systems are either categorical, as in the *International Classification of Mental and Behavioural Disorders*

(ICD–10; World Health Organization, 1992) and the *Diagnostic and Statistical Manual of Mental Disorders* (DSM–IV; American Psychiatric Association, 1994), or dimensional, as for example found in Achenbach & Edelbrock (1978). As the names suggest, categorical systems involve making a selection from a list of diagnoses where the symptoms and symptom timings have been specified, whereas dimensional systems look to see if behavioural symptoms cluster together statistically to form groups or characteristic patterns. In the dimensional approach, multivariate statistical methods such as factor analysis are used to uncover the tendency of specific types of behaviour to cluster in patterns (as the dimensions of illness).

Categorical approaches work best when the members of a diagnostic class are homogeneous, and where the classes themselves have clear boundaries, while also being mutually exclusive. Categorical systems often mirror the common clinical need to make dichotomous clinical decisions. Finally, categorical and dimensional systems are not necessarily contradictory. Constructs such as 'intelligence' may be conceptualised both as a dimension and a category. The same may also be true of conditions such as depression and behaviour difficulties.

Multi-axial classification

Being based on diagnosis, neither the categorical nor the dimensional approach comes close to describing the full complexity of an individual child's difficulties. The most widely used schemes (ICD–10 worldwide, DSM–IV in the USA, Canada and Australia) have thus developed a five-axis categorisation to broaden the descriptive power for any individual child. Clinicians are required to make judgements on each axis. The usage of these axes is handled rather differently between the two manuals (Table 5.1). The broad categories are:

- clinical disorders and other conditions
- personality disorders and mental retardation
- general medical conditions
- psychosocial and environmental problems
- global assessment of functioning.

Routine use of a multi-axial system provides for more comprehensive attention to these areas, in a convenient format for both recording and conveying clinical information. In addition, the complexity and hetero-geneity of the individual are more easily described, and a biopsychosocial model is emphasised.

There are numerous coarse and fine detail differences between the two classifications (Table 5.1): ICD–10 allows coding of self-harm and physical assault, whereas DSM–IV does not; DSM–IV has several scales for global assessment of functioning, whereas ICD–10 has none.

Table 5.1 Comparison of multi-axial assessment in DSM–IV and ICD–10

Axis no.	ICD–10	DSM–IV
I	Clinical psychiatric syndromes (F codes)	Clinical syndromes; other conditions that may be a focus of clinical attention
II	Developmental disorders (F80–F89)	Developmental disorders, personality disorders and mental retardation
III	Intellectual level (F70)	General medical conditions
IV	Other conditions from ICD–10 often associated with mental and behavioural disorders (A50–S06)	Psychosocial and environmental problems
V	Psychosocial stressors (Z00–Z99)	Global assessment of functioning
Self-harm	External causes of morbidity and mortality (X60–X84)	No equivalent
Assault	External causes of morbidity and mortality (X93–Y07)	No equivalent

The DSM–IV and ICD–10 systems

DSM–IV

The DSM–IV classification is available as a book, as a quick reference guide, as a brochure and in several electronic formats.

In DSM–IV the disorders are grouped into 16 major diagnostic classes (disorders usually first diagnosed in infancy, childhood or adolescence, mood disorders, schizophrenia and other psychotic disorders, and so on). There is one further class, 'other conditions that may be a focus of clinical attention'. The class of disorders usually first diagnosed in infancy, childhood and adolescence is a useful convenience, but is not intended to imply that children and young people can have only those disorders. All diagnostic classes may be used in this age group. The 'other conditions' class is divided into six categories with a rich variety of subtypes:

- psychological factors affecting medical condition
- medication-induced movement disorder
- other medication-induced disorder
- relational problems
- problems related to abuse or neglect
- additional conditions that may be a focus of clinical attention.

The definition of mental disorder includes the following features:

- clinically significant behavioural or psychological syndrome, or pattern, occurring in an individual;

- association with present distress or disability, or with a significantly increased risk of death, pain, disability or an important loss of freedom;
- syndrome or pattern not merely an expectable and culturally sanctioned response to a particular event, for example the death of a loved one;
- disorder currently a manifestation of behavioural, psychological or biological dysfunction, whatever the original cause;
- political, religious or sexually deviant behaviour, and conflicts between the individual and society shall not be seen as mental disorders unless they fulfil the above criteria.

The DSM–IV diagnostic codes are numeric codes of up to five digits separated by a decimal point. The first three digits specify the type of general disorder (e.g. '315' for developmental disorders of learning, motor skills and communication). Following the decimal point, the fourth, and sometimes fifth, digits are used to specify subtype.

Some diagnoses have specific criteria for mild, moderate and severe illness, for example conduct, manic episode, major depressive episode and mixed episode disorders. Others have specific criteria for partial remission. Finally, the issue of recurrence is considered. In clinical practice, it is often the case that individuals re-present with a partial set of symptoms of a previous disorder. In these cases, clinicians have the following options:

- to code the disorder as current or provisional;
- the 'not otherwise specified' category;
- the 'prior history' category.

Epidemiological data show that the co-occurrence of two or more separate child psychiatric conditions (comorbidity) is common (Caron & Rutter, 1991). The DSM–IV copes with this by coding a principal diagnosis or reason for visit, along with as many other diagnoses as are required to account for the full range of presenting symptoms. Multiple diagnoses may be listed in order, both multi-axially or non-axially. Where a multi-axial scheme is used, the principal diagnosis is assumed to be the first diagnosis on Axis I. If the principal diagnosis is on Axis II, the qualifying phrase 'principal diagnosis' is used next to it. There is also a provisional diagnosis specifier for those situations where only partial history is present but there is strong reason to suspect that full criteria will eventually be met.

In recognition of the diversity of clinical presentations, some of which do not meet explicit criteria for disorder, DSM–IV includes the 'not otherwise specified' category.

Although DSM–IV encourages multiple diagnoses, it discourages unnecessary coding of comorbidity, by setting rules for the formulation of a diagnostic hierarchy, and setting criteria to exclude other diagnoses and suggest a differential diagnosis for some disorders. This assists in the following situations:

- where mental disorder is induced by a general medical condition, or is substance-induced, when this diagnosis takes priority over the primary diagnosis for the same symptoms;
- where a more pervasive disorder (e.g. schizophrenia) includes the defining symptoms of the identified disorder, when the less pervasive disorder includes an exclusion criteria set showing that only the schizophrenia is diagnosed;
- where the boundaries between conditions are hard to call, when the phrase 'not better accounted for by' is used. In some situations, both diagnoses would be better coded.

ICD-10

The ICD-10 is available in two main forms: the traditional *Clinical Descriptions and Diagnostic Guidelines*, and the *Diagnostic Criteria for Research*; there is also a primary care version (*Diagnostic and Management Guidelines for Mental Disorders in Primary Care*). Mental and behavioural disorders are listed as a shortened glossary in Chapter V(F) of the ICD-10 itself, and is not recommended for mental health clinicians to use. The following description refers to the *Clinical Descriptions and Diagnostic Guidelines* version of ICD-10 only.

The ICD-10 has ten specific categories of mental illness, and one residual category for unspecified mental disorder:

- organic, including symptomatic, mental disorders
- mental and behavioural disorders due to psychoactive substance use
- schizophrenia, schizotypal and delusional disorders
- mood disorders
- neurotic, stress-related and somatoform disorders
- behavioural syndromes associated with physiological disturbances and physical factors
- disorders of adult personality and behaviour
- mental retardation
- disorders of psychological development
- behavioural and emotional disorders occurring in childhood and adolescence
- unspecified mental disorder.

In ICD-10 an alphanumeric code is used rather than the simple numeric code of DSM-IV. The initial character is a letter indicating the chapter of ICD-10 in use; the following characters are numeric, with a two-digit category code (e.g. F80, specific developmental disorders of speech and language), followed by an additional digit after a decimal point to denote a specific disorder, and a possible fifth digit to define further the individual disorder. The fourth and fifth character codes can be seen in action in F32.1 (moderate depressive disorder) and F32.11 (moderate depressive disorder with somatic syndrome).

The ICD–10 uses a similar definition of disorder to that in DSM–IV:

- implies the existence of a clinically recognisable set of symptoms or behaviour;
- associated with distress and interference in personal functioning;
- social deviance or conflict alone, without personal dysfunction, is not included.

Similarly, ICD–10 encourages the recording of as many diagnoses as are necessary to cover the clinical picture. Again, it is suggested that a main diagnosis is coded, where possible, as that best suited to the task in hand. In the clinical setting, this will be the diagnosis causing out-patient consultation, or day-patient or in-patient care. In other settings, the lifetime diagnosis (e.g. schizophrenia) may have primary impor-tance. Where there is uncertainty for the diagnostician, it is suggested that the list of disorders is based on the numeric order of the codes as presented in ICD–10.

Again, disorders from any category may present in childhood or adolescence, although the final three categories have particular relev-ance to the child and adolescent psychiatrist:

- mental retardation (F70–F79)
- disorders with onset specific to childhood (F80–F89)
- behavioural and emotional disorders with onset usually occurring in childhood and adolescence (F90–F98).

Examples of disorders occurring in other sections include mood, schizophrenia, gender identity and eating disorders.

Comparison between ICD–10 and DSM–IV

Clinical psychiatric syndromes

Both ICD and DSM classifications use a categorical system, based on an atheoretical approach, using specific diagnostic criteria arising from both the phenomenology of the case and the timing of the disorder's development, and its relationship to precipitating trauma. The ICD–10 differs from DSM–IV in having a conceptual description of each disorder category, as well as specific diagnostic criteria. The diagnostic criteria themselves are perhaps more rigorous in DSM–IV than in ICD–10, although neither specifies how the information is to be collected. The DSM–IV criteria are also less technical in some instances: for example, ICD–10 refers to the cardinal features of hyperkinetic disorder as overactivity and impaired attention, briefly describing them in separate paragraphs, whereas DSM–IV identifies inattention (nine criteria, e.g.

'often does not seem to listen when spoken to directly'), hyperactivity (six criteria, e.g. 'often fidgets with hands or feet or squirms in seat') and impulsivity (three criteria, e.g. 'often blurts out answers before questions have been completed'), as well as three more general criteria for fulfilment of the diagnosis.

Disorders of childhood and adolescence

The ICD–10 uses the F70–F79, F80–F89 and F90–F98 blocks to contain disorders usually first diagnosed in infancy, childhood or adolescence (mental retardation, disorders of psychological development, and behavioural and emotional disturbances with onset usually occurring in childhood and adolescence). Other disorders can occur in people of almost any age, and are coded elsewhere (for example eating, sleep and gender identity disorders in F50, F51 and F64, respectively). The DSM–IV takes the approach of a separate section devoted to the disorders usually first diagnosed in infancy, childhood or adolescence. This subsumes mental retardation and learning disorders, language and developmental disorders, attention-deficit and disruptive behaviour disorders, feeding and eating disorders of infancy or early childhood, tic disorders, elimination disorders, and other disorders of infancy, childhood or adolescence (Table 5.2).

Table 5.2 Disorders usually first diagnosed in infancy, childhood or adolescence

ICD–10	DSM–IV	
Mental retardation	**Mental retardation**	
F70 Mild mental retardation	317	Mild mental retardation
F71 Moderate mental retardation	318.0	Moderate mental retardation
F72 Severe mental retardation	318.1	Severe mental retardation
F73 Profound mental retardation	318.2	Profound mental retardation
F78 Other mental retardation	319	Mental retardation, severity unspecified
F79 Unspecified mental retardation	**Learning disorders**	
Disorders of psychological development	315.0	Reading disorder
F80 Specific developmental disorders of speech and language	315.1	Mathematics disorder
	315.2	Disorder of written expression
F81 Specific developmental disorders of scholastic skills	315.9	Learning disorder not otherwise specified (NOS)
F82 Specific developmental disorder of motor function	**Motor skills disorder**	
	315.4	Developmental coordination disorder
F83 Mixed specific developmental disorders	**Communication disorders**	
F84 Pervasive developmental disorder	315.31	Expressive language disorder
F88 Other disorders of psychological development	315.31	Mixed receptive-expressive language disorder
F89 Unspecified disorder of psychological development	315.39	Phonological disorder
	307.0	Stuttering
	307.9	Communication disorder NOS

Cont'd

There is considerable similarity and overlap between the two classifications, although it should be noted that in ICD–10, some disorders are effectively classified by first age of onset, for instance phobic anxiety.

Table 5.2 *Cont'd*

ICD–10	DSM–IV
Behavioural and emotional disturbances with onset usually occurring in childhood and adolescence	**Pervasive developmental disorders**
F90 Hyperkinetic disorders	299.00 Autistic disorder
F91 Conduct disorders	299.80 Rett's disorder
F92 Mixed disorders of conduct and emotions	299.10 Childhood disintegrative disorder
	299.80 Asperger disorder
F93 Emotional disorders with onset specific to childhood	299.80 Pervasive developmental disorder NOS
F94 Disorders of social functioning with onset specific to childhood and adolescence	**Attention-deficit and disruptive behaviour disorders**
	314.xx Attention-deficit/hyperactivity disorder
F95 Tic disorders	314.9 Attention-deficit/hyperactivity disorder NOS
F98 Other behavioural and emotional disorders with onset usually occurring in childhood and adolescence	312.xx Conduct disorder
	313.81 Oppositional defiant disorder
	312.9 Disruptive behaviour disorder NOS
F99 Mental disorder, not otherwise specified	**Feeding and eating disorders of infancy or early childhood**
	307.52 Pica
	307.53 Rumination disorder
	307.59 Feeding disorder of infancy or early childhood
	Tic disorders
	307.23 Tourette disorder
	307.22 Chronic motor or vocal tic disorder
	307.21 Transient tic disorder
	307.20 Tic disorder NOS
	Elimination disorders
	xxx.xx Encopresis
	787.6 With constipation and overflow incontinence
	307.7 Without constipation and overflow incontinence
	307.6 Enuresis (not due to a general medical condition)
	Other disorders of infancy, childhood, or adolescence
	309.21 Separation anxiety disorder
	313.23 Selective mutism
	313.89 Reactive attachment disorder of infancy or early childhood
	307.3 Stereotypic movement disorder
	313.9 Disorder of infancy, childhood or adolescence NOS

Table 5.3 Categories of intellectual functioning (IQ scores)

	ICD–10	DSM–IV
Mild	50 to 69	50–55 to 70
Moderate	35 to 49	35–40 to 50–55
Severe	20 to 34	20–25 to 35–40
Profound	<20	<20 or 25

Developmental disorders

Both language and learning disorders are frequently associated with impaired social skills, peer relationships and self-esteem (Cantwell & Baker, 1988). Axis I disorders are also frequently associated with developmental disorders.

Intellectual functioning

Both ICD–10 and DSM–IV divide mental retardation into the four categories of mild, moderate, severe and profound, according to IQ derived from standardised tests (Table 5.3). Both ICD–10 and DSM–IV include a 'severity unspecified' category (F79 and 319 respectively) for use where there is a strong presumption of mental retardation, but where the person is untestable by standard tests; ICD–10 also has a category F78 ('other mental retardation') for use where associated sensory deficits (e.g. blindness or deafness) makes testing difficult.

Associated medical conditions

The DSM–IV uses the ICD–9–CM codes for selected general medical conditions. These codes are presented in two parts: first, codes for general medical conditions over 18 separate categories, and second, codes for medication-induced disorders.

The ICD–10 has a similar list of conditions frequently associated with mental illness as an annex (the A to S codes), although there is nothing to stop you using any of the physical codes found in the complete ICD–10 listings; indeed, this is strongly recommended. Sixteen categories are provided.

Psychosocial stressors

In ICD–10, psychosocial stressors are expressed within factors influencing health status and contact with health services (Z codes). There are 27 categories and 91 sub-codes. The ICD–10 field trials showed poor inter-clinician agreement, which is reflected in the minimal instructions for use.

In DSM–IV, a psychosocial problem is defined as a negative life event, or an environmental difficulty or deficiency, a familial or other interpersonal stress, an inadequacy of social support or personal resources, or any other problem defining the context of the development of the person's difficulties. The categories are shown below:

I   problems with primary support group
II   problems related to the social environment
III educational problems
IV   occupational problems
V   housing problems
VI   economic problems
VII problems with access to health care services
VIII problems related to interaction with the legal system/crime
IX   other psychosocial and environmental problems.

Globa assessment of functioning

The DSM–IV uses the Global Assessment of Functioning (GAF) scale. The GAF is a derivation of the Global Assessment Scale (GAS), itself a derivation of the Health–Sickness Rating Scale (Luborsky, 1962). This observer-rated scale gives a score of between 1 and 100, with lower scores equating to more disability.

The ICD–10 does not include a global assessment of functioning, although the Children's Global Assessment Scale (CGAS; Shaffer *et al* 1983) has been developed for use with children between the ages of 4 and 16, and is now well validated for use within community and clinical populations (Bird *et al*, 1990; Weissman *et al*, 1990; Green *et al*, 1994).

Epidemiology of child and adolescent disorders

Epidemiological studies provide statistics on the extent of morbidity from specific disorders within a population, and attempt to relate these both to the environment and the population itself (e.g. age, social class, gender), with a view to detecting associations with possible causal factors. Epidemiological statistics are usually expressed as incidence and prevalence rates. The term 'incidence' relates to the number of new cases appearing in the defined population within a specified period (usually a year), and is normally written as the rate per 100 000 population. Prevalence refers to the actual number of cases in a community at the time of measurement. Rates may be adjusted for age or sex, or are expressed in 'crude' form.

Since 1970, a number of rigorous epidemiological surveys of prevalence rates of psychiatric symptoms and disorders have been published in the developed world. Differing aims, target populations, methods and completeness of data-sets have understandably led to different findings. Tables 5.4–5.7 provide illustrative prevalence rates for the more common child psychiatric disorders.

Table 5.4 Epidemiology of common child psychiatric disorders

Disorder	Prevalence (%)	Age (years)	Reference	Notes
Attention-deficit hyperactivity disorder	3–6	School age	Goldman et al (1998)	
Affective disorders				
Bipolar disorder	0.5 7.5 1	5–9 10–14 14–18	Loranger & Levine (1978) Lewinsohn et al (1995)	0.5% of an established adult sample had onset at age 5–9 and 7.5% at age 10–14 years
Depression	0.4–2.5 0.4–8.3	Children Adolescent	Birmaher et al (1996)	
Dysthymic disorder	0.6–1.7 1.6–8.0	Children Adolescent	Birmaher et al (1996)	
Anxiety disorders				
General	10–15 10–20	Children Adolescent	Black (1995) Pine (1997)	
Separation anxiety disorder	0.7–12.9 2.0–3.6 2.4	Pre-adol. Adolescent 12–16	Craske (1997) Craske (1997) Bowen et al (1990)	Has the highest recovery rate (96%) over 3 years
Over-anxious or generalised anxiety disorder	2.7–12.4 2.4–7 3.6	Children Adolescent 12–16	Craske (1997) Craske (1997) Bowen et al (1990)	Has the highest rate of comorbidity
Simple phobia	2.4–9.2 3.6	Children Adolescent	Craske (1997) Craske (1997)	Tend to be associated with the least additional pathology
Obsessive–compulsive disorder (OCD)	0.3 1.9–4.0 1.9	Children Adolescent Adolescent	Craske (1997) Craske (1997) Wallace et al (1997)	Juvenile OCD has a bimodal incidence, male preponderance and may occur with ADHD and other developmental disorders (Geller et al, 1998)
Social phobia	0.3 0.4 0.9–1.1 1.1	5–10 11–15 Children Adolescent	Meltzer et al (2000) Craske (1997) Craske (1997)	Experience more loneliness and depression
Panic disorder	0–1.1		Pine (1997)	
Chronic fatigue	Rare	Child and adolescent	Khawaja & Van Boxel (1998)	There is no community survey in this age group. Overall prevalence in primary care approx. 0.5–1.5% (Wessely, 1995)

Cont'd

Table 5.4 *Cont'd*

Disorder	Prevalence (%)	Age (years)	Reference	Notes
Conduct disorder	8.3	4–11	Offord et al	M:F=3.5:1
	14	12–16	(1987)	M:F=2.5:1
Eating disorders				
Anorexia nervosa	0.36–0.83	12–19 girls	Wallace et al	
	0.04–0.17	12–19 boys	(1997)	
Bulimia nervosa	2.5	12–19 girls	Wallace et al (1997)	
Binge eating disorder	1.7 normal weight 14.3 obese	16–35 females	Fairburn & Cooper (1993)	
Gender identity disorder	(1.3)	4–5 boys	Achenbach & Edelbrock (1983)	Clinic samples consistently have referral rates of boys to girls of around 7:1 (Zucker et al, 1997)
Schizophrenia	Very rare	Before 6	Werry (1996)	39% males and 23% females had their first symptoms before 19 years of age
Sleep disorders				
General	4	At 5	Anders &	Behavioural and
	1	At 9	Eiben (1997)	supportive measures
	<2	Childhood		remain the best methods of treatment
Nightmares	20	Childhood		
Sleepwalking	15	4–12	Anders & Eiben (1997)	
Night terrors	3	18/12–6	Anders & Eiben (1997)	
Narcolepsy	0.4–0.7	Early adolescent	Anders & Eiben (1997)	
Tourette disorder	2.99	13–14	Mason et al (1998)	Male to female risk varies from 1.6:1 to 10:1 (Tanner & Goldman, 1997)

Clinical disorders

There are broadening criteria for attention-deficit hyperactivity disorder (ADHD), with growing appreciation of its persistence into adulthood. Pre-pubertal bipolar disorder is often a chronic, rapid-cycling, mixed manic state that may be comorbid with, or have features of, ADHD and/ or conduct disorder. There is significant functional impairment with high rates of comorbidity, particularly with anxiety and behaviour disorders, suicide attempts and high usage of mental health services. Irritability, chronicity and mixed symptoms of mania and depression give an atypical picture compared with adults (Wozniak & Biederman, 1997).

Depression increases in frequency with age in children and adolescents, often coexisting with anxiety and behaviour disorders, and associated with long-term morbidity and risk of suicide (Pataki & Carlson, 1995). Children identify their depression more often than their parents. Early-onset major depressive disorder and dysthymic disorder are frequent, recurrent and familial disorders that tend to continue into adulthood (Chapter 11). These disorders have poor psychosocial and academic outcomes. Risk is increased for substance misuse, bipolar disorder and suicide. Rates of depression are probably increasing, and both major depression and bipolar disorder are occurring at a younger age (Bland, 1997); 70% of patients with early-onset dysthymic disorder have a superimposed major depressive disorder, and 50% have other psychiatric disorders, including anxiety disorders (40%), conduct disorder (30%), ADHD (24%), and enuresis or encopresis (15%), with 15% having two or more comorbid disorders.

Anxiety disorders are more common in girls than boys. Comorbidity is found in up to 39% of children with an anxiety disorder, and 14% of adolescents in the community have two or more anxiety disorders. Additional diagnoses may include depression, attention-deficit disorder and conduct disorder (Craske, 1997). There is high overlap between the presence of overanxious disorder (OAD) and separation anxiety disorder (SAD), externalising disorder and depression. Half with OAD and SAD have pure anxiety disorder. Those with OAD and SAD are as impaired as those with conduct disorder and depression, but they admit to less social isolation, and their schoolwork is less affected.

Common specific fears include fear of heights, the dark, loud noises, injections, insects, dogs and other small animals, and school. Obsessive–compulsive disorder may be comorbid with tic, anxiety and affective disorders (March & Leonard, 1996). When socially phobic and specifically phobic children are compared, socially phobic children report more fears and more commonly display multiple phobias. Atypical presentations of panic disorder include fainting, shortness of breath, palpitations, 'seizures', or other psychological or behavioural complaints, including fear of vomiting or choking (sometimes with weight loss), separation anxiety, school avoidance, tempers or disturbed sleep (Black, 1995).

In adolescent eating disorders, the prevalence of substance misuse or depression among family members is higher in purging anorexia than in the restricting form. Substance misuse occurs more frequently in purging anorexia and is associated with stealing, self-mutilation, suicidality, laxative misuse, diuretic misuse and impaired social relationships (Bailly, 1993). There is no formal epidemiological study of prevalence or incidence of gender identity disorder in children. The original child behaviour checklist standardisation sample gave mothers' reported rates for sometimes or frequently wanting to be the opposite gender. These figures may represent the upper limit of prevalence and hence are given in parentheses.

In schizophrenia there are at least two clinical phenotypes, one with long-standing neurobehavioural difficulties of early onset, the other developing in a normal personality. Sleep problems are said to be more common in children of Indian subcontinent descent than in White children, and in children whose mothers did not reach secondary education.

Developmental disorders

Fombonne's excellent review of the epidemiology of autism (Fombonne, 1999) has shown that intellectual functioning within the normal range

Table 5.5 Epidemiology of developmental disorders

Disorder	Prevalence	Age	Reference	Notes
Asperger syndrome	20/10 000	2–15	Wing & Gould (1979)	M:F=3:1
	36/10 000	7–16	Ehlers & Gillberg (1993)	Minimum figures; M:F=4:1
	4/10 000	2–9	Steffenburg & Gillberg (1986)	M:F=4:1
Autism				
Nuclear/Kanner type	10–30/ 10 000	2–15	Chakrabarti & Fombonne (2001)	M:F=3:1
Autistic-spectrum	60/10 000	3–27	Chakrabarti & Fombonne (2001)	M:F=3.8:1
Specific maths difficulty				
Pure SMD	1.3%	9–10	Lewis et al (1994)	M:F=1:1
SMD + SRD	2.3%			M:F=1:1
Pure SRD	3.9%			M:F=1:1
Specific reading difficulty	9.3%	8–18	Esser & Schmidt (1994)	No correlation with pre/perinatal complications
Specific spelling difficulty	6–9%	Adolescent & young adult	Haffner et al (1998)	Academic achievement is considerably affected despite sufficient non-verbal IQ
Speech articulation disorder	32.5%	At age 5	Luotonen (1995)	Boys have more articulation problems
	18%	At age 7		
	7.4%	At age 9		
Stuttering	2%	7–14	Ardila et al (1994)	

M:F, male-to-female ratio; SMD, Specific maths difficulty; SRD, Specific reading difficulty.

is found in about 20% of autistic children (Table 5.5). On average, medical conditions of potential causal significance are found in about 6% of those with autism, with tuberous sclerosis being particularly important. Conversely, no evidence has been found for an association with other disorders such as neurofibromatosis, Down's syndrome or cerebral palsy. Congenital rubella and phenylketonuria, which were associated with an increased incidence of autistic disorders in the 1970s, no longer account for more than a tiny number of cases, owing to prevention and screening programmes for these disorders. Neither social class nor immigrant status is a risk factor for autism.

In specific reading difficulty there is an association with lower maternal educational level. There is often comorbidity with specific maths difficulty (Lewis *et al*, 1994). School-identified samples are subject to referral bias in favour of boys, whereas research-identified cases show an equal gender distribution (Shaywitz *et al*, 1990). Early speech development is slower in boys than in girls. The prevalence of minor brain injury, a history of developmental dyslexia, word-finding difficulties and depressive symptoms is higher among those who stuttered than among those who did not.

Risk factors

Table 5.6 shows the prevalence rates for several common risk factors for child and adolescent psychiatric disorder. Examples include child sexual abuse as a risk factor for eating disorders, epilepsy for behaviour disorders and mental retardation for psychotic disorders.

It is widely recognised that psychiatric morbidity covaries with psychoactive substance use (Weinberg *et al*, 1998). Indeed, having a psychiatric disorder is associated with an increased risk of substance use, and more involvement with any one substance will increase the risk of other substances being used (Boys *et al*, 2003). Analysis of the Child and Adolescent Survey of Mental Health (Meltzer *et al*, 2000) showed that the relationship between substance use and psychiatric morbidity is largely explained by regular smoking and (less so) regular cannabis use. This may be due to a combination of individual constitutional factors and the effects of drug consumption over the period of adolescent development and growth (Boys *et al*, 2003). The majority of adolescents who use drugs do not progress to misuse or dependence. Adolescent substance misuse clusters with delinquency, early sexual behaviour and pregnancy. It may also be linked to accidents, violence and school drop-out, as well as engagement in risky sexual behaviour, and risk of contracting HIV (Weinberg *et al*, 1998).

The most frequently occurring seizure disorder is febrile convulsion, which shows a wide geographic variation and is usually benign. Epilepsy affects 1% of the population by age 20. Rates rise to 30% in patients

Table 5.6 Epidemiology of risk factors

Factor	Prevalence	Age (years)	Reference	Notes
Child sexual abuse	10% abused by age 16, i.e. 4.5 million adults were abused in childhood	15+	Baker & Duncan (1985)	2019 men and women aged 15 and over interviewed as part of a MORI survey of a nationally representative sample of Great Britain (8% of males, 12% of females). No increased risk by social class or area of residence
	7–36% women 3–29% men		Finkelhor (1994)	Review of studies from 19 countries. F:M= 1.5:3.1
	10–12% girls	<14	Feldman *et al* (1991)	Data from the 1940s compared with 1970s and 1980s. Prevalence has not changed, but increased reporting due to changes in legislation and social climate
Drug, alcohol and addictive disorders				
Alcohol in previous week	29.0%	13	Kurtz (1996)	
Solvents, illegal drugs	2.0%	11	Pearce & Holmes (1995)	
Regular drug use	8.0%	16	Light & Bailey (1992)	
Heroin and cocaine	0.9%	15–16	Wallace *et al* (1997)	
Epilepsy	4%	All children	Hauser (1995)	
Mental retardation	1%	Children	Gillberg (1997)	Rates depend on the inclusiveness of the criteria used
	5%	School-age children	Lyon (1996)	
Smoking	28%	17-year-old girls 19.9% White 10.9% Latino 7.2% African American	French & Perry (1996)	Highest rates among White people, lowest in African Americans and Asians. Adolescent girls who do not go to college are more likely to smoke than those who do. Effective school-based interventions exist, but are usually not appropriately implemented
Teenage pregnancy and sexual health				
Live births	1.1–9.9/1000	<16 girls	Nicoll *et al* (1999)	Rates by health district for girls under 16. Highest rates in urban districts. Teenage birth rates in Eng and and Wales are the highest in Western Europe
Terminations	2.2–10.5/1000	<16 girls		
Gonorrhoea	1.07/1000	16–19 girls		
	0.71/1000	16–19 boys		
Chlamydia	4.45/1000	16–19 girls		
	1.15/1000	16–19 boys		

Table 5.7   Epidemiology of suicidal behaviour

Type	Prevalence (%)	Age (years)	Reference
Attempted suicide	6.9	15–16	Hawton *et al* (2000)
	6.8	15–19	Hulton *et al* (2001)
1-year repeat	24	15–19	Hulton *et al* (2001)
Completed suicide	0.0075	15–19 Boys	Pearce & Holmes (1995)
Completed suicide	0.0025	15–19 Girls	Pearce & Holmes (1995)

with learning disabilities, and 50% of those with multiple disabilities in institutional settings (Sunder, 1997)

Epidemiology of risk factors

Suicide

The suicide rate in England and Wales in 15- to 24-year-old males rose by 80% between 1980 and 1992, although New Zealand currently has the highest rate in the world (Table 5.7; Hawton, 1998). Similarly, rates of self-harm rose by 194% in the same age group in an Oxford sample between 1985 and 1995, although rates in females changed very little. A self-report survey of pupils aged 15–19 years in 41 schools in England showed rates of self-harm of 6.9% (Hawton *et al*, 2002), which closely parallels rates of 6.8% for first-time self-harm in Europe (Hulton *et al*, 2001). Attempted suicide is the best predictor of future suicide, with 24% of European adolescents making a further attempt within 1 year. Use of 'hard' methods, such as attempted suffocation, hanging or jumping from a height, also significantly predicts repetition. The Oxford Monitoring System for Attempted Suicide showed substantial increases in self-poisoning with paracetamol and antidepressants between 1985 and 1997. The increase in antidepressant self-poisoning closely paralleled local prescribing figures, although overdoses with selective serotonin reuptake inhibitors (SSRIs) occurred more often than expected. Paracetamol overdoses were more common in first-time attempts and young people, whereas overdoses of antidepressants and tranquillisers were more common in repeat attempts and older people. Non-ingestible poisons and gas were used by those with high suicidal intent. The changes in substances used most probably reflect availability, age and repeater status, although the degree of suicidal intent may also influence the choice of method (Townsend *et al*, 2001).

Prevalence of psychopathology

Over 50 studies in the past 40 years have attempted to estimate the overall prevalence of childhood and adolescent psychiatric disorders

(Roberts *et al*, 1998). Over 20 countries have been involved, most frequently the USA and the UK. Participants' ages ranged from 1 year to 18 years, and the DSM criteria were most frequently used for case definition. The range of prevalence rates found by Roberts extended from 1% to 51%, with a mean of 15.8%. Median rates across the age range were:

- pre-school 8%
- pre-adolescent 12%
- adolescent 15%.

The evidence is less informative than expected because of the familiar issues of sampling differences, the definition of caseness, the data analyses and presentation. Since the early 1980s a new generation of studies has emerged using more systematic strategies aimed at minimising errors. Hence, more use has been made of standardised diagnostic criteria and structured diagnostic interviews such as the Diagnostic Interview Schedule for Children, to reduce information variance. As expected, these studies have produced more homogeneous results than earlier surveys, and have confirmed childhood and adolescent disorders as being relatively common. Externalising disorders such as disruptive behaviour are more prevalent among children in foster-family care, even compared with children from backgrounds of similar deprivation (Pilowsky, 1995).

Prevalence rates at different ages

In the pre-school period emotional and behavioural problems consist of symptoms varying in number and severity, most of which do not fall into clearly differentiated categories permitting classification. Richman *et al* (1975) interviewed more than 800 mothers of randomly selected 3-year-old children in a London borough with a social class distribution similar to that in the UK as a whole. Using a behaviour screening questionnaire of tested reliability, they interviewed mothers of about 100 high-scoring children and 100 controls matched for gender and social class. The most common individual items of difficult behaviour in the whole group were bedwetting (37%), daytime wetting (17%), poor appetite (17%), night waking at least three times weekly (14%), difficulty settling at night, soiling, fears and overactivity (13% each).

Psychosocial adversity appears to have an important role. For example, maternal depression or family discord at age 3 years predicts the development of child behaviour disorder by age 8 years, even in children who do not show disturbance at 3 years. Speech and language delay at 3 years is a similarly powerful predictor.

The classic study of middle childhood was carried out in the 1960s on the total 10- and 11-year-old population of the Isle of Wight, chosen because it was an easily defined, stable geographical and administrative unit, socially representative of England as a whole. Standardised measures of physical health, IQ, and educational and psychological status were obtained for more than 2000 children – more than 90% of the total (Rutter *et al*, 1970). Parent and teacher screening questionnaires identified similar proportions of children with deviant behavioural scores, but only 19 out of 271 were identified by both, emphasising that multiple sources of information are essential in epidemiological studies. Stage 2 involved interviewing parents and the diagnostic examination of children with deviant scores. An additional random sample was taken to estimate cases missed by the screening, to reduce interview bias and to provide normative data. Of the children screened, 5.7% had a psychiatric disorder, corrected to 6.8% for the missed cases. Boys were affected almost twice as often as girls. In most cases this disorder had been present for at least 3 years. Only 10% were attending a psychiatric clinic.

The Dunedin study (Silva, 1990), a large cohort study, followed up 1037 children at 2-yearly intervals from birth to age 15 years. As in all similar cohorts, the rates of psychiatric disorder among adolescents were higher than earlier in childhood, and as in the Isle of Wight study, following up the same cohort with the same measures showed an increase in prevalence between the ages of 11 years and 15 years.

All studies identify larger numbers of disturbed adolescents from individual interview than from data given by parents or teachers. The major differences between studies in criteria and populations make it difficult to be clear whether there are changes in overall prevalence rates with age during the course of adolescence.

The Office for National Statistics survey of child and adolescent mental health in Great Britain (Meltzer *et al*, 2000) deserves special mention. The survey set out to produce prevalence rates for conduct, emotional and hyperkinetic disorders based on ICD–10 and DSM–IV criteria, to determine the burden of children's mental health, and to examine the use of health, social, educational and voluntary services by this group. The survey looked at 5- to 15-year-olds living in private households in England, Scotland and Wales between January and May 1999. A one-step design ensured that all children were eligible for a full interview, without a screening stage, and data collection included information from parents, teachers and the young people themselves (if aged 11+). The sample was drawn from child benefit records. Thirty opt-out letters were sent to each of 475 postal sectors (*n*=14 250). Interviews were achieved with 83% of those who were eligible and opted in, giving 10 438 assessments. Eighty per cent of teachers also returned questionnaires. Cases were derived using ICD–10 research diagnostic criteria, the disorder causing distress to the child, or having a considerable impact on the child's day-to-day life. Using these criteria,

10% of 5- to 15-year-olds had a mental disorder. Five per cent had a clinically significant conduct disorder, 4% had an anxiety or depressive disorder and 1% were hyperactive. Autistic disorders, tics and eating disorders accounted for only 0.5% of the sampled population. In 5- to 10-year-olds, 10% of boys and 6% of girls had a mental disorder. In 11- to 15-year-olds, the proportions were 13% for boys and 10% for girls. Prevalence rates of mental disorders were greater in children who:

- were in single-parent rather than two-parent families (16% v. 8%);
- were in reconstituted families rather than families without step-children (15% v. 9%);
- were in families of five or more children compared with those with two children (18% v. 8%);
- had an interviewed parent with no educational qualification rather than degree-level qualification (15% v. 6%);
- were in families where neither parent worked compared with both working (20% v. 8%);
- were in families with a gross weekly income of less than £200 compared with one of £500 or more (16% v. 6%);
- were in families of social class V rather than I (14% v. 5%);
- had parents who were social sector tenants rather than owner-occupiers (17% v. 6%);
- were in households with a striving rather than thriving geo-demographic classification (13% v. 5%).

Thus, children with mental disorder are more likely to be boys living in a low-income household, in social sector housing, with a single

Table 5.8 Other findings from the Office for National Statistics survey (Meltzer *et al*, 2000)

Realm	Mental disorder *v.* no mental disorder
Mental disorders, physical complaints	• More likely to have general health ratings of fair, bad or very bad: 20% *v.* 6%
	• Bedwetting: 12% *v.* 4%; speech and language problems: 12% *v.* 3%; coordination difficulties: 8% *v.* 2%; soiling: 4% *v.* 1%
	• 17% (1 in 6) of children with a life-threatening medical condition, had a mental disorder. Accidental poisoning rates: 25% *v.* 12%
Use of services	• Contact with GP in the previous 12 months: 47% *v.* 35%
	• Accident and emergency department attendance: once, 26% *v.* 17%; more than once: 7% *v.* 4%
	• In-patient stay: 9% *v.* 5%
	• Out-patient department visit: 29% *v.* 18%
	• Half of the children with mental disorders had seen someone in education, a quarter had used specialist health services, and a fifth had had contact with social services

Cont'd

Table 5.8 *Cont'd*

Realm	Mental disorder *v.* no mental disorder
	• Two-thirds of young people with mental disorder were seen by secondary-level services in the previous year • Parents of children with emotional disorders were most likely to ask family or friends for advice, and least likely to seek professional services: 23% *v.* 63% • 25% of 11- to 15-year-olds reported being in trouble with the police: 43% *v.* 21%
Scholastic educational	• One in five children had officially recognised special achievement needs: 49% *v.* 15% • Stage 5 statement of educational needs issued: 28% *v.* 13% • Of children with special educational needs at stage 5, 40% had mental disorders • Of children without special educational needs at stage 5, only 6% had mental disorders • Specific learning difficulty found: 12% *v.* 4% • Absent from school 11 days or more in the past term owing to: emotional disorders 25%, conduct disorders 21%, hyperkinetic disorders 14% • Played truant: 33% *v.* 9%. Conduct disorders have the highest rates, at 44%
Family social functioning	• Parent scoring 3 or more on the 12-item General Health Questionnaire (GHQ): 47% *v.* 23% • Children with GHQ-positive parents: no disorder 23%, one disorder 44%, two disorders 50%, three disorders 67% • Unhealthy family functioning: 35% *v.* 17% • Frequently sent to their rooms: 18% *v.* 8% • Frequently grounded: 17% *v.* 5% • Frequently shouted at: 42% *v.* 26% • Parents separated on one occasion: 50% *v.* 29% • Problems with the police: 15% *v.* 5% • Parent or sibling dying: 6% *v.* 3% • A third of parents said their child's problems made their relationship strained • A fifth of single parents blamed their child's problems for contributing to the relationship break-up • A quarter of parents said their child's problems made difficulties with other family members • 87% of parents said their child's problems made them worried; 58% felt their child's problems made them depressed
Child social functioning	• Severe lack of friendships: 9% *v.* 5% • Sought help and advice: 41% *v.* 23% • 41% of 11- to 15-year-olds who regularly smoked had mental disorder: 28% conduct disorder, 20% emotional disorder, 4% hyperkinetic disorder • Of the young people drinking alcohol once per week, 3 times as many had mental disorder: 24% • Rate of mental disorder in young people using cannabis more than once a week: 49%, less than once a month: 21%, never: 10%

parent. They are less likely to be in social class I or II, or living with married parents.

Some more findings of the survey are shown in Table 5.8.

Racial differences

There has been little systematic study of the prevalence rates of psychiatric disorder among children from ethnic minorities within the UK. In the Waltham Forest pre-school study, a 7% subsample of 3-year-old children whose mothers were born in the West Indies showed the same prevalence rate of overall disorder as did indigenous (White British) children (Earls & Richman, 1980). There were some differences in the pattern of symptoms. West Indian children were more faddy eaters, more difficult to settle at night, more fearful and had more articulation problems. Indigenous children were more likely to soil, wet the bed and have tempers. These differences may reflect contrasting child-rearing practices, but not necessarily. West Indian mothers were more likely to have been educated beyond the age of 16, and to work longer hours. Among other disadvantages, their children were more poorly housed and had experienced more separations from their parents.

A sample of 13 000 children born during one week in 1970 were tested at 5 years of age using standardised questionnaires administered by health visitors (Butler & Golding, 1986). A subsample of 174 ethnic West Indian children were more likely to have tantrums and speech problems compared with the whole sample. The excess risk for these symptoms disappeared with adjustment for social advantage, but higher rates of bedwetting and feeding problems did not. In both this and the Waltham Forest study, West Indian children suffered on a wide range of social indices; they were more likely to live in a single-parent family, with more siblings, more overcrowding and lower social class. A subsample of 257 five-year-old children whose parents were of Indian, Bangladeshi or Pakistani origin showed fewer behavioural problems than the indigenous population, even after controlling for social class and maternal age. There were fewer sleeping problems and accidents. They too lived in larger families with overcrowding and lower income and of lower social class.

Hackett et al (1991) compared community samples of 4- to 7-year-old Gujerati children with indigenous English children. The Gujerati children had only a quarter (5%) of the rate of disorder of the English sample (21%) and this difference related to family structure (especially single parenthood) and child-rearing patterns.

Rutter et al (1974) found that 10-year-olds in inner London born to West Indian parents did not show more disorder on parent interview than indigenous children, but did show higher rates of disorder on teacher interview. The difference was largely due to higher rates of conduct problems. There were also higher rates of restlessness and poor concentration, but not of non-sanctioned school absence, which was higher in the indigenous pupils. Rutter put forward two probable explanations, namely racial discrimination (although not necessarily by teachers) and the educational abilities of West Indian pupils compared with indigenous pupils. Girls of West Indian origin differed from indigenous girls in having rates of disorder closer to that of boys and for the disorder to be antisocial rather than emotional.

Although little is known about ethnic differences in anxiety disorders of childhood, ethnicity does not appear to be a risk factor for depression in adolescence (Kandel & Davies, 1982). British teenagers are more likely to have used all categories of illicit drugs than those in any other European Union country. Fifteen-year-old boys living in Wales and Northern Ireland are most likely to drink alcohol at least weekly, with highest rates among girls in Wales and Scotland (McKee, 1999). Over a quarter of Welsh girls smoke at least once a week. The reasons for these differences remain to be clarified, although there may well be links with poverty, education and home life. Extended education appears to be a major factor in delaying pregnancy, and education level is important in smoking rates. Pre-school education may also reduce harmful behaviour in adolescence and early adulthood. Once again, Britain lags behind the rest of Europe at the bottom of the educational spectrum in terms of literacy, numeracy and basic skills, but compares more favourably at the top. Poverty rates have increased markedly over the past 20 years, with many more families living in poverty in the UK than in the rest of the EU. British parents also work the longest hours in Europe, alongside a trend towards more shift working with the growth in 24-hour service industries. In the USA, the highest rates of alcohol use are found in Native Americans, followed in decreasing order by Whites, Hispanics, African Americans and Asian Americans (Edwards et al, 1995). In non-Western cultures, the prevalence of eating disorders has increased where dieting behaviours have become more common. Within Western cultures, it may be that the children from different ethnic backgrounds who do develop eating disorders come from families that maintain their own beliefs and practices and socialise primarily with others of the same ethnic origin. In other words, it is children who struggle to accommodate their experience at school and elsewhere with their home life who are at greater risk, rather than those from more Westernised families (Bryant-Waugh, 1993).

International studies report prevalence rates of obsessive–compulsive disorder in juveniles of 2.3% in Israel, 3.9% in New Zealand and 4.1% in Denmark. Lifetime comorbidity rates for other psychiatric disorders were high at 75–84%. Obsessive–compulsive disorder is more common in White than in African American children in clinical samples, although epidemiological data suggest no difference in prevalence as a function of ethnicity or geographic region (March & Leonard, 1996). The incidence rates for schizophrenia appear stable across countries and cultures over time, at least for the past 50 years, when restrictive and precise definitions of schizophrenia and standardised assessment methods are used on large, representative populations (Häfner & Heiden, 1997). The UK had the highest teenage pregnancy rates in Western Europe throughout the 1990s, with birth rates seven times those in The Netherlands among 15- to 19-year-olds (McKee, 1999). Rates of sexual activity are comparable with those in The Netherlands, but adolescents there use more contraception. In ranked order, the live birth rates per 1000 women among 15- to 19-year-olds in Western European countries are England & Wales 29.8, Portugal 20.9, Ireland 16.1, Austria 15.6, Norway 13.5, Greece 13.1, Finland 9.8, Germany 9.4, Belgium 9.1, Denmark 8.3, Spain 8.2, Sweden 7.7, Italy 7.3, France 7, The Netherlands 4.1 and Switzerland 4 (Nicoll et al, 1999).

Urban v. rural differences

Few studies have investigated the impact of urban living, compared with that of rural life, on the prevalence of psychiatric disorder. It is known that child psychiatric referral rates tend to be higher in areas of low social status, although not whether these differences arise from prevalence differences, detection, or referral differences (Gath et al, 1972). Reading backwardness has also been associated with low social class areas. Work on delinquency in the field of criminology has repeatedly shown higher rates in urban environments, with the highest rates in industrial cities, followed by non-industrial towns. Suicide tends to be more frequent in socially disorganised and isolated areas, but not in overcrowded areas, or ones with high unemployment. Studies of young adults with schizophrenia have typically shown higher admission rates in poor working-class areas adjacent to business districts, and lower rates in middle-class suburbs. It is now apparent that these findings are largely due to selective migration and downward drift, as their fathers' social class does not differ from that of the general population. It is also currently thought premature to state that there is a social class bias in early-onset anorexia nervosa, although there are a number of small-scale studies showing an over-representation of social classes I and II (e.g. Gowers et al, 1991).

Rutter's important Isle of Wight study (Rutter et al, 1975) showed rates of psychiatric disorder in non-immigrant 10-year-olds to be twice as high in London as on the Isle of Wight, with similar results for both specific reading retardation and behavioural problems. Lavik's comparison of 15-year-olds living in a suburb of Oslo and a rural Norwegian valley found rates of 20% and 8% respectively for psychiatric disorder (Lavik, 1977). Most of this difference was due to cases of conduct disorder, and Oslo had a much higher rate of family breakdown. In the Isle of Wight study the higher urban rates were largely accounted for by the much higher levels of family and school disadvantage. Family disadvantage was reflected in lack of home ownership, overcrowding, family size, discord and breakdown, parental mental illness, criminal activity, and a care history. Educational disadvantage was indicated by high teacher and pupil turnover, pupil absenteeism, and a large proportion of children receiving free school meals.

Historical trends

Prospective, family and genetic studies, community, repeated cross-sectional surveys, and data from mortality and police statistics suggest that suicide, delinquency, addictive behaviours and depression are all increasing (Fombonne, 1998). Crime statistics have risen in most developed countries by a factor of 5 since the Second World War, with the exception of Japan. There has also been a steeper rise in females than in males committing crimes. Most crimes are committed by teenagers and young adults, who tend to stop criminal activities in their mid-20s. Rates of conduct disorder and antisocial personality seem to be rising over time, which may well also relate causally to the increasing crime rates.

Large family genetic studies, and community surveys in different countries, suggest increasing rates of depression with an earlier age of onset across the century. Repeat surveys of 7- to 16-year-old American children over a period of 13 years indicated increased parent and teacher reports of depressed mood and scores of depressive syndromes. Other cross-sectional surveys of mental health on representative samples of American adults in 1957 and 1976 showed that young adult respondents reported fewer feelings of happiness in the more recent survey. Levels of reported happiness in 15 surveys of nationally representative samples in the USA reduced between the late 1950s and early 1970s, particularly in young respondents. The trend appears to apply to mild and moderate depressions but not for more severe depressions, and has not been found in dysthymic disorder (Birmaher *et al*, 1996).

Most developed countries saw a rise in alcohol consumption between 1950 and 1980. Rates rise steadily throughout the adolescent years and tend to decline in early adulthood. Ninety per cent of teenagers have experienced alcohol by the age of 16. Even though the rates of underage drinking have not increased in the UK, they are associated with larger quantities of alcohol consumption in recent years (Newcombe *et al*, 1994) and a rise in official National Health Service statistics for hospital discharges of 11- to 17-year-olds with a diagnosis of non-dependent misuse of alcohol over the same period. The increasing popularity of 'designer' drinks, particularly among 14- to 16-year-olds, has led to a pattern of drinking in less secure environments, greater drunkenness and heavier consumption (Hughes *et al*, 1997). Similar rises in illicit drug use from the 1950s have been shown, with epidemiological data tending to show increasing rates of substance misuse, and misuse among young people, together with a trend towards a younger age of onset of addictive behaviours in most countries. The flattening of rates seen in the 1980s has been replaced by a further upward trend since the end of the 1990s.

Studies using a rigorous methodology have consistently reported a recent increase in the incidence of anorexia nervosa (Hsu, 1996). Other studies also support an increasing rate, but have been criticised for lack of diagnostic rigour, being based on only referred populations, demographic changes in the population, and erroneous inclusion of readmissions (Fombonne, 1995). Earlier reports that eating disorders might have reached epidemic proportions were based on questionnaire studies using over-inclusive diagnostic criteria, however. There is no compelling evidence for a rising rate of bulimia nervosa, although this conclusion is based on a limited number of studies (Fombonne, 1998). It is not likely that there will be a great variation in the rates of schizophrenia over time, given the even distribution of morbidity across countries and cultures. Such studies that have been performed on case register data in Norway, Iceland and Australia (Victoria) have found fairly stable rates (Häfner & Heiden, 1997).

Almost all European countries saw increased rates of suicide over the past century, with most of the increase in young men, since rates in older men have fallen. Suicide is the leading cause of death among 15- to 24-year-olds in the UK, France and North America, and there is evidence of increasing rates in 10- to 14-year-olds in the USA, where there was a 120% increase between 1980 and 1992. Black adolescents are catching up with Whites, and rates are also increasing in minority youth in the USA. Rates for girls vary much more by country. Para-suicide is also increasing. Fombonne's survey of 1300 male adolescents in a London hospital referred to psychiatric services for suicidal behaviours found an increase from 6.5% in 1970–1972 to 16% in 1988–1990, with most of the increase accounted for by greater misuse of substances, particularly alcohol. Female rates of suicidal behaviour were higher than those for males, but did not show an upward trend (Fombonne, 1998). In the early 1990s pregnancy rates and termination rates were both falling; more recent data for 1995–1996 show a rise of 14.5% for terminations among those under 16 years old and a rise of 12.5% for the group aged 16–19 years. Similarly, maternity rates rose by 6.7% and 4.6% respectively in the two groups. In 1996, teenage girls accounted for 20% of all terminations, though only 9% of the births, and had the second-highest termination rates, behind 20- to 24-year-olds (Nicoll *et al*, 1999).

85

References

Achenbach, T. M. & Edelbrock, R. C. (1978) The classification of child psychopathology: a review and analysis of empirical efforts. *Psychological Bulletin*, **85**, 1275–1301.

Achenbach, T. M. & Edelbrock, R. C. (1983) *Manual for the Child Behavior Checklist and Revised Profile*. Burlington, VT: University of Vermont Department of Psychiatry.

American Psychiatric Association (1994) *Diagnostic and Statistical Manual of Mental Disorders* (4th edn) (DSM–IV). Washington, DC: APA.

Anders, T. F. & Eiben, L. A. (1997) Pediatric sleep disorders: a review of the past 10 years. *Journal of the American Academy of Child and Adolescent Psychiatry*, **36**, 9–20.

Ardila, A., Bateman, J. R., Nino, C. R., *et al* (1994) An epidemiologic study of stuttering. *Journal of Communication Disorders*, **27**, 37–48.

Bailly, D. (1993) Epidemiological research, disorders of eating behaviour and addictive behaviour. *Encephale*, **19**, 285–292.

Baker, A. W. & Duncan, S. P. (1985) Child sexual abuse: a study of prevalence in Great Britain. *Child Abuse and Neglect*, **9**, 457–467.

Bird, H. R., Yager, T. J., Staghezza, B., *et al* (1990) Impairment in the epidemiological measurement of childhood psychopathology in the community. *Journal of the American Academy of Child and Adolescent Psychiatry*, **29**, 796–803.

Birmaher, B., Ryan, N. D., Williamson, D. E., *et al* (1996) Childhood and adolescent depression: a review of the past 10 years. Part I. *Journal of the American Academy of Child and Adolescent Psychiatry*, **35**, 1427–1439.

Black, B. (1995) Anxiety disorders in children and adolescents. *Current Opinion in Paediatrics*, **7**, 387–391.

Bland, R. C. (1997) Epidemiology of affective disorders: a review. *Canadian Journal of Psychiatry*, **42**, 367–377.

Bowen, R. C., Offord, D. R. & Boyle, M. H. (1990) The prevalence of overanxious disorder and separation anxiety disorder: results from the Ontario Child Health Study. *Journal of the American Academy of Child and Adolescent Psychiatry*, **29**, 753–758.

Boys, A., Farrell, M., Taylor, C., *et al* (2003) Psychiatric morbidity and substance use in young people aged 13–15 years: results from the Child and Adolescent Survey of Mental Health. *British Journal of Psychiatry*, **182**, 509–517.

Bryant-Waugh, R. (1993) Epidemiology. In *Childhood Onset Anorexia Nervosa and Related Eating Disorders* (eds B. Lask & R. Bryant-Waugh), pp. 55–68. London: Erlbaum.

Butler, N. & Golding, J. (1986) *From Birth to Five: A Study of the Health and Behaviour of Britain's 5-Year-Olds*. Oxford: Pergamon.

Cantwell (1988) DSM–III studies. In *Assessment and Diagnosis in Child Psychopathology* (eds M. Rutter, A. H. Tuma & I. S. Lann), pp. 3–36. New York: Guilford.

Cantwell, D. P. & Baker, L. (1988) Issues in the classification of child and adolescent psychopathology. *Journal of the American Academy of Child and Adolescent Psychiatry*, **27**, 521–533.

Caron, C. & Rutter, M. (1991) Comorbidity in child psychopathology: concepts, issues and research strategies. *Journal of Child Psychology and Psychiatry*, **32**, 1063–1080.

Chakrabarti, S. & Fombonne, E. (2001) Pervasive developmental disorders in preschool children. *JAMA*, **285**, 3093–3099.

Craske, M. G. (1997) Fear and anxiety in children and adolescents. *Bulletin of the Menninger Clinic*, **61** (suppl. A), A4–36.

Earls, F. & Richman, N. (1980) The prevalence of behaviour problems in three year old children of West Indian parents. *Journal of Child Psychology and Psychiatry*, **21**, 99–106.

Edwards, R. W., Thurman, P. J. & Beauvais, F. (1995) Patterns of alcohol use among ethnic minority adolescent women. *Recent Developments in Alcoholism*, **12**, 369–386.

Ehlers, S. & Gillberg, C. (1993) The epidemiology of Asperger syndrome. A total population study. *Journal of Child Psychology and Psychiatry and Allied Disciplines*, **34**, 1327–1350.

Esser, G. & Schmidt, M. H. (1994) Children with specific reading retardation: early determinants and long-term outcome. *Acta Paedopsychiatrica*, **56**, 229–237.

Fairburn, C. G. & Cooper, Z. (1993) The eating disorder examination. In *Binge Eating* (eds C. G. Fairburn & G. T. Wilson), pp. 317–360. New York: Guilford.

Feldman, W., Feldman, E., Goodman, J. T., *et al* (1991) Is childhood sexual abuse really increasing in prevalence? An analysis of the evidence. *Pediatrics*, **88**, 29–33.

Finkelhor, D. (1994) The international epidemiology of child sexual abuse. *Child Abuse and Neglect*, **18**, 409–417.

Fombonne, E. (1995) Anorexia nervosa. No evidence of an increase. *British Journal of Psychiatry*, **166**, 462–471.

Fombonne, E. (1998) Increased rates of psychosocial disorders in youth. *European Archives of Psychiatry and Clinical Neuroscience*, **248**, 14–21.

Fombonne, E. (1999) The epidemiology of autism: a review. *Psychological Medicine*, **29**, 769–786.

French, S. A. & Perry, C. L. (1996) Smoking among adolescent girls: prevalence and etiology. *Journal of the American Medical Women's Association*, **51**, 25–28.

Gath, D., Cooper, B. & Gattoni, F. E. G. (1972) Preliminary communication: child guidance and delinquency in a London borough. *Psychological Medicine*, **2**, 185–191.

Geller, D., Biederman, J., Jones, J., *et al* (1998) Is juvenile obsessive–compulsive disorder a developmental subtype of the disorder? A review of the pediatric literature. *Journal of the American Academy of Child and Adolescent Psychiatry*, **37**, 420–427.

Gillberg, C. (1997) Practitioner review: physical investigations in mental retardation. *Journal of Child Psychology and Psychiatry and Allied Disciplines*, **38**, 889–897.

Goldman, L. S., Genel, M., Bezman, R. J., *et al* (1998) Diagnosis and treatment of attention-deficit/hyperactivity disorder in children and adolescents. *JAMA*, **279**, 1100–1117.

Gowers, S. G., Crisp, A. H., Joughin, N., *et al* (1991) Pre-menarcheal anorexia nervosa. *Journal of Child Psychology and Psychiatry*, **32**, 515–524.

Green, B., Shirk, S., Hanze, D., *et al* (1994) The Children's Global Assessment Scale in clinical practice: an empirical evaluation. *Journal of the American Academy of Child and Adolescent Psychiatry*, **33**, 1158–1164.

Hackett, L., Hackett, R. & Taylor, D. (1991) Psychological disturbance and its associations in the children of the Gujerati community. *Journal of Child Psychology and Psychiatry*, **32**, 851–856.

Haffner, J., Zerahn-Hartung, C., Pfuller, U., *et al* (1998) Impact and consequences of specific spelling problems of young adults – results of an epidemiological sample. *Zeitschrift für Kinder und Jugendpsychiatrie und Psychotherapie*, **26**, 124–135.

Häfner, H. & Heiden, W. (1997) Epidemiology of schizophrenia. *Canadian Journal of Psychiatry*, **42**, 139–151.

Hauser, W. A. (1995) Epidemiology of epilepsy in children. *Neurosurgery Clinics of North America*, **6**, 419–429.

Hawton, K. (1998) Why has suicide increased in young males? *Crisis*, **19**, 119–124.

Hawton, K., Fagg, J., Simpkin, S., *et al* (2000) Deliberate self-harm in adolescents in Oxford 1985–1995. *Journal of Adolescence*, **23**, 47–55.

Hawton K., Rodham K., Evans E., *et al* (2002) Deliberate self-harm in adolescents: self-report survey in schools in England. *BMJ*, **325**, 1207–1211.

Hsu, L. K. (1996) Epidemiology of the eating disorders. *Psychiatric Clinics of North America*, **19**, 681–700.

Hughes, K., MacKintosh, A. M., Hastings, G., *et al* (1997) Young people, alcohol, and designer drinks: quantitative and qualitative analysis. *BMJ*, **314**, 414–418.

Hulton, A., Jiang, G. X., Wasserman, D., *et al* (2001) Repetition of attempted suicide among teenagers in Europe: frequency, timing and risk factors. *European Child and Adolescent Psychiatry*, **10**, 161–169.

Kandel, D. B. & Davies, M. (1982) Epidemiology of depressive mood in adolescents: an empirical study. *Archives of General Psychiatry*, **39**, 1205–1212.

Khawaja, S. S & Van Boxel, P. (1998) Chronic fatigue syndrome in children: seven-year follow-up study. *Psychiatric Bulletin*, **22**, 198–202.

Kurtz, Z. (1996) *Treating Children Well: A Guide to Using the Evidence Base in Commissioning and Managing Services for the Mental Health of Children and Young People*. London: Mental Health Foundation.

Lavik, N. (1977) Urban–rural differences in rates of disorder. A comparative psychiatric population study of Norwegian adolescents. In *Epidemiological Approaches in Child Psychiatry* (ed. P. Graham), pp. 184–196. London: Academic Press.

Lewinsohn, P. M., Klein, D. N. & Seeley, J. R. (1995) Bipolar disorders in a community sample of older adolescents: prevalence, phenomenology, comorbidity, and course. *Journal of the American Academy of Child and Adolescent Psychiatry*, **34**, 454–463.

Lewis, C., Hitch, G. J. & Walker, P. (1994) The prevalence of specific arithmetic difficulties and specific reading difficulties in 9- to 10-year-old boys and girls. *Journal of Child Psychology and Psychiatry and Allied Disciplines*, **35**, 283–292.

Light, D. W. & Bailey, V. (1992) *A Needs Based Purchasing Plan for Child Based Mental Health Services*. London: NW Thames Regional Health Authority.

Loranger, A. & Levine, P. (1978) Age at onset of bipolar affective illness. *Archives of General Psychiatry*, **35**, 1345–1348.

Luborsky, L. (1962) Clinicians' judgements of mental health. *Archives of General Psychiatry*, **7**, 407–417.

Luotonen, M. (1995) Early speech development, articulation and reading ability up to the age of 9. *Folia Phoniatrica et Logopedica*, **47**, 310–317.

Lyon, G. R. (1996) Learning disabilities. *Future of Children*, **6**, 54–76.

March, J. S. & Leonard, H. L. (1996) Obsessive–compulsive disorder in children and adolescents: a review of the past 10 years. *Journal of the American Academy of Child and Adolescent Psychiatry*, **35**, 1265–1273.

Mason, A., Banerjee, S., Eapen, V., *et al* (1998) The prevalence of Tourette syndrome in a mainstream school population. *Developmental Medicine and Child Neurology*, **40**, 292–296.

McKee, M. (1999) Sex and drugs and rock and roll: Britain can learn lessons from Europe on the health of adolescents. *BMJ*, **318**, 1300–1301.

Meltzer, H., Gatward, R., Goodman, R., *et al* (2000) *Mental Health of Children and Adolescents in Great Britain*. London: Stationery Office.

Newcombe, R., Measham, F. & Parker, H. (1994) A survey of drinking and deviant behaviour among 14/15 year olds in North West England. *Addiction Research*, **2**, 319–341.

Nicoll, A., Catchpole, M., Cliffe, S., *et al* (1999) Sexual health of teenagers in England and Wales: analysis of national data. *BMJ*, **318**, 1321–1322.

Offord, D. R., Boyle, M. H., Szatmari, P., *et al* (1987) Ontario Child Health Study II: six-month prevalence of disorder and rates of service utilization. *Archives of General Psychiatry*, **44**, 832–836.

Pataki, C. S. & Carlson, G. A. (1995) Childhood and adolescent depression: a review. *Harvard Review of Psychiatry*, **3**, 140–151.

Pearce, J. & Holmes, S. P. (1995) *Health Gain Investment Programme, Lead Document for People with Mental Health Problems (Part 4)*. Nottingham: NHS Executive (Trent).

Pilowsky, D. (1995) Psychopathology among children placed in family foster care. *Psychiatric Services*, **46**, 906–910.

Pine, D. S. (1997) Childhood anxiety disorders. *Current Opinion in Paediatrics*, **9**, 329–338.

Richman, N., Stevenson, J. & Graham, P. (1975) Prevalence of behaviour problems in 3-year-old children: an epidemiological study in a London borough. *Journal of Child Psychology and Psychiatry*, **16**, 277–287.

Roberts, R. E., Attkisson, C. C. & Rosenblatt, A. (1998) Prevalence of psychopathology among children and adolescents. *American Journal of Psychiatry*, **155**, 715–745.

Rutter, M. (1978) Family, area and school influences in the genesis of conduct disorders. In *Aggression and Antisocial Behaviour in Childhood and Adolescence* (eds L. Hersov, M. Berger & D. Scoffer), pp. 95–113. Oxford: Pergamon Press.

Rutter, M., Tizard, J. & Whitmore, K. (eds) (1970) *Education, Health and Behaviour.* London: Longman. (Reprinted, 1981. New York: Krieger).

Rutter, M., Yule, W., Berger, M., *et al* (1974) Children of West Indian immigrants – I. Rates of behavioural deviance and of psychiatric disorder. *Journal of Child Psychology and Psychiatry*, **15**, 241–262.

Rutter, M., Cox, A., Tupling, C., *et al* (1975) Attainment and adjustment in two geographical areas. I – The prevalence of psychiatric disorder. *British Journal of Psychiatry*, **126**, 493–509.

Shaffer, D., Gould, M., Brasic, J., *et al* (1983) Children's global assessment scale. *Archives of General Psychiatry*, **40**, 1228–1231.

Shaywitz, S. E., Shaywitz, B. A., Fletcher, J. M., *et al* (1990) Prevalence of reading disability in boys and girls. Results of the Connecticut Longitudinal Study. *JAMA*, **264**, 998–1002.

Silva, P. A. (1990) The Dunedin multidisciplinary health and development study: a 15 year longitudinal study. *Paediatric and Perinatal Epidemiology*, **4**, 76–107.

Steffenburg, S. & Gillberg, C. (1986) Autism and autistic-like conditions in Swedish rural and urban areas; a population study. *British Journal of Psychiatry*, **149**, 81–87.

Sunder, T. R. (1997) Meeting the challenge of epilepsy in persons with multiple handicaps. *Journal of Child Neurology*, **12** (suppl. 1), S38–S43.

Tanner, C. M. & Goldman, S. M. (1997) Epidemiology of Tourette syndrome. *Neurologic Clinics of North America*, **15**, 395–402.

Townsend, E., Hawton, K., Harriss, L., *et al* (2001) Substances used in deliberate self-poisoning 1985–1997: trends and associations with age, gender, repetition and suicide intent. *Social Psychiatry and Psychiatric Epidemiology*, **36**, 228–234.

Wallace, S. A., Crown, S., Cox, A., *et al* (1997) *Health Care Needs Assessment: Child and Adolescent Mental Health.* Oxford: Radcliffe Medical Press.

Weinberg, N. Z., Rahdert, E., Colliver, J. D., *et al* (1998) Adolescent substance abuse: a review of the past 10 years. *Journal of the American Academy of Child and Adolescent Psychiatry*, **37**, 252–261.

Weissman, M. M., Warner, V. & Fendrich, M. (1990) Applying impairment criteria to children's psychiatric diagnosis. *Journal of the American Academy of Child and Adolescent Psychiatry*, **29**, 789–795.

Werry, J. (1996) Childhood schizophrenia. In *Psychoses and Pervasive Developmental Disorders in Childhood and Adolescence* (ed. F. Volkmar), pp. 1–56. Washington, DC: American Psychiatric Press.

Wessely, S. (1995) The epidemiology of chronic fatigue syndrome. *Epidemiology Review*, **17**, 139–157.

Wing, L. & Gould, J. (1979) Severe impairments of social interaction and associated abnormalities in children. *Journal of Autism and Developmental Disorders*, **9**, 11–30.

World Health Organization (1992) *The ICD–10 Classification of Mental and Behavioural Disorders. Clinical Descriptions and Diagnostic Guidelines.* Geneva: WHO.

Wozniak, J. & Biederman, J. (1997) Childhood mania: insights into diagnostic and treatment issues. *Journal of the Association for Academic Minority Physicians*, **8**, 78–84.

Zucker, K. J., Bradley, S. J. & Sanikhani, M. (1997) Sex differences in referral rates of children with gender identity disorder: some hypotheses. *Journal of Abnormal Child Psychology*, **25**, 217–227.

CHAPTER 6

The law in relation to children

David M. Foreman

This chapter discusses the law on professional practice, consent, confidentiality and child welfare in children with mental health problems. It also extends the discussion of the criminal law in Chapter 21, describing the main legal sanctions against children who break the law. The law relating to children with respect to education, divorce, disability, fostering, child abuse and adoption is dealt with in the relevant chapters of this volume. While the UK Mental Health Bill's new proposals for children are considered, the rest of this Bill is not covered in detail here, as much (although not the child section) is contentious and liable to amendment, and the Mental Health Act 1983 receives extensive coverage in more general textbooks.

The law and our duty of care

As child and adolescent psychiatrists, we are responsible for the medical care of children with mental illness. The Children Act 1989 defines a child as anyone under 18 years old. However, the age of maturity refers largely to the ability to participate in public life (Cretney & Masson, 2000). Other statutes determine that from the age of 16, children may consent to medical treatment (Family Law Reform Act 1969), may marry with parental consent (Marriage Act 1949) and are no longer compelled to attend school (Education Act 1996). Parents are also relieved of their duty to maintain children over 16 if they are in the care of a local authority (Children Act 1989). Legal recognition of moral awareness of right and wrong is set even earlier, with the age of criminal responsibility being 10 years (Children and Young Persons Act 1963), and children of any age are liable for civil damages for harm (tort). The law has thus created various subclasses of children, with different freedoms and responsibilities determined by their age.

Two groups of people are responsible for the medical care of children. The first are doctors. Case law sets the medical standard: the current

'Bolitho' standard requires medical practice to be reasonable in terms of currently accepted medical knowledge, as well as conforming to a respected body of medical opinion (Bolitho v. City and Hackney Health Authority, 1997). If a child lacks the capacity for consent, then the doctor's duty of care is owed to those who are eligible to request care on the child's behalf (Kennedy & Grubb, 2000) – the parents or their statutory equivalents (e.g. social services for a child on a care order). So, a doctor cannot routinely care for a child incapable of consent without parental agreement. In English law, there is no requirement for doctors other than general practitioners (GPs) to act simply because they become aware of someone they might help. It follows that the psychiatrist's medical duty of care does not arise the moment the referral is made, but remains with the GP until an undertaking to treat is given. The initial undertaking is to do no more than manage the referral appropriately. Most child psychiatrists work within multi-disciplinary teams. As there is no relevant case law or statute, courts will make use of guidelines from official bodies as evidence for standards that meet the 'Bolitho' criterion for acceptable medical practice here. The General Medical Council (2001), Royal College of Psychiatrists (2000) and Royal College of Paediatrics and Child Health (2002) all make reference to the importance of effective teamwork. So when doctors work as part of a multidisciplinary team, good teamwork and conflict resolution will be judged part of a doctor's necessary medical skills. However, the doctor will only be presumed 'responsible' for cases referred to the team when the doctor is the team's leader (Kennedy & Grubb, 2000). The other group of people owing a referred child a duty of medical care are the 'hospital managers'. Within the National Health Service (NHS) this refers to the Health Service Trusts and their managers. Their duties of care can be summarised under four headings. First, they must select qualified and competent employees. Second, they have a duty to instruct and supervise them. Next, they have to provide proper facilities and equipment, and finally establish systems necessary to the safe running of their service (Picard, 1981).

Consent, capacity and confidentiality

Assessment or treatment can begin only when consent has been obtained to proceed. In general, consent has three components. Did the consenting person have capacity? Was the person who gave consent appropriately informed? And was the consent voluntarily given? (Kennedy & Grubb, 2000). The eponymous judgment that defined 'Gillick competence' (Gillick v. West Norfolk and Wisbech Area Health Authority and Another, 1986a) considered a situation where a teenager was trying to obtain treatment (contraception) from her doctor against the wishes of her mother. Under this judgment, a minor was given a right to consent to treatment against her parent's wishes, as soon as she is old enough to understand the treatment sufficiently for her consent to be informed. The standard set by Gillick is quite high, requiring understanding of the moral and social implications of a medical procedure, as well as its technical aspects. However, two subsequent cases (Re W, 1992; Re R, 1993) considered cases when a child with a mental health problem, but not under section, was refusing treatment for the disorder. In both cases, the judges concluded that the same high standard should be applied to refusal of treatment, and they had not shown this capacity in their refusal, i.e. demonstrating that they understood the treatments and what they were for did not mean that they understood the full implications of refusing them. The judges also stressed taking the child's wishes seriously, and using the Mental Health Act 1983 where appropriate. Although this separation of consent and refusal can be defended (Foreman, 1999; Mason & McCall-Smith, 1999), it is certainly counterintuitive and leaves ordinary teenagers effectively powerless to refuse medical interventions. This compares unfavourably with the Mental Health Act 1983, where there are extensive rights of appeal, and the Children Act 1989, which states that a child has the right to refuse a medical examination if offered as part of an order under the law. The law in Scotland also seems to be developing differently (Houston, 1996), with a capacity for consent taken to imply a capacity for refusal.

From a practical perspective, we need to consider using the Mental Health Act 1983 when a teenage patient refuses to see us, not as a means of coercing a recalcitrant patient, but to protect the proper autonomy of our child patients at a vulnerable time in their lives. The Mental Health Act 1983 has no lower age limit, and the Children Act 1989 will probably not serve for a child who is Gillick competent, as it actually confers the power of refusal in a manner analogous to Gillick (British Medical Association, 2001).

For children who are not Gillick competent, medical assessment may proceed without further ado if at least one parent (or an agency with parental authority) consents. If the situation is an emergency requiring immediate action, or where delay would be dangerous, then the assessment can begin anyway (Gillick v. West Norfolk and Wisbech Area Health Authority and Another, 1986b). Otherwise, the courts will need to be involved either directly or by enabling another agency (usually the local authority) that can validly consent on behalf of the child despite parental absence or resistance.

The assessment of Gillick competence is governed by the law on capacity, of which Gillick competence itself is simply one type. In general there is a presumption of capacity unless incapacity can be proved, although once incapacity has been established, proof will also be needed to change that judgment (British Medical Association & Law Society, 1995). Incapacity is recognised to be situational, contingent and fluctuating, and our own assessment needs to reflect this (Foreman, 2001). Failure to make a good decision is not, by itself, proof of incapacity (Sidaway v. Board of Governors of the Bethlem Royal Hospital and the Maudsley Hospital, 1985).

Although there is little research on consent in everyday child and adolescent mental health service practice, what there is suggests that the service often does not obtain properly informed consent from its patients, as opposed to their parents (Paul et al, 2000). However, current proposals for the new Mental Health Act specify that teenagers of 16 and above will be treated as adults, with a right of refusal, while children younger than 16 may be assessed compulsorily on parental consent alone for no longer than 28 days (Department of Health, 2002).

Once a child is Gillick competent, the right to confidentiality is recognised in English common law as arising out of the nature of the doctor–patient relationship (Hunter v. Mann, 1974), and statutorily through Article 8 of the European Convention of Human Rights. However, these can be overridden by the 'need to know', 'public interest' and 'best interests of the child' principles. The first operates primarily in connection with multidisciplinary or inter-agency working (Harbour, 2001) and can include all agencies involved in planning care (Department of Health, 1996). 'Public interest' has been interpreted by the General Medical Council as being synonymous with the 'duty to inform' when safety of the patient or others is endangered (General Medical Council, 2000), but recent case law (W v. Edgell, 1990) has extended it to investigations of any grave matter by a public body. Courts sitting under the Children Act 1989, and applying the 'best interests' test, are moving towards full disclosure of all materials to all parties, irrespective of consent (Re L, 1997).

Although court proceedings under the Children Act 1989 are confidential, the information disclosed to the parties, especially expert reports, might subsequently be used by those parties in other, more public settings, e.g. criminal trials (Hall, 2001). Mental health legislation includes certain specific statutory qualifiers to confidentiality: a nearest relative must be consulted, and therefore informed, irrespective of the patient's wishes, before an application can be made under the 1983 Act; and this is also required before applying for a supervision order under the Mental Health (Patients in the Community) Act 1995 (Harbour, 2001). As the law currently stands, confidentiality is a matter of avoiding the inadvertent, mendacious or gratuitous exposure of private material.

Consent is complex, and the law on it is in a state of flux. So, if the situation is confusing, and it is not an emergency, then legal advice may be necessary, and should be available through NHS Trusts.

93

Legal governance of children's welfare

Parens patriae theoretically gives the court unlimited control over the lives of children through its inherent jurisdiction over children. Wardship, where the court takes parental responsibility for a child, has been rendered largely redundant by the various powers and orders available under the Children Act 1989, and its use further inhibited by making it incompatible with care proceedings. However, the inherent jurisdiction is still used to allow a court to decide difficult single issues, especially difficult medical decisions (Bainham, 2000).

The Children Act 1989 was to integrate all statutory aspects of child welfare. Proceedings under the Act have to make the child's interests 'paramount', be free from delay, consider whether any order is necessary, and judge the value of any order against the 'welfare checklist' (Box 6.1).

Care and supervision orders

At present, only a local authority or the National Society for the Prevention of Cruelty to Children (NSPCC) can apply for a care order or a supervision order on a child. The grounds for both are essentially that the child risks significant harm attributable to upbringing or loss of parental control (Children Act 1989). The risk of significant harm is to be interpreted broadly (Newnham LBC *v.* AG, 1993) and may refer to circumstances before protective arrangements are established on either a voluntary or compulsory basis (re M, 1994). However, the standard of proof required is high, particularly regarding the risk of future harm as harm is in fact a rare event, and to show that a rare event has a greater than 50% chance of happening in a particular case is demanding (Bainham, 2000). For example, the siblings of a child who was probably abused by the mother's cohabitee, but where a prosecution for rape had failed, could not be made subject to care orders as the standard of proof had not been met (H and R, 1996). The determination of 'significant harm' is also a matter of factual proof, so it is not sufficient to claim merely that a child will do better, or even much better, under a care

---

Box 6.1 The Welfare Checklist

1. The ascertainable wishes and feelings of the child, considered in the light of the child's age and understanding.
2. The child's physical, emotional and educational needs.
3. The likely effect on the child of any change in circumstances.
4. The child's age, gender, background and any characteristics of his which the Court considers relevant.
5. Any harm suffered, or risk of harm.
6. The capacity of the relevant adults to meet the child's needs.
7. The range of powers available to the Court under the Act.

---

order (Humberside CC *v.* B, 1993). Similar rules, and difficulties, apply to establishing the criterion of inadequate parental upbringing, although the failure of upbringing needs only to be contributory, not causative (Cretney & Masson, 2000). Being beyond parental control is a non-exclusive alternative to a failure of upbringing, but neither is sufficient without the establishment of significant harm. Once grounds are established, the decision between a care order or a supervision order is based on which will best secure the needs of the child (Re V, 1996). A care order has the effect of giving the local authority parental responsibility alongside the parents, with the additional power of being able to restrict the parents' exercise of their responsibilities, if this would secure the child's welfare. This effectively makes the local authority the 'senior partner' among the child's caretakers, but the other caretakers are not automatically dismissed, and indeed have continuing rights of contact. Although the local authority controls a care order, anyone with parental authority (including the local authority itself) or the child may apply to have the care order rescinded.

A supervision order merely establishes, by consent, the right of a designated local authority, youth offending team worker (see Chapter 21) or probation officer to 'advise, befriend and assist' the child, to take steps to see that the order is complied with, and to return to court if the order seems ineffective. It lasts for a year in the first instance but can be extended for up to 3 years, although it automatically lapses when the child reaches 18. Conditions that involve the parents may be attached to the supervision order.

Secure care order

An ordinary care order does not give the local authority the right to detain a child. However, a separate section of the Children Act (Section 25) allows the child to be placed in secure accommodation if the child has a history of absconding, and is likely to abscond from any other placement. The alterative grounds are if the child is likely to injure him/herself or anyone else unless secure accommodation is used. The order can be made without a pre-existing care order, but in that case a parent can overrule it. Also, it can only be made if the child is legally represented, and a children's guardian needs to be appointed. Without application to the court, a child may be kept confined for no more than 72 hours in every 21 days (Department of Health, 1991*a*).

Child assessment order

The child assessment order is specifically designed to allow social services (or the NSPCC) to check the welfare of children where they have concerns about abuse, but where evidence is not available through lack of parental cooperation. Although a short-term order (7 days), it is not for use in emergencies, which should be dealt with by emergency protection orders. The Guidance suggests that it is appropriate where suspicions have been accumulating for some time (e.g. unexplained failure to thrive or, in psychiatry, a severe attachment disorder without explanatory history). It requires the caretakers to produce the child, and to cooperate with investigations, including medical investigations. For this order, the welfare checklist does not apply: the hurdles to be jumped are the presumption of no order and the welfare principle in its general form.

Emergency protection order

The emergency protection order (Department of Health, 1991a) serves to remove a child from a (potentially) dangerous environment, or keep a child in a safe place, in an emergency. The court (or justice) must satisfy itself that there is a likelihood of significant harm occurring unless the child either remains away from the situation or is removed from it promptly (although not necessarily immediately). Anyone may apply for one, but if the applicant is not the local authority, the local authority may take the order over if it considers it to be in the child's best interests. The parents, other carers of the child and the local authority need to be served the order within 48 hours of it being made. As well as authorising removal or retention of the child by the applicant, it also requires anyone with the child to produce the child to the applicant, and gives the applicant parental responsibility over the child. It lasts for 8 days, and can be extended once, for a further 7 days.

Interim care or supervision orders

Interim care orders (and interim supervision orders) are available for situations where care proceedings have to be adjourned or are in progress, or the courts have requested social services' investigations under Section 37 (child protection investigations). As many consecutive orders may be made as are consistent with the no-delay principle.

Family assistance orders

Like a supervision order, a family assistance order is made by consent; a social worker or probation officer has to advise, assist and befriend; and the order gives no powers other than to return to court. However, the criterion of significant harm does not apply, although the circumstances do have to be 'exceptional' and the order judged 'efficacious'. Its major use is in contentious divorce cases, and local authorities cannot apply for them (Cretney & Masson, 2000).

Being 'accommodated'

Children may also be 'accommodated' by the local authority without legal application. The provision of accommodation is a duty towards children who have been lost, abandoned, are without anyone with parental responsibility, or whose parents are incapable of looking after them – provided the local authority considers the child requires accommodation. Accommodation may not be offered if anyone with parental authority either offers or arranges accommodation, and the parent can withdraw the child at any time (Brayne *et al*, 2001).

Research and innovative treatments

Specific English legislation on medical research on humans is confined to work with embryos, medicinal products, gene therapy and xenotransplantation (Kennedy & Grubb, 2000). Even the Research Ethics Committee system is not set up in statute, but as statutory guidance to the NHS (Department of Health, 1991*b*), so they may not govern research outside NHS settings except by consent. It follows that the law on medical research and innovative treatment on children is ordinary medical law. So, current guidelines (Medical Research Council, 2000) have the legal status of potential benchmarks the courts may apply when considering individual cases. When applying the principles of medical law to research on children, a helpful distinction that can be drawn is between therapeutic and non-therapeutic research. The former increases knowledge in the context of a treatment, whereas the latter seeks only to increase knowledge about a condition, and does not help the patient directly. Apart from obvious 'pure research' paradigms, non-therapeutic research also takes place when controls or placebo treatments are used. It is generally agreed that parents may consent on behalf of non-competent children to both therapeutic and non-therapeutic research (Kennedy & Grubb, 2000). Consent issues are less clear for competent children, even for teenagers between the ages of 16 and 18 years, and matters are best judged on a case-by-case basis, taking legal and ethical advice as appropriate.

With therapeutic research, the harm that can be risked should be balanced against the likely benefit (Kennedy & Grubb, 2000). With non-therapeutic research, the harm that can be risked should be at worst minimal. Although hard to quantify, a rate of 0.1–1% for minor complications has been suggested (Nicholson, 1986). Several authorities now stress that the standard of explanation of research needs to be higher than for everyday clinical interventions (Kennedy & Grubb, 2000; British Medical Association, 2001). Randomised controlled trials (RCTs) pose particular problems. A researcher undertaking an RCT must, at the outset, have no proof that one condition in the trial is better than another – the 'principle of equipoise' – as to randomly fail to give treatment to a patient who needs it is negligence. Many believe that RCTs should have stopping criteria, so that all who would benefit can receive the treatments as soon as a clear benefit is established, and the control criteria must not deny alternative necessary treatments.

Medical law currently considers innovative treatments to be justifiable exercises of medical skill, but the innovation has to be medically reasonable (Hunter *v.* Hanley, 1955). This should be taken as a warning that innovative treatments are best implemented according to professional guidance. We have seen that the courts will use such protocols to benchmark whether reasonably appropriate care was offered. Both the Royal College of Paediatrics and Child Health and the Royal College of Psychiatrists offer guidance on research and innovative treatments with children, particularly regarding consent (Royal College of Paediatrics and Child Health, 2000; Royal College of Psychiatrists, 2002). Both of these sets of guidelines stress that parents must make reflective judgements about the best interests of their child, and substantive consent may need to be delayed until they can. The paediatric guidance also stresses the need to take the wishes of the child seriously, even if the child is not Gillick competent, and the Royal College guidance identifies the need to proceed with great caution (but not necessarily stop) if parents disagree with each other. Obtaining a further opinion can be a useful safeguard against the risk of excessive therapeutic enthusiasm (British Medical Association, 2001).

Practically, the development of clinical goverance procedures means that NHS Trusts now have policies covering these issues, and personnel to help clinicians in difficult cases. If in doubt, contacting the local research ethics committee for advice is a wise decision.

The criminal law and children

General principles of the criminal law in relation to children are covered in Chapter 21. Here I discuss legal interventions that may be made with children who break the law, but not the legal management of children who commit serious crimes. A wide range of such interventions exists, as shown in the following list.

- **Police reprimands** are typically for a first and minor offence. The reprimand usually involves the family, and may also include a confrontation with the victim.
- **Police final warning.** This is for a minor second offence, and includes a mandatory assessment by the youth offending team (YOT; see Chapter 21). Further offences must always lead to a court appearance.

- **Referral order.** This is the usual legal disposal for youngsters who appears in court for the first time (provided they plead guilty). Lasting 3–12 months, the order involves a specific plan, managed by the YOT and overseen by a panel, to make reparation and reduce recidivism.
- **Reparation orders** require the child to make reparation to the victim, in a way specified in the order.
- **Action plan orders** require the young offender to attend the YOT twice a week, to receive a short, focused programme of punishment, reparation and rehabilitation, closely tailored to the perceived needs of the offender and crime. There is a particular focus on preventing reoffending.
- **Parenting orders and bindovers.** Parents may be ordered to attend parenting courses, or meetings with the YOT workers, and be bound over to take proper responsibility for their children.
- **Fines** are usually levied against the parent if the child is under 16. Parents may also be fined for failing either a parenting order or failing to be 'bound over' (see above) to manage their offspring responsibly.
- **Attendance centre orders** require a specific number of hours of attendance at specified times – typically 2-hour slots at the YOT fortnightly at weekends. The time is spent in physical activity and learning.
- **Curfew and electronic curfew orders** also restrict the young offenders' liberty to a specific place, e.g. their parents' home, though for no more than 12 hours daily. Electronic curfew orders use an electronic tag to track the young offender's movements.
- **Drug testing and treatment orders** may be used on youngsters over 16 with drug problems. They are for a minimum of 6 months, and are run by the adult probation service.
- **Detention and training orders** are custodial sentences, half of which are served in a young offenders' institution, and half at home reporting to the YOT. They last up to 2 years.

Children's rights and the law

The UK has ratified several international conventions designed to define and protect children's rights, but only the European Convention on Human Rights has been incorporated into UK law, through the Human Rights Act 1998. Relevant articles include the right to life (Article 2), prohibition of inhuman or degrading treatment (Article 3), right to liberty and security (Article 5), respect for privacy (Article 8), the right to redress if the Articles are breached (Article 13), non-discriminatory application of the Convention (Article 14), and in the annexed protocols the right to education (Protocol 2). The courts' practical interpretation of these rights will consider whether the right conferred is absolute, has exceptions or is to be balanced against other rights or needs. When balancing is permitted, the courts will first consider whether law supports the infringement, whether it is directed towards a legitimate aim, and whether the breach is proportional to the aims pursued (Wadham & Mountfield, 1999). So far, English case law has been scanty, but it is already becoming clear that the Convention is likely to be interpreted restrictively. For example, it cannot be used to support a claim to resource any particular treatment (North West Lancashire HA *v.* A D & G, 1999).

Conclusion

The law is a critical component of the healthcare delivery system for child and adolescent mental health. It grants the powers and imposes the duties that allow us to work, and so influences the form of the service we deliver. Legal knowledge should be seen as part of our therapeutic armoury, not just as a way of avoiding claims of malpractice.

References

Bainham, A. (2000) *Children: The Modern Law*. Bristol: Family Law.

Brayne, H., Martin, G. & Carr, H. (2001) *Law for Social Workers*. Oxford: Oxford University Press.

British Medical Association (2001) *Consent, Rights and Choices in Health Care for Children and Young People*. London: BMA.

British Medical Association & Law Society (1995) *Assessment of Mental Capacity: Guidance for Lawyers and Doctors*. London: BMA.

Cretney, S. & Masson, J. (2000) *Principles of Family Law*. London: Sweet & Maxwell.

Department of Health (1991a) *The Children Act 1989: Guidance and Regulations*. London: Department of Health.

Department of Health (1991b) *Local Research Ethics Committees*. London: Department of Health.

Department of Health (1996) *The Protection and Use of Patient Information*. London: Department of Health.

Department of Health (2002) *Mental Health Bill: Consultation Document*. London: Department of Health.

Foreman, D. M. (1999) The Family Rule: a framework for obtaining consent for medical interventions from children. *Journal of Medical Ethics*, **25**, 491–496.

Foreman, D. (2001) Ethical and legal issues. In *Adolescent Psychiatry in Clinical Practice* (ed. S. Gowers), pp. 258–29. London: Arnold.

General Medical Council (2000) *Confidentiality: Protecting and Providing Information*. London: GMC.

General Medical Council (2001) *Good Medical Practice*. London: GMC.

Hall, A. (2001) Confidentiality: a legal view. In *Confidentiality and Mental Health* (ed. C. Cordess), pp. 137–149. London: Jessica Kingsley.

Harbour, A. (2001) The limits of confidentiality: a legal view. In *Confidentiality and Mental Health* (ed. C. Cordess), pp. 151–157. London: Jessica Kingsley.

Kennedy, I. & Grubb, A. (2000) *Medical Law*. London: Butterworth.

Mason, J. & McCall-Smith, R. (1999) *Law and Medical Ethics*. London: Butterworth.

Medical Research Council (2000) *Good Research Practice*. London: Medical Research Council.

Nicholson, R. (1986) *Medical Research with Children: Ethics, Law and Practice*, p. 119. Oxford: Oxford University Press.

Paul, M., Foreman, D. & Kent, L. S. (2000) Out-patient clinic attendence: Consent from young people: ethical aspects and practical considerations. *Clinical Child Psychology and Psychiatry*, **5**, 203–212.

Picard, E. (1981) The liability of hospitals in Common Law Canada. *McGill Law Journal*, **26**, 997.

Royal College of Paediatrics and Child Health (2000) Guidelines for the ethical conduct of research involving children. *Archives of Disease in Childhood*, **82**, 177–182.

Royal College of Paediatrics and Child Health (2002) *Good Medical Practice in Paediatrics and Child Health*. London: Royal College of Paediatrics and Child Health.

Royal College of Psychiatrists (2000) *Good Psychiatric Practice* (Council Report CR83). London: Royal College of Psychiatrists.

Royal College of Psychiatrists (2002) *Guidelines for Researchers and for Research Ethics Committees on Psychiatric Research Involving Human Participants* (Council Report CR82). London: Royal College of Psychiatrists.

Wadham, J. & Mountfield, H. (1999) *Blackstone's Guide to the Human Rights Act 1998*. London: Blackstone.

Bolitho *v.* City and Hackney Health Authority [1997] All ER(HL), p. 771.

Gillick *v.* West Norfolk and Wisbech Area Health Authority and Another [1986*a*] FLR (HL), vol. 1, p. 224.

Gillick *v.* West Norfolk and Wisbech Area Health Authority and Another [1986*b*] All ER, vol. 3, p. 402.

H and R [1996] FLR, vol. 1, p. 80.

Houston [1996] BMLR, vol. 32, p. 93.

Humberside CC *v.* B [1993] FLR, vol. 1, p. 257.

Hunter *v.* Hanley [1955] SC, p. 200.

Hunter *v.* Mann [1974] QB, p. 767.

Newnham LBC *v.* AG [1993] FLR, vol. 1, p. 281.

North West Lancashire HA *v.* A D & G (1999) Lloyd's Rep Med (CA), p. 399.

Re L (1997) AC(HL), p. 16.

re M (1994) WLR, vol. 3, p. 55.

Re R (1993) Fam, p. 11.

Re V (1996) FLR, vol. 1, p. 776.

Re W (1992) WLR, vol. 3, p. 358.

Sidaway *v.* Board of Governors of the Bethlem Royal Hospital and the Maudsley Hospital [1985] AC, p. 67.

W *v.* Edgell [1990] All ER, vol. 1, p. 835.

CHAPTER 7

Assessment in child and adolescent psychiatry

Mary Eminson

Performing the initial assessment for a child or adolescent mental health problem is among the most sophisticated and complex tasks that psychiatry provides. It includes the ability to hold together assessment skills for several people at different stages of development, and to synthesise much verbal and non-verbal information. A crucial skill is engagement with a child or young person, taking into account the child's anxiety or reluctance. There is a need to manage the time and interactions for a group of people rather than an individual, allowing for different individuals' needs and the time the interviewer has available. Finally, as in all psychiatric assessments, it is necessary to keep in mind one's subjective impressions: how the family make you feel, as well as noting what family members say and do.

Presentations in child psychiatry are distinguished from those in most adult services by the roles of parents and carers, who are often responsible for recognising the difficulties, alerting helping services, ensuring the young person reaches an appointment, and giving much of the description and the history. In the range of services that might be included within 'child and adolescent psychiatry', there is a range of difficulty – as is the case in the role of parents/carers, with much variation in the dependence of the child on the parents. This might range from a very young child with attachment difficulties or high levels of activity, through to a 17- or 18-year-old about to leave home who is suicidal, hallucinating or depressed. In between these extremes will be children or younger adolescents with mental health difficulties of many kinds: problems of anxiety, moods, behaviour, attention, eating, elimination, sleep and social relations. These difficulties will arise in children who also have significant physical ill health, in those who have physical symptoms but no evidence of organic disease, and in young people with a range of learning difficulties. In some of these presentations, it is likely that other professionals – paediatricians, social workers, education professionals – will be those who draw attention to the problems and make the referral, rather than a general practitioner who has been contacted by a parent. Nevertheless, in all these circumstances the role of parents (or those who hold parental responsibility) in ensuring the child reaches a service is a crucial one.

Whoever has initiated the referral, and whatever the problem, the overall aims of the initial assessment remain very similar.

Preparation for the assessment

Who does the assessment? All child and adolescent mental health service (CAMHS) professionals undertaking initial assessments will share a set of core skills, but different professional training and further experience will bring more specialist expertise with certain age groups, disorders or problems. The decision about who undertakes the assessment might depend on time and staff resources in the service. Ideally, the mix of skills should be tailored to the problem described, and the members of the CAMHS workforce best placed to provide them, with tasks being shared depending on the individual skills. Thus, psychiatrists, psychologists, social workers, nurses, occupational therapists and other child mental health workers may undertake, or share, assessments in CAMHS. Conversely, it is often necessary for one individual to complete the initial assessment, and all psychiatrists should be able to undertake this. This chapter describes the components of a comprehensive initial child and adolescent psychiatric assessment at a non-specialist level. Table 7.1 summarises the tasks of assessment.

Table 7.1 Assessment tasks

Task	Milestones for the psychiatrist
To engage the young person and family	*Make a successful rapport*
To gain sufficient information to evaluate the nature and seriousness of the difficulties, taking into account biological, psychological and social factors	*Make notes (see key areas in Box 7.1)*
To assess the young person's mental health and consider any attendant risk from that	*Decide if a diagnosis is applicable (see Box 7.2)*
To plan the next steps of assessment or treatment and to have consent to undertake them	*Undertake any necessary risk assessment, including physical examination*
To share and, hopefully, agree a formulation and plan with the family	*Draw up an outline plan. Ensure that the relevant consent forms are signed*
To record one's observations clearly and legibly, and sign them	*Multi-axial formulation (see Box 7.3). Complete a letter or summary*

It is important to think about the setting for the assessment, and its effect on the young person and the assessor: the clinic setting might be the place where the clinician feels most relaxed and efficient, but might be anxiety-provoking (or stigmatising) for the family. In the case of urgent assessments, a paediatric ward or accident and emergency department will have different constraints on everyone concerned (e.g. time, privacy). If the assessment is for a specialist purpose, such as for court, this places extra demands for precision in record-keeping and changes the situation about confidentiality for the report.

Previous assessments or information from other agencies or services may sometimes be usefully reviewed before the interview, and consent may need to be gained to obtain these (for example, in the case of paediatric notes).

The initial contact needs to be efficient in reaching its goals comprehensively, but flexible in the way those goals are attained. The age of the child and nature of the difficulties outlined will allow for preparation: of suitable play material, considering the age of the child (and perhaps siblings), to entertain, engage and evaluate; of the interviewer (reading about the condition and earlier assessments); and of any instruments (questionnaires, checklists). In preparing for the interview itself, there is a choice to be made between types of assessment: an unstructured assessment that covers key areas and is tailored individually, a standard interview schedule such as the Diagnostic Interview Schedule for Children (DISC; Schaffer *et al*, 2000), a purely verbal interview, which enquires about symptoms in the past month or year, or the Kiddie Schedule for Affective Disorders and Schizophrenia (K–SADS; Ambrosini, 2000), which examines current and lifetime histories of worst episodes. Computerised versions of some of these schedules are now becoming available, but none is applicable to children aged under 6 years or so. A compromise used in many non-specialist services is to use a broad standard questionnaire before the initial assessment, perhaps the Strengths and Difficulties Questionnaire (Goodman, 1997) and one or two more focused instruments relevant to the problems presented, during or after it. However, answers on the questionnaires may be inaccurate and scores should be used as an adjunct to the clinical interview, not a substitute for it. The assessment interview in ordinary clinical practice will follow a conventional structure similar to that outlined below, but not a strictly standardised format: the interview schedules require more time.

Use of interpreters or translators

Many communities now include families, either settled or refugees/asylum seekers, where some or all family members speak little English and where there are many vulnerabilities to mental health difficulties.

Where children speak little English, strenuous efforts should be made to find a child and adolescent mental health care professional who can communicate directly. Pragmatically, it may be necessary to go ahead with an interpreter for the appointment. Use of the child's parent or sibling as an interpreter has many drawbacks, and it is worth searching out someone independent of the family. It will be crucial to establish that you are asking for translation, rather than interpretation, of what is said, and important to know whether the interpreter has knowledge of mental health. In all circumstances, it is important to allow extra time for such assessments, not only to make your formulation but also to allow for explanations to those with no familiarity with UK services.

Introduction and engagement

Many services now have leaflets or other information for parents and young people, which are sent out before the appointment. These lay the ground for later explanations and for introducing yourself: wearing a badge is always good practice and in many settings mandatory. It is useful to begin observation of families in the waiting area, and to note their level of noise and organisation.

Explain the important basics about the assessment: how long you will be meeting for, how the time will be structured, if there is any equipment in the room the children should not touch. If there is a camera or one-way screen, explain, demonstrate and answer questions about any observers or videotapes, including gaining written consent where appropriate. The role of each professional involved in the assessment will need to be explained to the family, who may have assumptions about what is meant by involvement of a social worker ('taking children away') or psychiatrist ('he must be mad'). A common introduction is 'I am a doctor who sees young people with problems like yours. I will want to hear your point of view as well as your parents'.'

Because of the complexity of the assessment task, the space in which you undertake it is one of the key variables for non-urgent assessments. Ensure the room is big enough, at a reasonable temperature and that no one will be made uncomfortable by interruptions or feeling that they can be overheard. All young people need to be greeted and engaged appropriately and given permission or encouragement to use the toys. Everyone should feel 'safe' in terms of confidentiality. Mobile telephones should be switched off so that everyone can concentrate on the task at hand. The interview begins with a warm welcome to family members, a confirmation of why, at whose request and for whom they have attended, and a neutral, non-judgemental approach to the referral problem, especially when adolescents are being assessed or where 'disapproved' activities are involved.

The initial account

Parents or caregivers obviously have a crucial role in giving the initial account of the problems that have brought them to the service. It is important to understand the parental concerns and to clarify the family's attitude to psychiatric assessment. Equally, the young person who is the subject of the interview has a central role and must be engaged. A common practice is to invite all adolescents at the outset to say why they have been brought (or come willingly), and to ask all younger children if they know why their parents have brought them. Even when the young person is reluctant to talk and cedes the main account to their parents, he or she will have noted the importance placed on their contribution.

The current problem is the best place to start most assessments. Once this is adequately understood the structure may vary, but must include the relevant areas to achieve the interview's aims. Box 7.1 presents suggested headings for taking the history, which may be used as an *aide-mémoire*. Initially, it is important to orient oneself by checking the origin of the referral and gaining a quick understanding of family composition or carers' responsibilities. Open questions then establish the nature and range of difficulties about which the family is concerned. It is essential that this enquiry is wide and not restricted to what is first mentioned: the interviewer should keep checking. At this stage it is helpful to continue a dialogue with the young person about the difficulties being described, continuing to seek the individual's views and observe his or her reactions. This also provides an opportunity to study family relationships.

It is necessary to gain a detailed account to establish a comprehensive understanding of the presenting problems, their antecedents, consequences, associated factors and impairments, the chronicity and severity. Closed questions will often be required to gather an accurate and detailed

---

Box 7.1 Key components of the history

- Family composition
- A detailed account of symptoms (both parents' and young person's views)
- History of problems/symptoms
- Development history
- Temperament or personality
- Past medical history
- Medication
- Social/peer relationships
- Drug, alcohol and substance use and misuse
- School attendance, attainment, behaviour, relationships
- Family history and family psychiatric history
- Family relationships

---

picture, and targeted questions follow from details of what is presented and other coexisting problems. Thus, the major focus will be on the key psychiatric features, for example the precise form of the psychotic illness or eating disorder, with detailed enquiries about relevant symptoms, and the interviewer making use of detailed knowledge from other chapters in this book. Other problems often associated with such a diagnosis will then be enquired about carefully – for example, substance use or misuse, self-harm and social withdrawal in the case of psychosis. Finally, direct questions may be asked about other major areas of psychopathology that have not been mentioned so far – for example, behaviour or antisocial difficulties, or anxiety. It is a matter of judgement and experience to decide how much detail to gather at the outset, or whether to gain an overview and detail later. Whichever structure is chosen, the initial interview gives the opportunity to ask, however briefly, about the full range of child psychiatric difficulties (summarised in Box 7.2). Do not conclude your review too quickly and foreclose your thinking about other possibilities. Unexpected co-morbidity may be identified.

This conjoint part of the interview, to gain an overview of current problems, usually takes 15–30 minutes, and involves both parent and child. It is helpful for the interviewer then to summarise the current difficulties in a sentence or two, checking agreement. This provides punctuation in the interview, after which time everyone can be reminded of what will be included in later parts.

Box 7.2 ICD–10 diagnostic clinical psychiatric syndromes: major categories for children and adolescents (World Health Organization, 1996)

- Pervasive developmental disorders: autism, atypical autism, Asperger syndrome
- Hyperkinetic disorders, attention-deficit disorders
- Conduct and oppositional disorders
- Tic disorders
- 'Other' disorders including non-organic enuresis, encopresis, pica
- 'Social functioning' disorders – elective mutism, attachment disorders
- Mental and behavioural disorders due to psychoactive substances
- Schizophrenia, schizotypal and delusional disorders
- Mood (affective) disorders: depression, bipolar affective disorders, mania
- Stress and adjustment reactions
- Anxiety disorders, generalised and specific: separation anxiety, panic, phobias
- Obsessive–compulsive disorders
- Dissociative and somatoform disorders
- Eating disorders
- Sleep disorders
- Psychological factors affecting physical conditions
- Disorders of adult personality and behaviour

The next steps

The next stage is to gather background information and talk to the young person alone, to establish the child's views and assess his or her mental state. Deciding whether to continue with the family together, or to speak separately to parents or child, depends very much on the problem, age of child, how many people are undertaking the assessment and whether children can be supervised safely elsewhere. When an adolescent is the subject, there is a decision to be made about whether detailed background information needed from parents is gathered before interviewing the adolescent alone, or in the reverse order, which would give the benefit of letting the young person have 'first say'. In most circumstances, it is helpful to hear the background before spending time with the young person. With very young children, practical constraints in the clinic may limit the feasibility of seeing parents alone. In these circumstances, it may be best to give children explicit permission to 'play while listening' at this stage. There are some drawbacks to keeping the children within the room; parents will speak less freely about their own experiences and feelings in sensitive areas, and their sensitivities should be respected. Always ask parents if they would like an opportunity to speak without the children, which can be arranged if necessary for a subsequent occasion.

The background history

Background (the section following 'History of problems/symptoms' in Box 7.1) includes the child's development, the child's health and functioning in the past, and important information about family structure and relationships. Examine the milestones of physical and emotional development: motor, sensory and cognitive achievements; and the development of relationships. Ensure you have details of any significant physical health problems, current or past, and are clear which specialists are currently involved. Enquire about psychosocial aspects, but omit sensitive enquiries if children are still present. Was the pregnancy welcomed or otherwise? Highly precious, perhaps following loss of an earlier pregnancy? A discussion of attachment issues will arise naturally from these questions.

The account of family structure and relationships needs to encompass important issues which may be of aetiological significance and/or be relevant for intervention. The parents' history of their own childhood may be directly relevant to the child's own problems – learning, abuse, mood or eating difficulty or attention-deficit hyperactivity disorder (ADHD), for example, may all affect the risks of the child having difficulties in this area – and also have an impact on parenting. A three-generational family tree, a useful way to structure this section, can be gathered when parents and child are together. This allows enquiry about physical, psychological, social and relationship issues in each part of the family, usually starting with the referred child and siblings, then moving back to examine the parents' relationships and histories, including childhoods and families. Drawing this family tree is often a task in which children can be engaged, adding names and ages.

When acquiring this information, one is simultaneously taking note of the level and kind of emotion in the family, the complexity of language, and the nature and congruity of the account of family relationships and history. Are there discrepancies between the approaches of the parents? One needs to be alert to other factors in the account, for example the extent to which the family is critical and blaming of the young person, as this too may be relevant in understanding the aetiology or maintenance of the problems.

Functioning in other settings

The extent and pervasiveness of problems is important in judging severity, and may be essential for understanding aetiology and planning management. Therefore, enquiry is made about the extent to which difficulties are seen in other settings (with other family members, at school, at church or on holiday), where demands on the child or triggers for problems may be different. The secondary effects of problems will also be evaluated by these queries: how is the child functioning at school academically, behaviourally, with adults and with peers? Is there a lack of information about other settings because the child has no friends or is never asked to their homes? These enquiries need to be made with due account of cultural context.

Although most children attend school, the social context of the rest of their lives may differ markedly from the interviewer's own, or one's assumptions. Some questioning to clarify these family and social expectations may be helpful. How do the family usually spend their time at weekends and holiday times? Is the patient able to function in these circumstances in the same way as other children in the family or in the patient's culture?

Individual interview with a child or adolescent

The third section of the interview is usually the individual time spent with the child or adolescent. As when meeting any new patient or client, there are two key functions, which may sometimes be difficult to integrate in the time and setting. These tasks are to achieve a sympathetic understanding of the point of view and perspective of the young person and to make a full assessment of his or her current

109

mental state. For almost all disorders (ADHD is perhaps an exception), a full diagnostic assessment can only be made with knowledge of the child's own experience of the symptoms, description of how they feel and their account of problems – so a good rapport and communication are essential. The 'sympathetic understanding' aspect of the assessment should also facilitate engagement as a prelude to any future therapeutic work. It must be a cardinal skill of any child and adolescent mental health professional to maximise potential for any future individual or family work which may be required, and to ensure the experience of psychiatric assessment is a positive one, of being heard and understood.

The methods of carrying out this individual interview may differ widely between children at different ages, with different problems or disorders, and what follows is only a broad guide. Carrying out these interviews requires high levels of skill, and an ability to adjust to the child's cognitive level and developmental stage. This involves being warm and open, without being 'gossipy' and informal, or distant and patronising – a hard balance to achieve sometimes. Observing one or more experienced professionals undertake detailed assessment of a child and an adolescent before conducting an interview oneself is essential. Subsequently, reviewing a video of one's own performance can be very instructive. Jones (2003) gives a more detailed account of approaches and techniques used in communicating with vulnerable and abused children.

It is also helpful to be aware of normal developmental milestones, especially with young children, so that you can assess development informally against the normal milestones in terms of speech, coordination, motor skills (both gross and fine) and their social relating (Sheridan, 1980). This may alert you to the need for more formal evaluation later.

Confidentiality

A further complexity in the individual interview is the need to create an atmosphere of safety and privacy. One wishes to enable the child to explain private thoughts and perhaps distressing experiences without giving a false impression of complete confidentiality. Although very young children might be best assessed with their parents throughout (see below), the individual interview is otherwise an opportunity to understand the details of the child's own symptoms and to establish how the child relates and responds to an unfamiliar but interested and sympathetic adult. Explain to a child of any age that this is a 'private' interview and you want to know what they think and feel. Although their parents will want some feedback, you will not be telling them exactly what is said, but will agree with the young person, at the end, how best to summarise. If there is anything that you MUST tell their parents/carers, you will let them know what it is. Adolescents of normal intelligence may require a more detailed review of the issues involved, but confidentiality conflicts are less frequent than is sometimes feared. In principle, the detail of what is shared with a clinician is confidential, but if for any reason there are matters that the clinician thinks need to be discussed with parents, you will tell the young person what these are. It is almost always possible to agree a form of words about what needs to be shared.

Very occasionally, a clear conflict arises: the adolescent discloses serious abuse, suicidal plans or risk-taking (use of parental medication perhaps), which must be addressed with parents, and perhaps other authorities, immediately. Deciding how to handle such a disclosure may require a break to discuss this with a senior colleague. Although the relationship with the young person may be damaged as a result, in these circumstances child protection considerations have to take a higher priority than engagement and confidentiality. However ambivalent and angry the young person may be at the time, he or she often wishes for authoritative containment of the risks and will commonly acknowledge later that this disclosure was necessary.

Practicalities of individual interviews

There are four phases, each of which provides opportunity for observation, and which should run smoothly into each other. The first phase is the process of separating the child from the parents; the second is the development of trust and rapport, the 'warming up'; then the detailed review of thoughts, feelings and experience, with any pencil and paper tests or other assessments; and finally, rounding up and safe closure, before return to the family.

Pre-school and early school-age children

Children aged 2–3 years are uncommonly seen in child and adolescent mental health services, and in most cases attempting a separate interview at this age is probably unwise (as in a community paediatric or child development clinic). The parent's report of how the child will behave on separation may be more valuable than actually testing this out on a first occasion. With older pre-schoolers, particularly those who are used to time away from their parents, a short separation can usually be achieved once child and parent have relaxed. Explain to the child you would like to spend a little time on your own with them while their parents wait nearby. It is a good idea to describe what you will be doing ('We will be playing with these toys together', 'We'll be talking a bit and doing some drawing'), as these children are likely to have no previous experience to guide them. If the child has had much illness or healthcare, it might be appropriate to explain what you will *not* be doing, e.g. giving an injection.

Children at school are used to separating from their parents and should, by this stage of the assessment, be relaxed with the setting and the professional. Spending perhaps 15 minutes with an interested adult and a set of new toys is usually easily accepted and enjoyable to all but the most anxious or frightened child. This assumption depends of course on previous experiences and expectations, and the way the parent has prepared the child for your assessment. If, for whatever reason, the child becomes distressed when alone with you, it is best not to persist but to invite the parents to return.

With infants or young children, the 'interview' and/or mental state assessment is achieved through play rather than being focused on 'the problem'. What these children are able to tell you in response to your questions about their own experience is not likely to help you in deciding the diagnosis or severity, as they are unlikely to be able to contribute to your knowledge because of their developmental stage. However, this is an opportunity to observe, to assess development, and to examine capacity for interaction and relationships. Paper, crayons, felt-tip pens, and a doll's house or farm with family or animal figures will suffice as play materials: let the child take the lead in this. Try to respond and reflect on the child's play rather than ask a lot of questions. Observe the child's ability to handle crayons or a simple jigsaw; a simple test such as the Goodenough Draw a Man Test (Harris, 1963) may be incorporated. Observe how easily the child leaves the parent, how long before the child relaxes with you (which may be far too quickly with a disinhibited child with disrupted attachments or severe ADHD), how they approach a toy or game, including how long and effectively they concentrate. What is the content of the play and what themes appear? Are these areas typical ones for the developmental stage and this child's life experience, or more unusual? Some children's difficulties, assessed from the history, can quickly be confirmed in even a brief unstructured play assessment: for example, pervasive develop-mental difficulties such as autism are clearly evidenced by distorted social communication, avoidance of eye contact, and unusual play, perhaps an interest only in spinning the wheels of a toy car. Similarly, hyperactive children are often active, distractible and impulsive in the play session, confirming parental reports, and severely antisocial children might display persistently violent themes in aggressive play. It remains useful to spend time alone with them to see how they relate to an interested stranger, and to review coexisting problems and make a rough assessment of cognitive capacity.

Middle childhood

In this age group, it is a matter of judgement whether to open the individual interview by talking about 'the problems', to start with conversation about other topics, or to begin with play rather than talk for the 'warming-up' phase. Whichever is chosen, the principles of communication (summarised in Box 7.3) with young people are followed – there are distinct differences from interaction with an adult. Simple, clear questions (probably closed) are used, asking about one topic at a time and using comprehensible language. The grammatical structure must be simple and take into account the child's age and developmental level, and the family's verbal and psychological sophistication. It is important for children that one's non-verbal communication and facial expressions are warm and sympathetic: they should give very clear signals of interest and acceptance, more overt signals than used with adults, and congruent with what is being said.

The kind of broad, open questions that might be suitable for adults ('Tell me about the problem...') will cause anxiety in young people. Children will not tell you if they do not understand what you have asked: they may simply give the answer they think is wanted. With pre-adolescents, it is better to begin with direct, closed enquiries about neutral and reassuring topics, covering areas from the earlier part of the interview: perhaps family members, pets or the journey to the appointment. If strong views and emotions have already been expressed, a reassuring comment about this will acknowledge any distress and be supportive ('You've been having a very tough time at school, I think?'). Remember when asking questions about thoughts and feelings that one must be careful always to tailor one's language to the child's level of understanding and to check you have been understood. Emotional difficulties, in general, have a detrimental effect on previously achieved levels of emotional maturity. A further key issue is to be clear about whether you are speaking about recent or more remote feelings and experiences. Children's concepts of time are strongly affected by development, so asking about 'when' or 'how often' may not produce accurate information unless there is corroboration.

For many children, it will be possible, either in direct interaction or by talking alongside play, to move on to talk about the problem areas. Toys to engage children aged 5–12 years need not be sophisticated. Clean paper, good-quality felt-tip pens, a doll's house, farmyard and some construction materials will suffice. It is useful to have access to some toys that involve either greater dexterity (e.g. a marble run) or more interaction. (These toys may be different from those in the waiting room, which might include magazines or computer games, which are less helpful for examining interaction.) Talking about the problem is more likely to be successful for problems such as fears and anxieties. It is likely to be difficult when it is something like soiling that is denied by the child, and perhaps impossible with a severely autistic child, when one can simply offer an opportunity for interaction where one observes the child's functioning.

Box 7.3 Principles of communicating with children

This advice is given for interviews with young children, and the change to a more 'adult' style occurs gradually through adolescence, depending on the young person, their level of emotional distress, their cognitive capacity, and family and social factors. It is always best to start with simple language; a common mistake is assuming greater sophistication than exists. Simple language need not be patronising.

Your affect
- Warm and friendly – clearer signals of interest than usual with adults. Neutral or serious, not disapproving, about accounts of 'undesired' behaviours.

Warming up
- Simple, closed questions, e.g. on family, school, pets – use the family's vocabulary if possible.

Throughout
- Simple language and grammar, easy vocabulary, short words.
- Single questions.
- No subsidiary clauses or double questions.
- If no response, ask questions using simpler vocabulary or grammatical construction.
- Always check you have been understood by summarising and reflecting back.

Describing episodes or events
- Use direct, open enquiries for a range of behaviours – with examples ('I wanted to talk to you about what's been happening at school/when you've been playing out/at home…').
- After a broad review of the area concerned, with open questions, change to simple, closed enquiries to define exactly what is being described. For example, if parents describe the child setting fires, and the child acknowledges this, ask about the detail of the last time this happened. 'When exactly?' (last week, yesterday, in the holidays – *see time concepts section below*). 'Where?' (at home, in the park). 'Who with?' 'Can you tell me all about that day?'
- Once it is understood that you are really interested in the detail of the events, you will be able to go back over the account to examine feelings, fears, worries and sense of responsibility, to build up a picture of both risk and development of conscience.
- Leading questions about someone else may have a place in developing a more fluent conversation about a difficult area. 'I knew a boy once who ran away… He wanted to… Have you ever done something/felt like that?'

Asking about emotions at any age
- Open questions, one at a time. Remember that the child probably cannot distinguish between 'think' and 'feel'. If there is no clear response to an open question about feelings, offer a closed question for a yes/no answer. 'Did you feel angry/upset/sad?'
- If there is still no response, consider offering pictures of faces, or illustrations from books, to see if the child can identify someone experiencing a similar emotion.

Cont'd

Box 7.3 *Cont'd*

- Don't use more complex words for emotions until you are sure you have been understood. Check with another open question.
- To explore intensity of feelings, introduce scaling using a range of 4–6 points, or more for older children (4 or top = 'the most frightened I've ever been'; 3 or next = 'very frightened'; 2 = 'a bit frightened'; 1 = 'not frightened at all'). Make comparison with, for example, how frightened the child was about coming to the clinic.

Time concepts

- Children's sense of time – how long symptoms lasted, how long ago or how long for – is very inaccurate (as for many adults). Use parents and other informants for details of timing and frequency.
- Children can give measures of intensity for recent events, but be clear exactly what you are asking about. 'When you were frightened on that day? How bad was it?'

Don't...

- ask leading questions such as 'You felt angry about that, didn't you?'. If the the child looks miserable, try a more open approach: 'Were you upset?' or if the child looks sullen, 'Were you angry?'

If a discussion about the problem area, or about the child's thoughts and feelings, is possible, then the assessment of mental state may be as comprehensive as with an adolescent or adult, and it is now evident that many of the phenomena are very similar, for example in depression. However, although the content is the same, language and concepts require careful adjustment. For example, it is difficult to ask children about whether they feel guilty or have poor concentration and be confident of an accurate answer. When asking about suicidal thoughts or feelings, one may often need to ask about the general area of difficult, angry and upset feelings first. Then ask for more specific examples. Have they felt like hurting themselves? Or running away (which may have many explanations, but is a marker of distress, and possibly a primitive, quasi-suicidal behaviour)? Or dying? If verbal explanations falter, it may be helpful to proffer someone else's thoughts. 'One boy I saw said he felt like running away when... Have you ever felt like that?'

With a pre-adolescent child, 15–20 minutes are usually sufficient for an initial interview. This can be rounded off by thanking the child for telling you about him/herself, summarising what you think you have understood and reminding the child what you will say to the parents.

Adolescents

As with younger children, the approach to an individual interview with an adolescent must be interested and sympathetic, encouraging of openness, demonstrating concern, and explaining and acknowledging

115

any worries about the appointment. The 'communication principles' still apply. A detailed understanding of adolescents' views of their problems is essential. It must be clear you do not necessarily expect their views to be the same as their parents'. Enquiries cover the broad areas of emotions and behaviour, including a clear idea of the adol-escent's views on any difficulties at school or elsewhere – do not assume that you know what he or she is thinking and feeling. If the individual's non-verbal communication is clear, but expression is difficult, it is worth reflecting what you see: 'You look quite upset/angry/sad...'. An interested but also neutral approach allows explor-ation of activities that are frowned upon or illegal, and where the young person may be taking risks. It is important to ask directly not only about moods, feelings, suicidality and other aspects of mental state, for example hallucinations, but also about sexual behaviour, and nicotine, alcohol and other substance use. Common sense should be applied in using this advice: it is unlikely to be appropriate to ask detailed questions about injected drug use of a shy and overprotected school refuser who has not left home for weeks. After a careful review of the adolescent's symptoms or difficulties, lead into enquiries about friendships (or lack of, or change in these), about school and how it is viewed, and a review of the adolescent's life in general.

Physical examination

It is not routine to carry out a full physical examination of a child during an initial psychiatric assessment, but it should always be considered. This means the decision about examination needs to be made actively on each occasion, and depends on the history, type of problem and the clinic setting. The psychiatrist should be competent in assessing basic physical and neurological signs. It is necessary to be confident in examination skills and in performing a basic neurological examination, including coordination. Help (and further training) should be sought from paediatric colleagues to improve skills and confidence in this area if previous experience is limited. Facilities for such an examination should be available (including a chaperone if necessary) to include as a minimum the examination of all body systems and facilities, to record and plot height, weight, head circumference and blood pressure. Permission to carry out the examination should be obtained from both child and parent, and both should be given an explanation, in appropriate language, of the nature and purpose of the examination. The findings should be fed back to both parent and child, and in language appropriate to each with an explanation about further investigations. Basic general paediatric (e.g. Campbell & McIntosh, 1992) or paediatric neurology (Newton, 1995) textbooks provide information on which practical experience is built.

Brief neurodevelopmental assessment

A brief neurodevelopmental assessment can be completed quite quickly in the course of an initial assessment. Observation of the child's skill in dressing and undressing may alert one to the need for a neurological examination later by an appropriately skilled person. Note the child's hand preference, the degree of clumsiness, lack of coordination or unsteadiness; look carefully for asymmetrical physical development, unusual facial appearance and any skin blemish (pigmented or depigmented patches, naevi, unusual nails or hair texture, and bruising or scars).

Children generally find it entertaining to perform for 'Fog testing' (Fog & Fog, 1963) (walking in a straight line, heel-toe walking, and walking on tiptoes, on heels, and on the outer edge of the foot); asymmetry in and extent of overflow movements are relatively easily seen. Concentrating on the activities will display neurodevelopmental immaturity or asymmetry, which may require further physiotherapy, occupational therapy or neurological assessment. Coordination of hands and arms can be assessed by asking to see the child's handwriting, drawing and copying of figures; then with the child standing, eyes shut, arms outstretched and watch for tremor or drifting of one arm. This may be followed by 'finger to nose' testing (for dysdiodochokinesis) with eyes still closed. Rapid finger-thumb opposition and tapping the back of the opposite hand complete a brief examination.

Findings in the history or examination may prompt a request for more expert paediatric (or paediatric neurological) assessment. Details are beyond the scope of this chapter, but some special investigations are quite common. Neurological and neuropsychiatric disorders may require investigation by electroencephalography, brain scans and blood investigations of drug levels. Genetic and chromosomal investigations may be required where there is developmental delay, a suspicion of a disintegrative condition, a significantly related condition in the family pedigree, or the child's appearance is unusual. There may be a local protocol for investigation of children with developmental delay, and discussions with a paediatric colleague with interest or responsibility for children with genetic or learning disorders is useful – or a joint appointment perhaps. A joint appointment with a paediatrician may be required if there are unresolved issues about investigations or findings in an adolescent with a somatising presentation or fatigue.

Information from others

Although it is normal to have information from parents or carers as well as from the young person, it may also be useful to know about the perspectives of others. A non-custodial parent or grandparents may also offer a useful perspective. For the assessment of some conditions, such

117

as hyperkinesis, the extent to which the symptoms are pervasive is essential diagnostic information. It is common to need more information about relevant physical health issues, school attainments, performance and behaviours, before firm conclusions are drawn. There may be more assessments to be considered, including standardised schedules such as the ADOS (autism). At this point it may be useful to gain permission to contact the school and other agencies involved, and usually a consent form for these contacts is signed. A school visit may be appropriate. Schools (with parental consent) will contribute details of a child's behaviour, psychological and social functioning, as well as their educational potential and attainment. The school will report on any assessments that have been made – numeracy, literacy, standardised assessment tests – and provide a copy of any educational statement (although parents have their own copy). Teachers will have a different perspective on a child's peer relationships from that which may be presented by parents and the child themselves. Depending on the problem, it may be useful to ask teachers to complete a standard questionnaire, for example those of Conners (1997) for ADHD.

Other assessments

Children and adolescents' cognitive ability is a key part of their functioning, and may require more formal assessment than the superficial impression of an interview. The school's report has already been mentioned. A formal assessment may have already been undertaken by an educational psychologist. The indication for more formal assessment by a clinical psychologist should be discussed with the psychologist to clarify whether, and by whom, this should be undertaken. Indications vary with the problem, resources and setting, but may be because of expertise in particular areas (for example, to explore specific neurocognitive deficits), and to identify children who are performing beyond their potential as well as below it.

Although indications for psychometric assessment may have been evident at the referral stage, the initial history and examination is often the point where it is clear that this should be considered, because of the suggestion of inconsistencies in the child's cognitive performance or the possibility of a learning disability. The three most common indications in ordinary practice are when:

1. Developmental delay, either specific or generalised, is suspected in young children who have not been assessed before. (The local community paediatrician will probably have a part to play here, and may undertake some assessments.) If there seems to be a specific language delay, however, or other issues such as unusual language expression, it would be reasonable to ask a speech and language therapist for an assessment.

2. There are discrepancies in educational attainment between the child's apparent potential and achievement, including the possibility of specific learning disorders. These discrepancies may operate in either direction; that is to say, low attainment may be because the child's potential is much less than expected or achievements are greater than expected. If the difficulties are likely to result in 'statementing' procedures under the Education Act 1981, or in the need for remedial intervention, any testing should be done in active collaboration with psychologists responsible for education provision.

3. Neuropsychiatric deficits are suspected; that is, there are large discrepancies between verbal and performance skills, and problems with memory, visuospatial ability, and speed in psychomotor tasks. When a deteriorating condition is under consideration, serial testing may be required. Special circumstances, for example to identify specific deficits following head injury or performance after psychiatric illness, may justify assessment.

Even when the child's primary difficulty is evident (e.g. severe attention deficit) it can be useful to see what can be achieved under optimal conditions.

In any of these circumstances, the report of the child's behaviour in the test situation is a useful addition to test results. The psychologist's experience in how children approach tests parallels the psychiatrist's in judging how children respond to an interview. The degree of organisation, concentration and anxiety about tests, the extent of fear of failure, the type of problem-solving approach and response to difficult items all increase the understanding of the child's functioning and difficulties. Sergeant & Taylor (2002) provide a substantial review of the psychological assessment and testing of children. The more commonly used basic cognitive tests at different ages are listed in Box 7.4.

Formulation

Formulation of child and adolescent mental health problems, and reaching a decision about possible interventions, involves a synthesis of information from several domains of the child's functioning, with a range of relevant psychosocial and contextual issues. The initial interview must have ranged sufficiently widely, and in adequate depth, to allow this initial conceptualisation to be made securely. A preliminary understanding should be reached by the end of the first assessment, so that this can be shared with the young person and their family, and provide ample opportunity for questions from all parties.

It is conventional to organise the psychiatrist's own thoughts under the headings of the ICD–10 multi-axial classification (see Box 7.2),

Box 7.4   Commonly used basic cognitive tests

British Ability Scales – Revised, 2.5–17 years (Elliott, 1996)
Standardised on a British population, the scales were designed to assess a broader range of competencies than just IQ. Sub-scales are speed, reasoning, spatial imaging, perceptual matching, short-term memory, retrieval and application of knowledge. For each, a percentile rank is given and an overall IQ calculated.

Griffiths Mental Development Scales (revised), 0–8 years (Griffiths, 1996)
This test has four sub-scales: locomotor, personal/social, hearing/speech, and hand/eye coordination. It yields a quotient for each sub-scale and a general quotient which has a mean of 100 and a standard deviation of 12. It has been standardised on a British population and is used often by medical personnel with appropriate training, for example community paediatricians and child psychiatrists working with young children and those with learning disabilities. It is used less commonly in the upper age range, except in those with learning disabilities.

Wechsler Intelligence Scale for Children (WISC–IV), 6–17 years (Wechsler, 2003)
Verbal and performance sub-scales yield a verbal, performance, and full-scale IQ; there is a short form of four sub-tests. Probably still the most commonly used intelligence test, it is lengthy and was standardised on an American sample, although a British version of the test is normally used in the UK. It is helpful as a first-line neuropsychiatric assessment to indicate the need for more specific tests.

Wechsler Objective Reading Dimensions (WORD) (Wechsler, 1992)
This tests reading accuracy, comprehension and spelling, giving age scores.

Wechsler Objective Numerical Dimensions (WOND) (Wechsler, 1996)
This tests a child's progress in acquiring fundamental numeracy skills.

although other conceptual and explanatory frameworks (psychodynamic, systemic) will often be incorporated in thinking, explanation and deciding how to intervene. The multi-axial system most commonly used in the UK conceptualises disorders using ICD–10 categories for the first axis – any psychiatric disorder within the child – although DSM–IV categories are also sometimes used for this axis. The next three axes also code 'within child' conditions – specific (Axis II) and generalised (Axis III) learning difficulties (using defined categories) and concurrent physical health conditions (Axis IV), which also includes descriptions of specific types of self-harm – the codes allow one to distinguish poisoning with different types of medication, for example, and 'maltreatment syndromes'. Axis V uses a set of broad categories to describe psychosocial situations. Many clinicians now supplement these axes by a marker of severity, such as the Global

Assessment of Severity, Child version (CGAS; Schaffer *et al*, 1983) or a global measure of functioning, such as the Health of the Nation Outcome Scales for Children and Adolescents (HoNOSCA; Gowers *et al*, 1999a,b). Chapter 5 contains a fuller discussion of comparative diagnostic classifications and their use.

The feedback to the family is usually a succinct summary of the problems and how these have been conceptualised by the interviewer. This will include a psychiatric diagnostic label if relevant, and an explanation of what this label or description means to the psychiatrist in terms of intervention or treatment. Options for further assessment and treatment may then be sketched out. The family should know what will happen next, which clearly depends on the nature and severity of the psychiatric issues, and how further appointments will be initiated. It may be reassuring to explain who will receive a copy of any letter (it is envisaged in the NHS plan that patients will in future receive copies of correspondence). If treatment is to begin immediately, for example with medication or an admission, this will require considerably more explanation and discussion time, perhaps taking the interview to 2 hours or more in length – by which time families are likely to be tired and slow to absorb new information. If there are small or very active children present, it might be better to meet again to go into such issues in detail when all are fresh. The confidence with which this formulation is reached and delivered will depend on many issues, including the level of experience of the interviewer, and whether there has been an opportunity to punctuate the assessment with discussions with a senior colleague.

Notes from the assessment will normally be completed both during and after the process – using standardised headings and considering legibility, any abbreviations, and the evidence needed for any conclusions and treatment plan. This is the basis for the letter, and the foundation for future plans.

Vignette 1 – Kyle: ADHD

Kyle is a 7-year-old referred by his general practitioner; the referral letter explains that the school's special educational needs coordinator (SENCO) has encouraged Kyle's mother to seek help. Kyle is the eldest of three children from a single-parent family.

Kyle's mother says she 'thinks he has ADHD'. At home his behaviour is very difficult. He never concentrates on anything, is aggressive to his younger sister and his mother, and is the main reason that his mother's partner decided to leave. Kyle has been excluded from school on a couple of occasions because of his behaviour and the SENCO has requested help from specialist educational services, who have also assessed Kyle and support his referral as they think his concentration is very poor. Kyle is active and distractible in the initial conjoint part of the appointment, smashing up toys and rushing around the room, pinching and pushing his sister.

Key points to consider in this assessment

- The history needs to take into account biological, social, developmental and temperamental factors.
- Extra resources will be needed to supervise Kyle and his sister, if you need to talk to Kyle's mother alone.
- Information will be required from the school and the behaviour support services.
- Kyle's interactions with you when alone will enable assessment of his capacity to relate, focus his attention and respect boundaries. It is unlikely to make a difference to the diagnosis, but will help with assessment of attachment issues and understanding the extent of behavioural difficulties and how best to address them.
- His mother's management of him in the appointment is an example of their interactions and will be important in deciding the sort of help she might need.

Vignette 2 – Angela

Angela is a 13-year-old referred by the school nurse with the general practitioner's agreement. Angela came to the attention of the school nurse because she was found to be cutting her arms and stomach with glass and razors: school friends were concerned. She also admitted to the nurse having taken several small overdoses of paracetamol (which she has not reported otherwise). Angela comes to the appointment with both her parents, although they are divorced and live separately. Angela is quiet with no eye contact and is very reluctant to speak in the initial conjoint part of the interview. She looks both sad and annoyed as her parents describe her increasingly difficult behaviour over the past two or three years, with withdrawal, moodiness, 'unsuitable' friends and some alcohol use. They think she made herself sick on one occasion. The parents' relationship is obviously still acrimonious and they argue vehemently in the room.

Key points to consider in this assessment

- Will you see Angela before you take the history from her parents, or do you need to hear from them first?
- Do you need to separate the parents to enable them to concentrate on Angela rather than criticisms of each other?
- It transpires that Angela has been seeing the school counsellor. Although her parents are happy for you to contact this person, Angela does not want you to speak to him. What will you do?
- When you see Angela on her own, after initial reluctance she is easily engaged. She feels very lonely and unloved, and tells you about extensive arguments. She has many symptoms of depression, has some suicidal intent and has a collection of tablets; how much of this do you need to share with her parents?
- Do you need to discuss the level of risk with a senior person during the appointment?

References

Ambrosini, P. J. (2000) Historical development and present status of the schedule for affective disorders and schizophrenia for school-age children (K–SADS). *Journal of the American Academy of Child and Adolescent Psychiatry*, **39**, 49–58.

Campbell, A. G. M. & McIntosh, N. (1992) *Forfar & Arneil's Textbook of Pediatrics*. Edinburgh: Churchill Livingstone.

Conners, C. K. (1997) *Conners' Rating Scales Revised: Instruments for Use with Children and Adolescents*. North Tonawanda, NY: Multi-Health Systems.

Elliott, C. D. (1996) *British Ability Scales: BAS–II* (2nd edn). Windsor, Berks: NFER-Nelson.

Fog, E. & Fog, M. (1963) Cerebral inhibition examined by associated movements. In *Minimal Cerebral Dysfunction. Papers from the International Study Group held at Oxford, September 1962* (eds R. C. Mackeith & M. Bax). London: National Spastics Society Medical Education and Information Unit/William Heinemann.

Goodman, R. (1997) The Strength and Difficulties Questionnaire: a research note. *Journal of Child Psychology and Psychiatry*, **38**, 581–586.

Gowers, S. G., Harrington, R., Whitton, A., *et al* (1999*a*) A brief scale for measuring the outcomes of emotional and behavioural disorders in children: HoNOSCA. *British Journal of Psychiatry*, **174**, 413–416.

Gowers, S. G., Harrington, R., Whitton, A., *et al* (1999*b*) Health of the Nation Outcome Scales for Children and Adolescents (HoNOSCA). Glossary for HoNOSCA Score Sheet. *British Journal of Psychiatry*, **174**, 428–431.

Griffiths, R. (1996) *The Griffiths Mental Developmental Scales* (revised by M. Huntley). High Wycombe, UK: The Test Agency.

Harris, D. B. (1963) *Children's Drawings as Measures of Intellectual Maturity: A Revision and Extension of the Goodenough Draw-a-man Test*. New York: Harcourt, Brace & World.

Jones, D. P. H. (2003) *Communicating with Vulnerable Children: A Guide for Practitioners*. London: Gaskell.

Newton, R. W. (ed.) (1995) *Color Atlas of Pediatric Neurology*. London: Mosby-Wolfe.

Schaffer, D., Gould, M. S., Brasic, J., *et al* (1983) A children's global assessment scale (CGAS). *Archives of General Psychiatry*, **40**, 1228–1231.

Schaffer, D., Fisher, P., Lucas, C. P., *et al* (2000) NIMH Diagnostic Interview Schedule for Children version IV (NIMH DISC–IV): description, differences from previous versions, and reliability of some common diagnoses. *Journal of the American Academy of Child and Adolescent Psychiatry*, **39**, 28–38.

Sergeant, J. & Taylor, E (2002) Psychological testing and observation. In *Child and Adolescent Psychiatry* (2nd edn) (eds M. Rutter & E. Taylor), pp. 97–102. Oxford: Blackwell.

Sheridan, M. D. (1980) *From Birth to Five Years: Children's Developmental Progress*. Windsor: NFER-Nelson.

Wechsler, D. (1992) *Wechsler Objective Reading Dimensions (WORD)*. London: Psychological Corporation.

Wechsler, D. (1996) *Wechsler Objective Numerical Dimensions (WOND)*. London: Psychological Corporation.

Wechsler, D. (2003) *Manual for the Wechsler Intelligence Scale for Children* (4th edn). London: Psychological Corporation.

World Health Organization (1996) *Multi-axial Classification of Child and Adolescent Psychiatric Disorders*. Cambridge: Cambridge University Press.

CHAPTER 8

Developmental disorders

Paul Tiffin and Ann Le Couteur

Brain development and maturation are a complex and sensitive process. It is therefore of little surprise that developmental disorders are a common finding within the general population. Workers in child and adolescent mental health services (CAMHS) will frequently encounter children affected by a developmental disorder, either as the presenting problem or comorbid with emotional or behavioural disturbance. This comorbidity was first reported in the Isle of Wight study (Rutter *et al*, 1970). Among the 4% of 9- to 10-year-olds with a specific reading delay, a third also had a definite conduct disorder. These findings have been replicated in numerous studies. However, it is important to remember that there is no specificity for particular child and adolescent mental disorders.

The nosology of developmental disorders has been problematic and the validity of many of the syndromes has been questioned. Current classification systems are based on patterns of behavioural characteristics and developmental profile. It is likely that as our understanding increases, existing classification will be modified. This chapter focuses primarily on the presentation of pre-school and school-aged children. It does not deal with the needs of older adolescents and young adults (see Chapter 3 for a discussion of normal development).

The ICD–10 (World Health Organization, 1992) divides developmental disorders into specific disorders and pervasive disorders (Box 8.1). These disorders are characterised by a history of delay or deviant development identified in infancy or early childhood, an increased prevalence in males, and often a family history of similar or related disorders.

F80–83   Specific developmental disorders

The specific developmental disorders are of both theoretical and practical importance to those working in CAMHS, since children with specific developmental disorders show high rates of comorbidity with psychiatric disorders (Williams & McGee, 1994; Davison & Howlin, 1997). Further, increased prevalence of almost all specific developmental disorders has

---

Box 8.1 Disorders of psychological development[1] (ICD–10, World Health Organization, 1992)

Specific developmental disorders of speech and language
Specific speech articulation disorder
Expressive language disorder
Receptive language disorder
Acquired aphasia with epilepsy (Landau–Kleffner syndrome)
Other developmental unspecified disorders of speech and language

Specific developmental disorders of scholastic skills
Specific reading disorder
Specific spelling disorder
Specific disorder of arithmetical skills
Mixed disorder of scholastic skills

Specific developmental disorders of motor function

Pervasive developmental disorders
Childhood autism
Atypical autism
Rett syndrome
Other childhood disintegrative disorder
Overactive disorder associated with mental retardation and stereotyped movements
Asperger syndrome

1. This list omits some other and unspecified categories.

---

been found in children presenting with a psychiatric disorder (Rutter *et al*, 1970; Cohen *et al*, 1998; Blomquist, 2000).

The specific developmental disorders are differentiated from both the pervasive developmental disorders and learning disabilities by the presence of an overall standardised IQ above 70 (or non-verbal IQ above 70 for developmental disorders of speech and language). They are characterised by an impairment or delay in the development of functions that are strongly related to biological maturation of the central nervous system. Specific developmental disorders may affect language, visuo-spatial skills and/or motor coordination. The presence of organic or medical disorders, such as deafness, neurological conditions or in some cases a pervasive developmental disorder, may exclude the diagnosis.

In practice, children with one identified specific developmental disorder often have several areas of delayed skill (Manor *et al*, 2001).

F80 Specific developmental disorders of speech, language and communication

'Specific' language impairment is likely to be caused by a variety of underlying problems ranging from difficulties with auditory perception to deficits in conceptual development (Bishop, 1992). Bishop emphasised that the validity of language impairment as a specific and valid diagnostic category remains uncertain. Twins data suggest that specific language impairment is not genetically distinct from less specific disorders, where delayed language function occurs in conjunction with a low performance IQ (Bishop, 1994).

The ICD–10 classification system for specific developmental disorder of speech, language and communication relies solely on the pattern of deficits observed. There is a wide variation in the normal development of speech and language skills. To meet diagnostic criteria, there needs to be evidence of language delay of sufficient severity to be 'outside the limit of two standard deviations' but not secondary to a recognised neurological abnormality, mental retardation, significant environmental factors or structural abnormalities such as hearing loss, cleft palate or cerebral palsy. These disorders of speech, language and communication are often associated with academic, social, emotional and behaviour problems (Cantwell & Baker, 1991). In one study, for example, language impairment was detected in 64% of children aged 7–14 years referred to a psychiatry service. In 40% of these children the language impairment had never been suspected (Cohen *et al*, 1998).

F80.0 Specific speech articulation disorder

Specific speech articulation disorder is characterised by a lag in the child's ability to produce speech sounds competently in relation to the child's chronological age. Other language skills should fall within the normal range.

F80.1 Expressive language disorder

Expressive language disorder occurs when there is a significant delay in language production, although comprehension falls within the normal range. As a result vocalisations are generally impaired, although verbal fluency may be sparse, normal or even increased, depending on the precise deficit. There are often accompanying articulation difficulties (Rapin & Allen, 1983; Rapin, 1996). Children with expressive language disorder tend to use non-speech means to communicate, e.g. gestures, smiles and demonstration mime. Imagination and make-believe play skills should be relatively intact. The condition tends to improve with age, but often problems in organising discourse (such as relaying a story) persist (Rapin, 1996). It has been suggested that children with predominantly expressive language disorders should not receive therapy until after the age of 4 years because of the high rate of spontaneous improvement (Whitehurst & Fischel, 1994). However, affected children often experience difficulties in peer relationships, emotional disturbance and conduct problems. Inattention and overactivity are reported, particularly in school-aged children.

F80.2   Receptive language disorder

The young child who fails to respond to familiar names or follow simple instructions by the age of 2 years may have a delay in the ability to understand language, once a primary sensory impairment has been excluded. Children with receptive language deficits have difficulty in analysing and recognising the different sound components of spoken words (Worster-Drought & Allen, 1930).

There is usually some degree of accompanying expressive language difficulties and high rates of associated social-emotional behaviour problems. Affected children often benefit from being taught using visual methods of communication, such as computers and 'flash cards'. Autism and other pervasive developmental disorders should always be considered in individuals presenting at a young age with apparent receptive language delay.

F80.3   Acquired aphasia with epilepsy (Landau–Kleffner syndrome)

Acquired aphasia with epilepsy is a rare syndrome of unknown aetiology characterised by a previous period of normal language development until the onset of the disorder, usually at the age of 3–7 years. Expressive language skills are then lost but with a preservation of general intellectual function (Landau & Kleffner, 1957). The onset is accompanied by epileptic seizures in most cases, although in some only paroxysmal abnormalities on electroencephalography (EEG) will be apparent. Deterioration in language function tends to occur over days or weeks. The temporal association between the seizures and the loss of function is somewhat variable, with up to 2 years separating the two events either way.

In children presenting with a history of possible regression and epilepsy, assessment is required to exclude possible autistic-spectrum disorder. In a magnetoencephalography study investigating children with Landau–Kleffner syndrome and children with a history of autistic regression, 82% of the children with autism demonstrated epileptiform activity similar to that of those with Landau–Kleffner syndrome (Lewine et al, 1999).

Anticonvulsant treatment, sometimes in combination with high-dose corticosteroids, has been reported to be effective in treating seizure activity (Sikic et al, 2001) and has a more variable effect on the aphasia (Marescaux et al, 1990). Little is known about the long-term outcome in these children, but it is likely that most will have a persistent significant language deficit.

F80.8   Other developmental disorders of speech and language

Lisping (a tendency to pronounce 's' as 'th' sounds) is placed in this diagnostic category.

Stuttering (stammering) is classified within F98 of ICD–10 ('other behavioural and emotional disorders with onset usually occurring in childhood and adolescence'), although there is no established link with mental health problems.

F81   Specific developmental disorders of scholastic skills

Specific developmental disorders of scholastic skills, like specific developmental disorders of speech and language, are more common in boys, have high rates of comorbid disorders (e.g. attention-deficit hyperactivity disorder and conduct disorder) and are of unknown aetiology. It is likely to be a biological dysfunction rather than a consequence of early experience, brain trauma or disease. This diagnosis requires evidence of significant scholastic underachievement relative to the child's mental age, i.e. underachievement that is usually evident during the early years of schooling and is not explained by other individual external factors, such as educational experience. 'Dyslexia' is a popular term for impaired reading ability, but lacks a precise and universally accepted definition.

F81.0   Specific reading disorder

Reading difficulties (not due to inadequate education) are present in 4–5% of the population (Yule & Rutter, 1976). The relationship between conduct disorder, other child and adolescent mental health disorders and specific reading disorder is complex. Maughan (1995) suggested that early reading difficulties in boys – but not in girls – may serve as a 'gateway' to later conduct disorder, whereas poor reading ability developing at a later age in conduct-disordered children is secondary to disrupted schooling. Another study reported that 43.5% of children exhibiting 'pervasive hyperactivity' had a specific reading disorder, compared with 15.6% of children without hyperactivity (Goodman & Stevenson, 1989). Low self-esteem, poor peer relationships and problems with school adjustment are also common. Some individuals with specific reading disorder will also exhibit difficulties in spelling (Warnke, 1999).

F81.1   Specific spelling disorder

To diagnose an individual as having specific spelling disorder there must be significant difficulties with spelling while reading ability falls within the normal range. Difficulties include letter reversal and unusual spelling of even common words. One study demonstrated that the rate of specific spelling disorder in children with 'pervasive hyperactivity' was 43.5%, compared with 12.8% in non-hyperactive children (Goodman & Stevenson, 1989).

F81.2 Specific disorder of arithmetical skills

This is a specific impairment of arithmetic functions such as addition or multiplication (not secondary to learning disability or poor schooling). Around 3–6% of school children will exhibit significant difficulties with numeracy skills, and most also have problems with speech, language or reading delay (Padget, 1988; Shalev *et al*, 2000).

F82   Specific developmental disorder of motor function

This developmental disorder of fine and (usually) gross motor skills is due to impairment of coordination and motor planning. Other terms used include 'dyspraxia', 'clumsy child syndrome' and 'developmental coordination disorder'. There is no universally accepted definition of this term (Dewey, 1995).

Parents and carers of children with specific developmental disorder of motor function might give a history of delay in walking and other motor milestones. The child may be described as 'clumsy' or 'accident-prone'. Teachers may comment on poorly formed handwriting and untidy work. The child may be awkward in gait, and have difficulty with ball skills, drawing skills, completion of jigsaw puzzles, building models and so on.

The tendency for motor delay to accompany problems of attention and scholastic skills has led to the concept of a disorder of attention, motor control and perception ('DAMP'; see Blomquist, 2000).

F84   Pervasive developmental disorders

There are some important areas of overlap in the clinical pictures of pervasive developmental disorders and specific developmental disorders that may be of aetiological significance. For example, disorders of language skills and motor control are common in individuals with a pervasive developmental disorder and normal IQ (Gilchrist *et al*, 2001; Green *et al*, 2002). There may be continuities and discontinuities in adult outcome (see Chapters 3 and 4).

Relatives of individuals who have a specific developmental disability sometimes manifest a range of other neurodevelopmental problems (Elbert & Seale, 1988).

Pervasive developmental disorders are characterised by the triad of impairment in reciprocal social interactions, communication and a restricted, often stereotyped, repetitive repertoire of non-adaptive interests and activities (World Health Organization, 1992). Onset is usually in infancy or early childhood, although, as in childhood disintegrative disorder, a period of normal development may occur prior to regression or loss of skills. Although 'pervasive developmental disorder' is the term used in ICD–10, 'autistic-spectrum disorder' is increasingly used by professionals, families and voluntary agencies. This 'autistic spectrum' spans a range of disorders from the severely learning-disabled and handicapped child with autism, to the academically able child with impaired social skills.

There is a strong association between autism and learning disability (ICD–10 'mental retardation'). Seventeen per cent of individuals with learning disabilities have a diagnosis of autism and 80% of people with narrowly defined autism have a full-scale IQ below 70 (Deb & Prasad, 1994). Most individuals with pervasive developmental disorders are likely to have an uneven cognitive profile, with areas of significant cognitive deficit and some areas of relative strength. A frequently reported profile is one of relative strength in performance IQ compared with verbal IQ (Rumsey & Hamburger, 1990). Indeed, it has been reported (Rimland, 1978) that 10% of individuals with autism have a special skill, out of keeping with their overall functioning ('savantism').

Pervasive developmental disorders and autistic-spectrum disorders affect about 60 children per 10 000 under 8 years of age; between 10 and 30 children per 10 000 have more narrowly defined autism (Baird *et al*, 2000*a*; Chakrabarti & Fombonne, 2001). These reported rates have increased over recent years (Fombonne, 2001). It is likely that at least part of the explanation lies in the broadening of diagnostic concept and a growing awareness and recognition of autistic-spectrum disorders. Around 3–4 times as many males as females are diagnosed with autistic-spectrum disorders, although this gender difference diminishes with increasing level of global intellectual disability (Volkmar *et al*, 1993).

Presentation of the autistic-spectrum disorders

It is important that all child health professionals have an awareness of autistic-spectrum disorder and a clear picture of this group of disorders so that early concerns can lead to a multidisciplinary assessment of need and an appropriate family care plan. The diagnosis relies heavily on a detailed developmental history as well as specific observations and assessments. There are three key aspects of development and behaviour, but not all children show all behaviours.

Communication

Language delay is usual, with around half of those with a diagnosis of autism never achieving useful speech (Prizant, 1983). Children who do develop speech have difficulties with the social use of language (conversation) and speech abnormalities, such as stereotyped phrases or pronoun reversal. There are also likely to be deficits in aspects of non-verbal communication, such as reduced gesture and pointing to express interest (Stone *et al*, 1997).

Deficits in imitation, social play (peek-a-boo or hide-and-seek) and imaginative play also occur (Lewis & Boucher, 1995).

Social interaction

Deficits in reciprocal (two-way) social interaction are a core feature of autistic-spectrum disorder (Wing & Gould, 1979). Affected infants and young children may not respond in an expected manner to comfort or physical contact with the caregiver. Social use of smiling and other facial expressions may not develop, or may appear inappropriate or incongruous. Young children may not react to the sound of their carer's voice and it may be difficult to catch their attention.

With increasing age, the social deficits may become more obvious – a child who lacks interest in other children can play successfully alongside other children (parallel play), but will experience problems as the social expectations for shared play become more complex. Children with autistic-spectrum disorders often become isolated, are at risk of being bullied and lack the social skills to develop successful friendships.

Restricted, repetitive behaviours and interests

The ICD–10 focuses on four behavioural areas for a diagnosis of pervasive developmental disorder/autistic-spectrum disorder:

(a) encompassing preoccupation with one or more circumscribed interests;
(b) compulsive and rigid adherence to routines and rituals;
(c) stereotyped and repetitive motor mannerisms;
(d) preoccupations with 'part-objects' or 'non-functional' qualities of play materials (such as texture or smell).

The form these behaviours take and their level of sophistication will depend in part on the overall intellectual function of the child. However, even able individuals can exhibit simple stereotyped movements (Turner, 1999; Gilchrist et al, 2001).

Interests are often expressed in inanimate or mechanical objects or there is a circumscribed interest, such as in train timetables. The interests often have an intense, concrete quality that severely limits the social opportunity for the child.

Autistic individuals are typically inflexible. Change can be very unsettling, resulting in anything from mild anxiety to catastrophic outbursts. Although obvious parallels with obsessive–compulsive disorder have been drawn, there are key qualitative differences in the phenomenology of the rituals and behaviours seen in both conditions (McDougle et al, 1995).

Repetitive movements seen in autism can include characteristic hand and finger mannerisms, repetitive manipulation of objects, repeated self-injury, repetitive vocalisations and even syncope (fainting)

131

due to respiratory stereotypy (Gastaut *et al*, 1987). Repetitive movements can be disabling, and, in the case of self-injury, may be the most pressing clinical problem presented.

A preoccupation with 'part objects' and/or non-functional qualities of play material would include a child who turns a toy car upside down and repeatedly spins its wheels or who sits and flaps the pages of a book, rather than using the objects as intended. Many children will also show at least one non-specific, unusual sensory response, such as a startle reflex to anticipated skin contact (O'Neill & Jones, 1997; Baranek, 1999).

F84.0   Childhood autism

Since Kanner's original description (Kanner, 1943), a diagnostic consensus has emerged for the diagnosis of narrowly defined autism and standardised interviews and observation schedules have been developed (Lord *et al* 1994, 2000; Leekam *et al*, 2002; Le Couteur *et al*, 2003).

Twin and family studies have provided support for the validity of autism and highlight the importance of genetic factors. It is likely that the phenotype results from a moderate number of genes acting together. The British twin study estimated broad heritability at 91–93%, with a concordance rate of 69% in monozygotic twins and around 5% in dizygotic twins (Bailey *et al*, 1995). This genetic liability almost certainly extends to a broader phenotype characterised by similar, but milder, deficits than those seen in autism (Le Couteur *et al*, 1996; Bailey *et al*, 1998). More recent genetic studies of autism link the autistic phenotype to susceptibility loci on at least four separate chromosomes, including 7q and 2q (Monaco & Bailey, 2001). Further work is under way to replicate these findings and identify candidate genes (see Chapter 4).

Most parents of autistic children suspected problems in the months leading up to the child's second birthday. A quarter to a third report loss of speech and/or play and social skills in early childhood.

Despite the pioneering work of O'Connor & Hermelin (1971), uncertainty remains about whether one primary deficit could account for all the features associated with the autistic phenotype. Disorders of mentalising skills (a lack of the so-called 'theory of mind'; Baron-Cohen, 1993), the lack of an ability to use context in executive planning (Klinger & Renner, 2000), weak central coherence and facial processing deficits have all been implicated either individually or in combination as possible psychological mechanisms underlying autistic-spectrum disorders (Happe & Frith, 1996).

Like most medical conditions, autism and autistic-spectrum disorder are likely to be genetically heterogeneous. A number of individuals with autism have an increased head circumference (Woodhouse *et al*, 1996). This finding may be a familial feature. Approximately 10–15% of cases of autism are associated with currently identifiable medical disorders (Rutter *et al*, 1994; Barton & Volkmar, 1998). This association is more marked in individuals with a somewhat atypical clinical picture and more severe learning disability (Fombonne *et al*, 1999). Around 20% of individuals with tuberous sclerosis will have autism (Baker *et al*, 1998). A wide range of chromosomal abnormalities have been associated with autistic-spectrum disorder (Gillberg, 1998). The most commonly reported is on chromosome 15: affected individuals have autistic-spectrum disorder, severe mental retardation and seizures. The fragile-X anomaly occurs in approximately 4% of individuals with autism (Bailey *et al*, 2001). Further evidence of the organic basis of autism is the high prevalence of seizures in the disorder; at least a third of individuals with autism will develop epilepsy. There are two peaks in age of onset of seizures: early childhood, and adolescence/early adulthood.

Post-mortem studies, mainly with severely affected individuals, have reported abnormalities in the cerebellum and structures deep in the cerebral cortex together with changes in cell density and brain volume. This work needs replication (Pierce & Courchesne, 2001). There has been recent interest in physiological abnormalities affecting the gastrointestinal tract and the immune system (Wakefield *et al*, 1998; Torrente *et al*, 2002). Much media coverage has been given to the proposed link between the combined measles, mumps and rubella (MMR) vaccination, bowel disorders and autism (Wakefield *et al*, 1998). Current epidemiological evidence does not support this proposed link (Ashraf, 2001; Medical Research Council, 2001). Casein- and gluten-free diets have been tried, with some reports of improvement, for both autistic and bowel symptoms. To date, no properly controlled study has been published. The most consistent finding is the non-specific one of raised levels of blood serotonin (5-hydroxytryptamine, 5-HT), particularly in pre-pubertal individuals (Anderson *et al*, 1987; McBride *et al*, 1998); this has also been reported in other neuropsychiatric disorders.

F84.5   Asperger syndrome

Although Asperger drew attention to what he called 'autistic psychopathy' in a group of children in 1944, similar case reports date from earlier in the 20th century (Wolff, 1996). Wing's seminal paper was published in 1981 (Wing, 1981), but it is only in ICD–10 and DSM–IV (World Health Organization, 1992; American Psychiatric Association, 1994) that Asperger syndrome is separately defined. The nosological validity of Asperger syndrome remains uncertain (Szatmari, 2000; Volkmar *et al*, 2000; Gilchrist *et al*, 2001). The patterns of neuropsychological deficits yield conflicting results (Ozonoff *et al*, 1991).

For an ICD–10 diagnosis of Asperger syndrome, individuals need to show abnormalities that are qualitatively similar to those seen in autism, but to a less extreme extent. There should be no clinically significant general delay in language or cognitive development. Self-help skills, curiosity regarding the environment and adaptive behaviour should fall within the normal range during the first 3 years.

With the increasing recognition of a spectrum of autistic disorders, there is inevitably a diagnostic debate about the current subgroups. However, it is important to note that individuals with pervasive developmental disorder/autistic-spectrum disorder are much more common than individuals with narrowly defined autism (Fombonne, 1999).

The diagnosis of F84.1, 'atypical autism', can be applied when onset is after the age of 3 years and/or there are insufficient observable deficits in the key areas for a diagnosis of childhood autism. This category may be most applicable in cases of profound learning disability or severe receptive language disorder. Children with milder or atypical presentations of autistic symptoms can also be categorised as F84.8 (other pervasive developmental disorders) and F84.9 (pervasive developmental disorder, unspecified).

F84.2   Rett syndrome

Rett syndrome is an X-linked, dominant progressive neurodevelopmental disorder that affects girls almost exclusively. It is characterised by normal development in the first year or two of life, followed by loss of skills gained, deceleration in head growth, characteristic midline hand-wringing movements and trunk ataxia. Affected individuals become profoundly learning disabled, although some mild improvement in function is sometimes seen in late childhood. Complications include contractures and kyphoscoliosis, due to the abnormal posture and immobility (Hagberg, 1993). Mutations in the *MECP2* gene on the X-chromosome, responsible for DNA methylation, have recently been described in 65–80% of typical cases and have also been found in male relatives with profound mental retardation (Orrico *et al*, 2000; Armstrong, 2001).

F84.3   Other childhood disintegrative disorder

This category is reserved for children who exhibit a normal developmental pattern until the age of at least 2 years before losing acquired skills such as language ability, bladder control and social development (Volkmar & Rutter, 1995). The final picture may be similar to that of childhood autism. In most cases the aetiology is unknown, although some have been due to cerebral lipoidoses or leukodystrophy. Heller's syndrome is included in this category. It is a rare and poorly understood condition in which an encephalopathy is postulated to be the cause of the regression observed (Corbett *et al*, 1977).

Case example 1

Stuart, aged 4 years, was born at term by normal delivery. He was described as a very placid, easy baby, who did not cry and was a slow eater.

His parents became concerned when he was approximately 2 years old because he was not developing speech and showed no interest in play. At 4 years, his non-verbal cognitive skills were within the average range but he showed marked delay in language development.

Motor development was within normal limits. As a baby he made no communicative sounds, but enjoyed being cuddled and sitting on his parents' lap. By the age of 3, although he made some attempt at pointing, his parents had to guess all his needs. He made two sounds, one happy and the other distressed. He would take an adult's hand when he wanted something but made no clear communicative gestures. He showed over-sensitivity to household noises. It was always difficult to get his attention. He had no understanding of stories, preferring to flick the pages and pick out his favourite picture.

He showed no wariness of strangers and would simply wander off if something took his interest. He would approach his parents for some comfort but showed little interest in other people or their activities. His facial expressions were often inappropriate and his behaviour markedly dis-inhibited. He had no understanding of shared interests or enjoyment, and no creative or imaginative play.

He also had many unusual, repetitive preoccupations. These included a fascination with water (he would watch water flowing down the plughole or toilet and would lie down in puddles); he repetitively turned light switches on and off, tore paper into strips and lined it up on the floor. He became distressed if interrupted. He had a variety of attachments to unusual objects, such as a bottle of lentils. Finally, he had an unusual sensory interest in the feel of hair and plastic, and some maneristic behaviour including finger flapping at the edge of his peripheral vision and spinning in a complicated way. He was diagnosed as having childhood autism.

Case example 2

Gordon, a 13-year-old boy, presented to child psychiatry services after two incidents at school when he had assaulted fellow pupils following only minor provocation. His parents were concerned regarding Gordon's lack of friends and felt that his aggressive outbursts were in response to bullying. He achieved well academically, except at English and art which he found difficult, and he was otherwise very well-behaved and compliant. Like his father, an accountant, Gordon was very rigid and found any change in routine extremely anxiety-provoking.

His parents remembered that Gordon had exhibited some mild language delay, beginning to speak only by the end of his second year. There was no reported delay in gross motor skills, with Gordon taking his first steps at the age of one. However, he was reported to be a rather accident-prone child, a very untidy writer and still struggled to tie his shoelaces.

For much of his earlier childhood, play had been solitary, although he later played alongside other children. His parents could not recall any imaginative play such as role-play or dressing up, with Gordon preferring to arrange toy cars or play on his computer. He was interested in science fiction and had a large collection of annuals that he had virtually committed to memory. Gordon had one main friend, whom he saw outside of school hours; this was a slightly younger boy who shared Gordon's interest in video games. Gordon was described by his parents as being a serious young man, who was generally very quiet and kept himself to himself. He was perplexed by humour, often took things that people said to him literally, and rarely made direct eye contact with others.

With parental permission, Gordon's school was contacted and provided a report. This detailed that although Gordon was generally a 'loner', there was no evidence of serious bullying. Two recent violent incidents had occurred: one when Gordon thought a boy had been making fun of him and the other while he had been working with another boy on a science project. In the latter, Gordon had become frustrated at his partner's inability to follow his instructions exactly and had pushed him off his chair. Although not considered academically gifted, Gordon worked very hard and achieved well in most subjects. However, he struggled and would become anxious when asked to create artwork or writing from his imagination.

A formalised structured assessment interview was performed and a diagnosis of Asperger syndrome made. An additional diagnosis of 'disorder of development of motor function' was also made, in view of his fine motor clumsiness.

Assessment

Since 60% of parents of children with a pervasive developmental disorder recognise a problem in the first 18 months (English & Essex, 2001), it is important both to elicit parental concerns and to take them seriously. In all age groups, diagnosis depends heavily on a developmental history and focused observations across more than one setting. Diagnosis in younger children is difficult, although feasible from around 2 years onwards. Delay or deviance in communication or social skills, or the observation of unusual behaviour (e.g. repetitive behaviours), should lead to a general developmental assessment. This should identify concerns and explore any relevant family history, the developmental milestones and the progress of the child. A physical and neuro-developmental examination should take place, in particular to identify any dysmorphic features, neurocutaneous markers, neurological signs or abnormal growth trajectories. The child's visual and hearing acuity should also be assessed.

If an autistic-spectrum disorder is suspected a keyworker should be appointed for the child/family and a referral made for a multi-agency assessment (National Initiative for Autism: Screening and Assessment, 2003). This may include assessment using a standardised instrument such as the Autism Diagnostic Interview – Revised (ADI–R; Lord *et al*,

1994; Le Couteur *et al*, 2003), or the Diagnostic Interview for Speech and Communication Disorders (DISCO; Leekam *et al*, 2002), and direct observational assessments such as the Autism Diagnostic Observation Schedule (ADOS; Lord *et al*, 2000). Cognitive, speech and language, motor, behavioural, educational, mental state evaluations and a family assessment must also be performed. In addition to the full physical examination, chromosome karyotype and fragile-X DNA analysis, other investigations should take place where clinically indicated. This may include neuroimaging if tuberous sclerosis is suspected, or an EEG when there is a history of regression or seizures. For further guidance on assessment see the guidelines of the National Initiative for Autism: Screening and Assessment (2003).

Management

Effective management of any childhood disability begins with an honest and sensitive approach to diagnosis (North Western Regional Advisory Group for Learning Disability Services, 1992; Baird *et al*, 2000*b*). Access to practical support, such as financial benefits and parental support groups, should be facilitated and appropriate educational material provided, with opportunities for discussion given.

For a child or young person with an autistic-spectrum disorder, an individual coordinated intervention plan is required for the child and for the family (family care plan). Research has supported the effectiveness of a range of intervention approaches, but there is no evidence that one approach is more effective than others (Rogers, 1996; Dawson & Osterling, 1997; Jordan *et al*, 1998). The emphasis has been on behavioural and educational approaches. Teaching parents to understand and communicate more successfully with their child may enhance parental self-esteem and their ability to cope. This involvement of parents/families as 'co-therapists', to foster social communicative interactions and develop appropriate management strategies, may well prevent the development of secondary behavioural problems (Schopler *et al*, 1986; Runco & Schreibman, 1987; Koegel, 1995).

There is good evidence that specific behaviours and skills can be taught to children and adults with autism, although there are limitations to the generalisation and spontaneous usage of the skills learned (Howlin & Rutter, 1987; Lord, 2000). Positive behaviour support systems (Carr *et al*, 1999) focus on positive aspects of both the child's behaviour and environment, so that appropriate rather than problem behaviours are encouraged. It is important that behaviour problems are not seen as separate from the needs of the child/individual as a whole.

A specific individual educational plan should be developed for all pre-school and school-aged children with autistic-spectrum disorder (ASD).

'Education has been the most powerful source of improvement for children and adolescents with ASD in the past 30 years' (National Research Council, 2001). However, there have been few direct comparisons of different teaching strategies. Most programmes have many features in common. How best to combine the 'active ingredients' of well-known programmes such as Applied Behaviour Analysis (ABA; Leaf & McEachin, 1999) and Treatments and Education of Children, Adolescents and Adults with Autism (TEACCH; Mesibov, 1997; Marcus et al, 2000) with other specific strategies for this disorder (National Initiative for Autism: Screening and Assessment, 2003) is not a matter that has yet been evaluated.

Although some studies have shown that non-autistic peers can be employed to assist autistic children in gaining social skills in group settings (Wolfberg & Schuler, 1993; Laushey & Heflin, 2000), there is no evidence that access to mainstream provision is beneficial to all children with autistic-spectrum disorder. Each child needs to be considered individually and the educational settings planned accordingly.

Specific therapies and treatment of comorbidity

A range of therapies have been promoted for individuals with autistic-spectrum disorder. Most of these therapies have lacked experimental evidence of effectiveness, although some such as secretin injections and facilitated communication have been shown to have no effect or to be contraindicated, respectively (Mostert, 2001; Levy et al, 2003). To date, there is little evidence that any treatment alters the core symptomatology (du-Verglas et al, 1988).

However, medication and other targeted interventions (such as augmented communication programmes, physiotherapy and occupational therapy) should be used to treat specific symptoms and/or as adjuncts to the behavioural and educational components of an individual care plan. There are recent reports of promising trials with newer antipsychotic medication and selective serotonin reuptake inhibitors (SSRIs) (McDougle et al, 1995; Fatemi et al, 1998; Lord & Bailey, 2002).

Comorbid mental health problems such as anxiety, depression and obsessive–compulsive disorder should be treated (Gordon et al, 1993; Ghaziuddin & Greden, 1998). There are also some reports of the use of SSRIs and naltrexone in reducing the frequency of self-injurious behaviour.

Individuals with autistic-spectrum disorder and epilepsy may require anticonvulsant therapy. However, EEG abnormalities in the absence of an appropriate history are not an indication for treatment.

Conclusion

There is a growing awareness of both specific and more pervasive developmental disorders as a major source of impairment and handicap in children presented for help to professionals. Professionals of all disciplines have a role in the early identification and appropriate assessment of neurodevelopmental vulnerability. The managing clinician must then coordinate a multi-agency response that is sensitive to the needs of carers and children, irrespective of diagnostic labelling (Cass *et al*, 1999).

References

American Psychiatric Association (1994) *Diagnostic and Statistical Manual of Mental Disorders* (4th edn) (DSM–IV). Washington, DC: American Psychiatric Association.

Anderson, G. M., Freedman, C. X., Cohen, D. J., *et al* (1987) Whole blood serotonin in autistic and normal subjects. *Journal of Child Psychology and Psychiatry*, **28**, 885–900.

Armstrong, D. D. (2001) Rett syndrome neuropathology review 2000. *Brain and Development*, **23** (suppl. 1), S72–76.

Ashraf, H. (2001) US expert group rejects link between MMR and autism. *Lancet*, **357**, 1341.

Bailey, A., Le Couteur, A., Gottesman, I., *et al* (1995) Autism as a strongly genetic disorder: evidence from a British twin study. *Psychological Medicine*, **25**, 63–77.

Bailey, A. Palferman, S., Heavey, L., *et al* (1998) Autism: the phenotype in relatives. *Journal of Autism and Developmental Disorders*, **28**, 369–392.

Bailey, D. B., Hatton, D. D., Skinner, M., *et al* (2001) Autistic behavior, FMR1 protein and developmental trajectories in young males with fragile X syndrome. *Journal of Autism and Developmental Disorders*, **31**, 165–174.

Baird, G., Charman, T. & Baron-Cohen, S. (2000a) A screening instrument for autism at 18 months of age: a six-year follow-up study. *Journal of the American Academy of Child and Adolescent Psychiatry*, **39**, 694–702.

Baird, G., McConachie, H. & Scrutton, D. (2000b) Parents' perceptions of disclosure of the diagnosis of cerebral palsy. *Archives of Disease in Childhood*, **83**, 475–480.

Baker, P., Piven, J. & Sato, Y. (1998) Autism and tuberose sclerosis complex: prevalence and clinical features. *Journal of Autism and Developmental Disorders*, **28**, 279–285.

Baranek, G. T. (1999) Autism during infancy: a retrospective video analysis of sensory-motor and social behaviors at 9–12 months of age. *Journal of Autism and Developmental Disorders*, **29**, 213–224.

Baron-Cohen, S. (1993) From attention-goal psychology to belief-desire psychology: the development of a theory of mind and its dysfunction. In *Understanding Other Minds: Perspectives from Autism* (eds S. Baron-Cohen, H. Tager-Flusberg & D. J. Cohen). Oxford: Oxford University Press.

Barton, M. & Volkmar, F. (1998) How commonly are known medical conditions associated with autism? *Journal of Autism and Developmental Disorders*, **28**, 273–278.

Bishop, D. V. (1992) The underlying nature of specific language impairment. *Journal of Child Psychology and Psychiatry and Allied Disciplines*, **33**, 3–66.

Bishop, D. V. (1994) Is specific language impairment a valid diagnostic category? Genetic and psycholinguistic evidence. *Philosophical Transactions of the Royal Society of London – Series B: Biological Sciences*, **346**, 105–111.

Blomquist, H. K. (2000) The role of the Child Health Services in the identification of children with possible attention deficit hyperactivity disorder/deficits in attention, motor control and perception (ADHD/DAMP). *Acta Paediatrica Supplementum*, **89**, 24–32.

Cantwell, D. P. & Baker, L. (1991) *Psychiatric and Developmental Disorders in Children with Communication Disorders*. Washington, DC: American Psychiatric Press.

Carr, E. G., Horner, R. H., Turnbull, A. P., et al (eds) (1999) *Positive Behavior Support in People with Developmental Disabilities: A Research Synthesis*. Washington, DC: American Association on Mental Retardation.

Cass, H., Price, K., Reilly, S., et al (1999) A model for the assessment and management of children with multiple disabilities. *Child: Care, Health and Development*, **25**, 191–211.

Chakrabarti, S. & Fombonne, E. (2001) Pervasive developmental disorders in preschool children. *JAMA*, **285**, 3093–3099.

Cohen, N. J., Menna, R., Vallance, D. D., et al (1998) Language, social cognitive processing, and behavioral characteristics of psychiatrically disturbed children with previously identified and unsuspected language impairments. *Journal of Child Psychology and Psychiatry and Allied Disciplines*, **39**, 853–864.

Corbett, J., Harris, R., Taylor, E., et al (1977) Progressive disintegrative psychosis of childhood. *Journal of Child Psychology and Psychiatry*, **18**, 211–219.

Davison, F. M & Howlin, P. (1997) A follow-up study of a primary-age language unit. *European Journal of Disorders of Communication*, **32**, 19–36.

Dawson, G., & Osterling, J. (1997) Early intervention in autism: effectiveness and common elements of current approaches. In *The Effectiveness of Early Intervention: Second Generation Research* (ed. M. Guralnick). Baltimore: Brookes.

Deb, S. & Prasad, K. B. G. (1994) The prevalence of autistic disorder among children with a learning disability. *British Journal of Psychiatry*, **165**, 395–399.

Dewey, D. (1995) What is developmental dyspraxia? *Brain and Cognition*, **29**, 254–274.

du-Verglas, G., Banks, S. R., & Guyer, K. E. (1988) Clinical effects of fenfluramine on children with autism: a review of the research. *Journal of Autism and Developmental Disorders*, **19**, 297–308.

Elbert, J. C. & Seale, T. W. (1988) Complexity of the cognitive phenotype of an inherited form of learning disability. *Developmental Medicine and Child Neurology*, **30**, 181–189.

English, A. & Essex, J. (2001) *Report on Autistic Spectrum Disorders. A Comprehensive Report into Identification, Training and Provision Focusing on the Needs of Children and Young People with an Autistic Spectrum Disorder and their Families within the West Midlands Region*. Birmingham: West Midlands SEN Regional Partnership. http://www.westmidlandsrcp.org.uk/report_on_asds.htm.

Fatemi, S. H., Realmuto, G. M., Khan, L., et al (1998) Fluoxetine in treatment of adolescent patients with autism: a longitudinal open trial. *Journal of Autism and Developmental Disorders*, **29**, 303–307.

Fombonne, E. (1999) The epidemiology of autism: a review. *Psychological Medicine*, **29**, 769–786.

Fombonne, E. (2001) Is there an epidemic of autism? *Pediatrics*, **107**, 411–412.

Fombonne, E., Roge, B., Claverie, J., et al (1999) Microcephaly and macrocephaly in autism. *Journal of Autism and Developmental Disorders*, **29**, 113–119.

Gastaut H., Zifkin, B. & Rufo, M. (1987) Compulsive respiratory stereotypies in children with autistic features: polygraphic recording and treatment with fenfluramine. *Journal of Autism and Developmental Disorders*, **17**, 391–406.

Ghaziuddin, M. & Greden, J. (1998) Depression in children with autism/pervasive developmental disorders: a case-control family history study. *Journal of Autism and Developmental Disorders*, **28**, 111–115.

Gilchrist, A., Green, J., Cox, A., et al (2001) Development and current functioning in adolescents with Asperger syndrome: a comparative study. *Journal of Child Psychology and Psychiatry and Allied Disciplines*, **42**, 227–240.

Gillberg, C. (1998) Chromosomal disorders and autism. *Journal of Autism and Developmental Disorders*, **28**, 15–25.

Goodman, R. & Stevenson, J. (1989) A twin study of hyperactivity I. An examination of hyperactivity scores and categories derived from Rutter teacher and parent questionnaires. *Journal of Child Psychology and Psychiatry and Allied Disciplines*, **30**, 671–689.

Gordon, C. T., State, R. C., Nelson, J. E., *et al* (1993) A double-blind comparison of clomipramine, desipramine, and placebo in the treatment of autistic disorder. *Archives of General Psychiatry*, **50**, 441–447.

Green, D., Baird, G., Barnett, A. L., *et al* (2002) The severity and nature of motor impairment in Asperger syndrome: a comparison with specific developmental disorder of motor function. *Journal of Child Psychology and Psychiatry and Allied Disciplines*, **43**, 655–668.

Hagberg, B. (ed.) (1993) Rett syndrome – clinical and biological aspects. *Clinics in Developmental Medicine* (no. 127). Cambridge: Cambridge University Press.

Happe, F. & Frith, U. (1996) The neuropsychology of autism. *Brain*, **119**, 1377–1400.

Howlin, P. & Rutter, M. (1987) *Treatment of Autistic Children*. Chichester: John Wiley.

Jordan, R., Jones, G. & Murray, D. (1998) *Educational Interventions for Children with Autism: A Literature Review of Recent and Current Research* (Research Report 77). London: Department for Education and Employment.

Kanner, L. (1943) Autistic disturbance of affective contact. *Nervous Child*, **2**, 217–250.

Klinger, L. G. & Renner, P. (2000) Performance-based measures in autism: implications for diagnosis, early detection, and identification of cognitive profiles. *Journal of Clinical Child Psychology*, **29**, 479–492.

Koegel, L. K. (1995) Communication and language intervention. In *Teaching Children with Autism: Strategies for Initiating Positive Interactions and Improving Learning Opportunities* (eds R. L. Koegel & L. K. Koegel), pp. 17–32. Baltimore: Paul H. Brookes.

Landau, W. & Kleffner, F. (1957) Syndrome of acquired aphasia with convulsive disorder in children. *Neurology*, **7**, 523–530.

Laushey, K. M. & Heflin, L. J. (2000) Enhancing social skills of kindergarten children with autism through the training of multiple peers as tutors. *Journal of Autism and Developmental Disorders*, **30**, 183–193.

Leaf, R. & McEachin, J. J. (eds) (1999) *A Work in Progress: Behavior Management Strategies and a Curriculum for Intensive Behavioral Treatment of Autism*. New York: Different Roads to Learning.

Le Couteur, A., Bailey, A., Goode, S., *et al* (1996) A broader phenotype of autism: the clinical spectrum in twins. *Journal of Child Psychology and Psychiatry*, **37**, 785–801.

Le Couteur, A., Lord, C. & Rutter, M. (2003) *Autism Diagnostic Interview – Revised*. Los Angeles, CA: Western Psychological Services.

Leekam, S., Wing, L., Libby, S., *et al* (2002) The Diagnostic Interview for Social and Communication disorders: algorithms for ICD–10 childhood autism. *Journal of Child Psychology and Psychiatry and Allied Disciplines*, **43**, 327–342.

Levy, S. E., Souders, M. C., Wray, J., *et al* (2003) Children with autistic spectrum disorders. I: comparison of placebo and single dose of human synthetic secretin. *Archives of Disease in Childhood*, **88**, 731–736.

Lewine, J. D., Andrews, R., Chez, M., *et al* (1999) Magnetoencephalographic patterns of epileptiform activity in children with regressive autism spectrum disorders. *Pediatrics*, **104**, 405–418.

Lewis, V. & Boucher, J. (1995) Generativity in the play of young people with autism. *Journal of Autism and Developmental Disorders*, **25**, 105–121.

Lord, C. (2000) Achievements and future directions for intervention research in communication and autism spectrum disorders. *Journal of Autism and Developmental Disorders*, **30**, 391–396.

Lord, C. & Bailey, A. (2002) Autism spectrum disorders. In *Child and Adolescent Psychiatry* (4th edn) (eds M. Rutter & E. Taylor), pp. 636–663. Oxford: Blackwell Science.

Lord, C., Rutter, M. & Le Couteur, A. (1994) Autism Diagnostic Interview – Revised: a revised version of a diagnostic interview for caregivers of individuals with possible pervasive developmental disorders. *Journal of Autism and Developmental Disorders*, **24**, 659–685.

Lord, C., Risi, S., Lambrecht, L., *et al* (2000) The Autism Diagnostic Observation Schedule – Generic: a standard measure of social and communication deficits associated with the spectrum of autism. *Journal of Autism and Developmental Disorders*, **30**, 205–223.

Manor, O., Shalev, R. S., Joseph, A., *et al* (2001) Arithmetic skills in kindergarten children with developmental language disorders. *European Journal of Paediatric Neurology*, **5**, 71–77.

Marcus, L., Howlin, P. & Lord, C. (2000) TEACCH services for preschool children. In *Preschool Education Programs for Child with Autism* (eds J. Handleman & S. L. Harris). Austin, TX: Pro-Ed Inc.

Marescaux, C., Hirsch, E., Finck, S., *et al* (1990) Landau–Kleffner syndrome – a pharmacologic study of 5 cases. *Epilepsia*, **31**, 768–771.

Maughan, B. (1995) Annotation: long-term outcomes of developmental reading problems. *Journal of Child Psychology and Psychiatry and Allied Disciplines*, **36**, 357–371.

McBride, P. A., Anderson, G. M., Hertzig, M. E., *et al* (1998) Effects of diagnosis, race and puberty on platelet serotonin levels in autism and mental retardation. *Journal of the American Academy of Child and Adolescent Psychiatry*, **37**, 767–776.

McDougle, C. J., Kresch, L. E., Goodman, W. K., *et al* (1995) A case-controlled study of repetitive thoughts and behavior in adults with autistic disorder and obsessive-compulsive disorder. *American Journal of Psychiatry*, **152**, 772–777.

Medical Research Council (2001) *Review of Autism Research, Epidemiology and Causes*. London: Medical Research Council.

Mesibov, G. (1997) Formal and informal measures of the effectiveness of the TEACCH Programme. *Autism*, **1**, 25–35.

Monaco, A. P. & Bailey, A. J. (2001) Autism. The search for susceptibility genes. *Lancet*, **358** (suppl.), S3.

Mostert, M. P. (2001) Facilitated communication since 1995: a review of published studies. *Journal of Autism and Developmental Disorders*, **31**, 287–313.

National Initiative for Autism: Screening and Assessment (2003) *National Autism Plan for Children (NAPC)*. London: National Autistic Society. Also at http://www.rcpsych.ac.uk/college/faculty/niasa.htm

National Research Council (2001) *Educating Children with Autism*. Washington, DC: National Academies Press.

North Western Regional Advisory Group for Learning Disability Services (1992) *Breaking the News: A Resource for Developing Guidelines for Good Practice, Procedures and Training in Informing Parents of Diagnosis of a Child's Impairment*. Calderstones, Blackburn: NWRHA.

O'Connor, N. & Hermelin, B. (1971) Cognitive deficits in children. *British Medical Bulletin*, **27**, 227–231.

O'Neill, M. & Jones, R. S. (1997) Sensory-perceptual abnormalities in autism: a case for more research? *Journal of Autism and Developmental Disorders*, **27**, 283–293.

Orrico, A., Lam, C., Galli, L., *et al* (2000) MECP2 mutation in male patients with non-specific X-linked mental retardation. *FEBS Letters*, **481**, 285–288.

Ozonoff, S., Pennington, B. & Rogers, S. (1991) Executive function deficits in high-functioning autistic individuals: relationship to theory of mind. *Journal of Child Psychology and Psychiatry and Allied Disciplines*, **32**, 1081–1105.

Padget, S. (1988) Speech- and language-impaired three and four year olds: a five-year follow-up study. In *Pre-school Prevention of Reading Failure* (eds R. Masland & M. Masland), pp. 52–77. Timonium, MD: York Press.

Pierce, K. & Courchesne, E. (2001) Evidence for a cerebellar role in reduced exploration and stereotyped behavior in autism. *Biological Psychiatry*, **49**, 655–664.

Prizant, B. M. (1983) Language acquisition and communicative behaviour in autism: toward an understanding of the 'whole' of it. *Journal of Speech and Hearing Disorders*, **48**, 296–307.

Rapin, I. (1996) Practitioner review: developmental language disorders: a clinical update. *Journal of Child Psychology and Psychiatry*, **37**, 643–655.

Rapin, I. & Allen, D. A. (1983) Developmental language disorders: nosologic considerations. In *Neuropsychology of Language, Reading and Spelling* (ed. U. Kirk), pp. 155–184. New York: Academic Press.

Rimland, B. (1978) Savant capabilities of autistic children and their cognitive implications. In *Cognitive Defects in the Development of Mental Illness* (ed. G. Serban), pp. 43–65. New York: Brunner/Mazel.

Rogers, S. (1996) Early intervention in autism. *Journal of Autism and Developmental Disorders*, **26**, 342–346.

Rumsey, J. M. & Hamburger, S. D. (1990) Neuropsychological divergence of high-level autism and severe dyslexia. *Journal of Autism and Developmental Disorders*, **20**, 155–168.

Runco, M. A. & Schreibman, L. (1987) Socially validating behavioural objectives in the treatment of autistic children. *Journal of Autism and Developmental Disorders*, **17**, 141–147.

Rutter, M., Tizard, J. & Whitemore, K. (1970) *Education, Health and Behaviour*. London: Longman.

Rutter, M., Bailey, A., Bolton, P., *et al* (1994) Autism and known medical conditions: myth and substance. *Journal of Child Psychology and Psychiatry and Allied Disciplines*, **35**, 311–322.

Schopler, E., Reichler, R. J. & Renner, B. R. (1986) *The Childhood Autism Rating Scale*. New York: Irvington.

Shalev, R. S., Auerbach, J., Manor, O., *et al* (2000) Developmental dyscalculia: prevalence and prognosis. *European Child and Adolescent Psychiatry*, **9** (suppl. 2), II58–64.

Sikic, N., Ivicevic-Desnica, J., Vrca, A., *et al* (2001) Importance of early drug treatment in prognosis of the Landau–Kleffner syndrome. *Collegium Antropologicum*, **25**, 529–534.

Stone, W. L., Ousley, O. Y., Yoder, P. J., *et al* (1997) Nonverbal communication in two- and three-year-old children with autism. *Journal of Autism and Developmental Disorders*, **27**, 677–696.

Szatmari, P. (2000) The classification of autism, Asperger's syndrome, and pervasive developmental disorder. *Canadian Journal of Psychiatry*, **45**, 731–738.

Torrente, F., Ashwood, P., Day, R., *et al* (2002) Small intestinal enteropathy with epithelial IgG and complement deposition in children with regressive autism. *Molecular Psychiatry*, **7**, 375–382.

Turner, M. (1999) Annotation: repetitive behaviour in autism: a review of psychological research. *Journal of Child Psychology and Psychiatry and Allied Disciplines*, **40**, 839–849.

Volkmar, F. R. & Rutter, M. (1995) Childhood disintegrative disorder: results of the DSM–IV autism field trial. *Journal of the American Academy of Child and Adolescent Psychiatry*, **34**, 1092–1095.

Volkmar, F. R., Szatmari, P. & Sparrow, S. S. (1993) Sex differences in pervasive developmental disorders. *Journal of Autism and Developmental Disorders*, **23**, 579–591.

Volkmar, F. R., Klin, A., Schultz, R. T., *et al* (2000) Asperger's disorder. *American Journal of Psychiatry*, **157**, 262–267.

Wakefield, A. J., Anthony, A., Schepelmann, S., *et al* (1998) Persistent measles virus (MV) infection and immunodeficiency in children with autism, ileocolonic lymphonodular hyperplasia and non-specific colitis. *Gut*, **42** (suppl. 1), A86.

Warnke, A. (1999) Reading and spelling disorders: clinical features and causes. *European Child and Adolescent Psychiatry*, **8** (suppl. 3), 2–12.

Whitehurst, G. J. & Fischel, J. E. (1994) Practitioner review: early developmental language delay – what, if anything, should the clinician do about it? *Journal of Child Psychology and Psychiatry*, **35**, 613–648.

Williams, S. & McGee, R. (1994) Reading attainment and juvenile delinquency. *Journal of Child Psychology and Psychiatry*, **35**, 441–459.

Wing, L. (1981) Asperger's syndrome: a clinical account. *Psychological Medicine*, **11**, 115–129.

Wing, L. & Gould, G. (1979) Severe impairments of social interaction and associated abnormalities in children: epidemiology and classifications. *Journal of Autism and Developmental Disorders*, **9**, 11–30.

Wolfberg, P. J. & Schuler, A. L. (1993) Integrated play groups: a model for promoting the social and cognitive dimensions of play in children with autism. *Journal of Autism and Developmental Disorders*, **23**, 467–489.

Wolff, S. (1996) The first account of the syndrome of Asperger described. Translation of a paper entitled 'Die Schizoiden Psychopathien im Kindesalter' by Dr G. E. Sucharewa, 1926, *Monatsschrift für Psychiatrie und Neurologie*, **60**, 235–261. *European Child and Adolescent Psychiatry*, **5**, 119–132.

Woodhouse, W., Bailey, A. & Rutter, M. (1996) Head circumference and pervasive developmental disorders. *Journal of Child Psychology and Psychiatry and Allied Disciplines*, **37**, 665–671.

World Health Organization (1992) *Tenth Revision of the International Classification of Diseases and Related Health Problems* (ICD–10). Geneva: WHO.

Worster-Drought, C. & Allen, I. M. (1930) Congenital auditory imperception (congenital word-deafness) and its relation to idioglossia and other speech defects. *Journal of Neurology and Psychopathology*, **10**, 193–236.

Yule, W. & Rutter, M. (1976) Epidemology and social implications of specific reading retardation. In *The Neuropsychology of Learning Disorders* (eds R. Knight & D. Bakker), pp. 25–39. Baltimore, MD: University Park Press.

CHAPTER 9

Disorders of conduct

Paul McArdle

Not least because of uncertainty about whether it is the responsibility of healthcare, social care or criminal justice, conduct disorder is a controversial phenomenon. However, families frequently consult health services for help with children who display symptoms of conduct disorder. Schools and social services may ask for health contributions to management of children and young people with conduct disorder, and the condition itself may present risks that are unequivocally within the arena of health. This chapter concerns some of the issues that conduct disorder raises, terminology and definitions, origins, prognosis, public health implications, and treatment.

The World Health Organization's ICD–10 (World Health Organization, 1992) characterises conduct disorder as 'a repetitive and persistent pattern of dissocial, aggressive, or defiant conduct'. It lists behaviours that are very similar to those in the American Psychiatric Association's DSM–IV (American Psychiatric Association, 1994). The DSM–IV further specifies that 'the basic rights of others or major age appropriate societal norms or rules are violated (criterion A)'. Criterion B requires that 'this disturbance in behaviour causes clinically significant impairment in social, academic or occupational functioning'. Criterion C requires that in older individuals, the criteria for antisocial personality disorder are not met. In order to make the diagnosis, and since the young person concerned might minimise symptoms, it is generally recommended that information is obtained from different sources, such as the school and young person's parents.

Criterion A includes 15 possible symptoms divided into four groups. The young person must have manifested at least three of these symptoms in the previous 6 months. The first group concerns aggression:

1. often bullies, threatens or intimidates others;
2. often initiates physical fights;
3. has used a weapon that can cause serious physical harm to others;
4. has been physically cruel to people;

5. has been physically cruel to animals;
6. has stolen while confronting a victim;
7. has forced someone into sexual activity.

The second group concerns destruction of property:

8. has deliberately engaged in fire-setting with the intention of causing serious damage;
9. has deliberately destroyed others' property (other than by fire-setting).

The third concerns 'deceitfulness or theft':

10. has broken into someone else's house, building or car;
11. often lies to obtain goods or favours or to avoid obligations (i.e. 'cons' others);
12. has stolen items of non-trivial value without confronting a victim (e.g. shoplifting).

The final group refers to 'serious violations of rules':

13. often stays out at night despite parental prohibitions, beginning before age 13 years;
14. has run away from home overnight at least twice while living in the parental home or parental surrogate home (or once without returning for a lengthy period);
15. often truants from school, beginning before age 13 years.

It further sub-classifies conduct disorder into adolescent-onset disorder, in which no symptom was apparent before 10 years of age, and childhood-onset disorder, in which at least one symptom was present before 10 years of age. As early-onset conduct disorder may be associated with aggression, impaired peer relationships and higher risk of adult antisocial personality disorder, this distinction may be important for prognosis (Moffitt et al, 2002). It differs from the sub-classification in ICD–10, which focuses on socialised and non-socialised conduct disorder. However, it is likely that there is overlap between the socialised and adolescent-onset disorder, probably attended by lower rates of impairment, and the non-socialised and childhood-onset varieties, with their greater neurodevelopmental vulnerability and probably poorer prognosis.

Whether early- or late-onset, conduct disorder is associated with an increased risk of school failure and drop-out, drug and alcohol misuse (Mannuzza et al, 1998), cigarette smoking (Lynskey et al, 1998) and dependence (Bardone et al, 1998), early sexual behaviour and teenage pregnancy (Kessler et al, 1997), crime, completed suicide (Brent et al, 1999) and a range of long-term costs to society (Knapp et al, 2002). It is also responsible for the disappearance from the education, training and ultimately the labour force of a significant group of physically fit young people (Scott et al, 2001a). This is in an era of ageing population when young workers, especially those with skills, are in great demand in

Western countries. Furthermore, there is evidence that conduct disorder is increasing in Western societies (Smith & Rutter, 1995). Consequently, some argue that it is a considerable public health challenge (Angold & Costello, 2001). However, it is more than this, perhaps a social, economic and ultimately a political challenge.

Yet as a concept, conduct disorder almost does not feature in public debate, and undergraduate medical curricula almost totally ignore it. Even child and adolescent psychiatrists avoid discussion of conduct disorder. This may be due to a residual notion that it remains a 'social' and even perhaps a moral rather than a psychiatric disorder, and perhaps also to a sense of hopelessness about treatment.

Aetiology

The term 'conduct disorder' is of relatively recent origin, at least in its current meaning. However, Still (1902) described something akin to the modern syndrome early in the 20th century. Interestingly, although he is credited with identifying attention-deficit hyperactivity disorder (American Psychiatric Association, 1994), Still hardly mentioned inattention and did not specifically mention impulsivity or hyperactivity. However, he did describe defiance, aggression, destructiveness and stealing, disturbed sexual behaviour and harsh punishment. The last was in his view justifiably, if ineffectively, elicited by the deviant behaviour of the children he saw. He referred to a moral disorder– in the sense of genetically determined failure of identification of right and wrong that was located in the child – as central to the condition. Interestingly, the notion of a moral disorder has re-emerged more recently in a description of remarkably similar cases attributable to early damage to the prefrontal cortex (Anderson et al, 1999). Still also recognised links with learning disability, brain dysfunction (at least as manifested by epilepsy) and development. However, he did not consider the role that environment might have in the genesis of the conditions that he described.

In contrast, consideration of environmental factors as of overwhelming importance in the genesis of conduct disorders was a dominant view in the latter part of the 20th century, and in the training of many currently practising child and adolescent mental health specialists. For instance, although the Isle of Wight survey (Rutter et al, 1970) described developmental abnormalities among conduct-disordered children, it was the link with paternal unemployment and criminality, overcrowding, 'broken homes' and maternal mental illness that influenced thinking. Patterson (cited in Keisner et al, 2001) discussed cycles of escalating coercive interactions as typical in the homes of aggressive children. These harsh, abrasive and inconsistent parenting practices show a strong correlation with child antisocial behaviour. In particular, if a child responds to a parental command with an aversive behaviour such as refusal, and if the parent then drops the demand, the child's aversive behaviour has been negatively reinforced. According to the model, the parent's demands became more imperative and coercive, mirrored by the child's increasingly determined defiance. Ultimately, the parent retires defeated but furious, the conflict unresolved. A version of this view is the role of parental expressed emotion, especially hostility and criticism, in the genesis of behavioural disturbance (Peris & Baker, 2000). For instance, Schachar et al (1987) reported that in a clinical sample, parental criticism and hostility were more significantly associated with conduct disorder than with hyperactivity.

Nevertheless, when early childhood behaviour and maternal stress are accounted for statistically, expressed emotion accounts for only a modest proportion of the variance of behaviour problems 3 years later (Peris & Baker, 2000). Furthermore, twin studies suggest that shared environmental effects account for only approximately 30% of the variance in childhood behaviour disorders (Jaffee et al, 2002). Other environmental influences reflect the capacity of neighbourhoods to buffer or exacerbate the impact of individual traits (Sampson et al, 1997; Caspi et al, 2000) or changes in family structure, and the capacity to supervise adolescents (Costello et al, 2003).

The lack of distinction between childhood- and adolescent-onset disorders is a problem in genetic studies, which tend to show significant contributions from genetic and, as far as they can be ascertained, family and non-family environment. It may be that the childhood-onset or unsocialised disorders that persist into adulthood and, according to DSM–IV, are 'symptomatic of an underlying dysfunction' are more likely to have a genetic component than the adolescent-onset or socialised variety (Langbehn et al, 1998). In the latter, other mechanisms, such as poor supervision, peer influences and neighbourhood problems may predominate (Fergusson & Horwood, 1999; Fergusson et al, 2002; Costello et al, 2003).

Nevertheless, extreme forms of unresponsive or hostile care may be associated with disorganised attachment (Lyons-Ruth, 1996) linked to 'anger [as]…a chronic experience'. Ingrained defensive strategies may emerge from these early experiences. These are said to include an emotionally insulated, disconnected affect, and behaviour that is characteristically hostile, aggressive and antisocial (Sroufe, 1995). In this way, the scene is set for the emergence of deviant social behaviour. Hence, it is probable that maternal criticism or certain types of interaction within families that are relatively common in clinical practice can contribute to deviant child behaviour (Meyer et al, 2000). However, in order to lead to extreme deviance alone, it is likely that the abnormality in relationships must also be extreme. These circumstances are uncommon and at least among younger children are probably not the usual route to conduct disorder (O'Connor & Rutter, 2000; McArdle *et al*, 2002). Hence, focusing on environmental factors, the relative importance of and links between intra-familial behaviours, family structure (for instance, as it affects supervision) and the neighbourhood quality are not well known. However, it is clear that all relevant environmental aspects of conduct disorder are not captured by examination of family 'dynamics' alone.

Comorbid difficulties

Most pre-pubertal children diagnosed with conduct disorder show predictable comorbidity (Moffitt *et al*, 2002). Deficits in verbal skills have also been long recognised among children with conduct disorders (Rutter *et al*, 1970; Lynam & Henry, 2001). These can commonly manifest as specific reading difficulty or as problems in language development. Indeed, Tomblin *et al* (2000) argue that early language impairment is 'a manifestation of the same problem that later presents as reading delay'. They further argue that 'the behaviour problems... arise from the presence of limited language skills and the (inability to meet) demands...for performance that requires verbal skills'. As the school curriculum progresses, these demands escalate, contributing to a breakdown of the relationship between the child and school. It appears that either a generalised language delay or a delay in comprehension of receptive language is most associated with disturbed behaviour (Beitchman *et al*, 1996*a,b*). Indeed, a study of adolescent 'delinquents' (the great majority of whom are likely to have conduct disorders) reported 'general verbal deficits encompassing problems of language and literacy' (Snowling *et al*, 2000). Whether language impairment, literacy delays or comorbid hyperactivity are the key precursors of conduct disorder remains unclear (Maughan *et al*, 1996).

Specific language impairment may be also associated with impairments in social cognition. These include the inability to understand humour or sarcasm, or understand another's mental state or intentions. It may be that an underlying deficit in social cognition may create difficulties in the development of language and difficulties in social interaction (Farmer, 2000). These deficits are similar to but more restricted than those seen in autistic children and may be manifestations of the broader phenotype of autism now known to be relatively common (Pickles *et al*, 2000). Indeed, clinical observation suggests that children with these social difficulties are often accused of aggression, often reactive to perceptions of victimisation that occur, particularly during unstructured school breaks (Hawker & Boulton, 2000). These character-istics might underlie the rejection by peers of childhood-onset or unsocialised conduct disordered children (McArdle *et al*, 2000). Conduct disordered children face misunderstanding, rejection, punishment and failure; it is no surprise that there is a high rate of comorbidity with major depression (Greene *et al*, 2002).

Attention-deficit hyperactivity disorder and hyperkinetic disorder are key differential diagnoses of conduct disorder, and may reflect abnormalities or immaturity of prefrontal cortical functioning (Barkley, 1997). It is because of this deficit that the child appears, for instance, distractible, subject to the 'contingencies of the minute'. So-called 'life-course persistent' conduct disorder of early onset and sustained course may be characteristically linked to this deficit (Moffitt *et al*, 2002). Indeed, some symptoms of hyperactivity are usual among preadolescent children with conduct disorder (McArdle *et al*, 1995), and Greene *et al* (2002) argue that at least 80% of younger children referred with conduct disorder (mean age 10.7 years) merit a further diagnosis of ADHD. Since affected individuals do not see the consequences of their actions, serious offences may result if the deficit persists, partly because consequences may be wildly misjudged.

Hence, a pattern of developmental vulnerability, including hyperactivity, developmental language disorders, abnormalities in social cognition and specific learning disabilities, represents a common or even necessary developmental background upon which childhood-onset or life-course persistent conduct disorders develop. This was first described by Rutter *et al* (1970), but perhaps we are only now beginning to give it due weight.

Oppositional defiant disorder

Oppositional defiant disorder is symptomatically a close relative of conduct disorder and, according to DSM–IV, is characterised by at least four of the following symptoms. The child:

- loses temper;
- argues with adults;
- actively denies or refuses adult requests;
- deliberately does things that annoy other people;
- blames others for his or her mistakes or misbehaviour;
- is touchy or easily annoyed by others;
- is angry and resentful;
- is spiteful or vindictive.

These symptoms need to be present for at least 6 months and be sufficiently severe to impair social or school functioning. Oppositional defiant disorder has similar correlates to conduct disorder (Burt *et al*, 2003) and may be an early manifestation of childhood-onset conduct disorder, perhaps before antisocial behaviour spills into the community (Beiderman *et al*, 1996; Burke *et al*, 2002). It has been included in ICD–10 'because of its predictive potential for later conduct problems'. Also, it 'is often found in other types of conduct disorder', clearly subsuming it within the overall conduct disorder category. Oppositional defiant disorder and aggression (Lahey *et al*, 1998) tend both to be of early onset and to predict adult antisocial behaviour (Langbehn *et al*, 1998). This suggests that oppositional defiant disorder with its 'personality-like' (Langbehn *et al*, 1998) characteristics, as well as aggressive conduct disorder, may be synonymous (or at least overlap) with Moffitt's life-span-persistent or DSM's childhood-onset conduct disorder.

According to a developmental psychopathology model of deviance, it is likely that an array of developmental vulnerabilities renders a child difficult to raise, educate and relate to. Especially if parents are vulnerable, such a child can elicit ineffectual coercive discipline, negatively reinforcing his or her aversive behaviour. This effectively trains the child in defiance. The quality of the attachment to parents in the first place and subsequently to other adults deteriorates, leading to a disorder of attachment superimposed upon an array of developmental deficits. Interestingly, this gene–environment interaction may be particularly important in determining adverse consequences for girls (Langbehn *et al*, 1998).

Angold *et al* (2002) argue that the prevalence of childhood-onset conduct disorder is 4.2% and that of adolescent onset is much less (1.3%). The total rate of 5.4% appears low, but includes only those that show impairment (i.e. that significantly or substantially interfere with quality of life), and is compatible with a number of other studies in Europe and the USA (McArdle *et al*, 2004). The key point is that most young people with conduct disorder are likely to exhibit complex comorbidity that affords opportunities for in-depth assessment, comprehensibility, explanation and intervention based on a compassionate and potentially helpful, rather than condemnatory, framing of their presentation.

Management

A number of treatments for conduct disorder that target aspects of the syndrome or correlates of the syndrome have emerged. These include school-based groups (Kolvin *et al*, 1981; McArdle *et al*, 2002), parenting (Scott *et al*, 2001*b*), cognitive–behavioural (Kazdin, 1997) and psychodynamic (Target & Fonagy, 1994) interventions. Also, there is some evidence that combinations of interventions can be synergistic and that some form of long-term intervention is important in maintaining gains (Kazdin, 1997).

Multimodal approaches that aim at different aspects of the disorder appear to have the greatest potential (Grizenko *et al*, 1993; Myers *et al*, 2000; Liddle *et al*, 2001; Swanson *et al*, 2001; Henggeler *et al*, 2003) and probably resemble the inter-agency interventions that emerge pragmatically in the UK (at least on those occasions when conduct disorder is energetically managed). Multisystemic therapy (MST) is particularly interesting: its efficacy with severely conduct disordered young people has been demonstrated (Henggeler *et al*, 2003). It is a complex intervention focused on 'the individual, family, peer, school, and social network variables that are linked with identified problems... MST adapts techniques from strategic and structural family therapy, behavioral parent training and cognitive–behavioral therapies'. It also allows for pharmacological interventions as appropriate. Hence it is an operationalised multimodal intervention which aims to 'enhance caregivers' capacity to effectively monitor adolescent behavior and whereabouts and to provide positive consequences for responsible youth behavior and sanctions for irresponsible behavior'. Similarly, at the peer level a frequent goal of treatment is to decrease the youth's involvement with delinquent and drug-using peers, and to increase his or her association with pro-social peers. Therapists place emphasis on improving links with school. The therapists are supervised by professionally trained personnel, but are themselves not necessarily so. The intervention is delivered at home, which virtually eliminates drop-out (Henggeler *et al*, 1996). The case-loads are low (four to six families per clinician), allowing for intensive contact (an average of 46 hours) over 5 months or so with an on-call commitment.

Multidimensional family therapy is a further family-based approach developed as a treatment for substance misuse (Liddle *et al*, 2001). However, it also is effective in reducing symptoms of conduct disorder. It resembles multisystemic therapy in that it targets a range of areas of the young person's life: family, education and peers, and in that it deploys techniques that individually appear to be well within the capability of UK services. It differs from multisystemic therapy in being 'office-based', and so risks the attrition inherent in clinic-based treatments for this group of children and young people. However, it might be possible to regard multidimensional family therapy as a less intensive form of intervention but similar in principle to multisystemic therapy. Other interventions have been reviewed by Kazdin (1997).

One of the puzzles of intervention research is that even effective interventions do not translate rapidly or even at all into practice (Weisz, 2000). This relates to the debate concerning efficacy (does it work under experimental conditions?) and effectiveness (does it work in the field?). Effectiveness studies (the few that exist) tend to show weaker effects than efficacy studies. Also, the effect sizes to be expected from even statistically significant change are not necessarily substantial.

Attrition and suitability are also relevant in the clinic setting. For instance, Scott *et al* (2001*b*) described the statistically significant effect of a group parenting intervention on the behaviour of children with 'antisocial behaviour'. However, approximately a quarter of the referred children were not entered in the trial, mainly because of comorbidity. Of those who took part in the trial, almost a fifth dropped out, and of those who persisted, a third continued to meet criteria for oppositional defiant disorder. Hence, this treatment would not have been suitable or would not have been the answer for the majority of the referred children. A third problem is case-load: for instance, multisystemic therapy relies on case-loads in single figures. Hence, it cannot be a widely disseminated intervention in child and adolescent mental health services in the UK as currently commissioned, where case-loads are often unavoidably substantial.

Finally, Kazdin (2000) has argued that intervention should be informed by our developing understanding of the psychopathology underlying disorders. None of the treatment approaches that have been developed distinguishes explicitly between childhood-onset and adolescent-onset conduct disorder, even though this seems to be an important demarcation. It may be that interventions focused on the former would emphasise careful developmental assessment and an informed multimodal intervention, e.g. psychoeducation and support for parents and schools, education in the broadest sense (focusing on identified problems with language and literacy, coping with peers) and pharmacological interventions for hyperactivity and aggression. For selected children, especially among those referred to services and whose cases are often very complex, parenting interventions would represent important components of such a multimodal programme, but might be sufficient treatment for only a minority. A further point is the need to sustain interventions for these chronic conditions, either through extended follow-up or booster doses, in order to maintain gains (Kazdin, 1997).

For those with adolescent-onset disorder, the emphasis might be more on promoting their association with pro-social peers, child–carer relationships and supervision. Whether differentiating the interventions for these two subgroups in this way will determine outcome is not yet known, but it may be one way that research should develop in the future.

Whatever approach is adopted, it is becoming increasingly important, indeed perhaps critical, for the credibility of mental health services that they demonstrate that their interventions are effective and cost-effective. Randomised controlled trials will be beyond the resources of most services, but studies using waiting list controls (Scott et al, 2001b), or even before-and-after studies using published data as comparisons, may well be feasible.

Conduct disorder is a common root of a range of problems that are often identified as social in nature and addressed by government as if they were entirely separate and unlinked. A strategic targeted approach to 'conquer conduct disorder' might not only reduce rates of conduct disorder, but could also improve the quality of life and life chances of large numbers of young people, reduce wasted effort on a whole range of developmentally uncomprehending initiatives, and reduce substance misuse, teenage pregnancy, suicide and crime.

References

American Psychiatric Association (1994) *Diagnostic and Statistical Manual of Mental Disorders* (4th edn) (DSM–IV). Washington, DC: American Psychiatric Association.

Anderson, S., Bechara, A., Damasio, H., *et al* (1999) Impairment of social and moral behavior related to early damage in human prefrontal cortex. *Nature Neuroscience*, **2**, 1032–1037.

Angold, A. & Costello, E. (2001) The epidemiology of disorders of conduct: nosological issues and comorbidity. In *Conduct Disorders in Childhood and Adolescence* (eds J. Hill & B. Maughan), pp. 126–168. Cambridge: Cambridge University Press.

Angold, A., Erkanli, A., Farmer, E., *et al* (2002) Psychiatric disorder, impairment, and service use in rural African American and white youth. *Archives of General Psychiatry*, **59**, 893–901.

Bardone, A., Moffitt, T., Caspi, A., *et al* (1998) Adult physical health outcomes of adolescent girls with conduct disorder, depression, and anxiety. *Journal of the American Academy of Child and Adolescent Psychiatry*, **37**, 594–601.

Barkley, R. (1997) *ADHD and the Nature of Self-control*. London: Guilford Press.

Beiderman, J., Faraone, S., Milberger, S., *et al* (1996) Is childhood oppositional defiant disorder a precursor to adolescent conduct disorder? Findings from a four year follow-up study of children with ADHD. *Journal of the American Academy of Child and Adolescent Psychiatry*, **35**, 1193–1204.

Beitchman, J., Brownlie, E., Inglis, A., *et al* (1996*a*) Seven-year follow up of speech and language impaired and control children: psychiatric outcome. *Journal of Child Psychology and Psychiatry*, **37**, 961–970.

Beitchman, J., Wilson, B., Brownlie, E., *et al* (1996*b*) Long-term consistency in speech/language profiles: II. Behavioural, emotional and social outcomes. *Journal of the American Academy of Child and Adolescent Psychiatry*, **35**, 815–825.

Brent, D., Baugher, M., Bridge, J., *et al* (1999) Age- and sex-related risk factors for adolescent suicide. *Journal of the American Academy of Child and Adolescent Psychiatry*, **38**, 1497–1505.

Burke, J., Loeber, R. & Birmaher, B. (2002) Oppositional defiant disorder and conduct disorder: a review of the past 10 years, part II. *Journal of the American Academy of Child and Adolescent Psychiatry*, **41**, 1275–1293.

Burt, S., Krueger, R., McGue, M., *et al* (2003) Parent–child conflict and the comorbidity among childhood externalizing disorders. *Archives of General Psychiatry*, **60**, 505–513.

Caspi, A., Taylor, A., Moffitt, T., *et al* (2000) Neighborhood deprivation affects children's mental health: environmental risks identified in a genetic design. *Psychological Science*, **11**, 338–342.

Costello, E., Compton, S., Keeler, G., *et al* (2003) Relationships between poverty and psychopathology: a natural experiment. *JAMA*, **290**, 2023–2029.

Farmer, M. (2000) Language and social cognition in children with specific language impairment. *Journal of Child Psychology and Psychiatry*, **41**, 627–636.

Fergusson, D. M. & Horwood, L. J. (1999) Prospective childhood predictors of deviant peer affiliations in adolescence. *Journal of Child Psychology and Psychiatry and Allied Disciplines*, **40**, 581–592.

Fergusson, D., Swain-Campbell, N. & Horwood, L. (2002) Deviant peer affiliations, crime and substance use: a fixed effects regression analysis. *Journal of Abnormal Child Psychology*, **30**, 419–430.

Greene, R., Biederman, J., Zerwas, S., *et al* (2002) Psychiatric comorbidity, family dysfunction and social impairment in referred youth with oppositional defiant disorder. *American Journal of Psychiatry*, **159**, 1214–1224.

Grizenko, N., Papineau, D. & Sayegh, L. (1993) Effectiveness of a multimodal day treatment program for children with disruptive behavior problems. *Journal of the American Academy of Child and Adolescent Psychiatry*, **32**, 127–134.

Hawker, D. & Boulton, M. (2000) Twenty years' research on peer victimisation and psychosocial maladjustment: a meta-analytic review of cross-sectional studies. *Journal of Child Psychology and Psychiatry*, **41**, 441–456.

Henggeler, S., Pickrel, S., Brondino, M., *et al* (1996) Eliminating (almost) treatment dropout of substance abusing or dependent delinquents through home-based multisystemic therapy. *American Journal of Psychiatry*, **153**, 427–428.

Henggeler, S. W., Rowland, M. D., Halliday-Boykins, C., *et al* (2003) One-year follow-up of multisystemic therapy as an alternative to the hospitalization of youths in psychiatric crisis. *Journal of the American Academy of Child and Adolescent Psychiatry*, **42**, 543–551.

Jaffee, S., Moffitt, T., Caspi, A., *et al* (2002) Influence of adult domestic violence on children's internalizing and externalizing problems: an environmentally informative twin study. *Journal of the American Academy of Child and Adolescent Psychiatry*, **41**, 1095–1103.

Kazdin, A. (1997) Treatment of conduct disorder. *Journal of Child Psychology and Psychiatry*, **38**, 161–178.

Kazdin, A. (2000) Developing a research agenda for child and adolescent psychotherapy. *Archives of General Psychiatry*, **57**, 829–835.

Keisner, J., Dishion, T. & Poulin, F. (2001) A reinforcement model of conduct problems in children and adolescents: advances in theory and intervention. In *Conduct Disorders in Childhood and Adolescence* (eds J. Hill & B. Maughan). Cambridge: Cambridge University Press.

Kessler, R., Berglund, P., Foster, C., *et al* (1997) Social consequences of psychiatric disorders, II: Teenage parenthood. *American Journal of Psychiatry*, **154**, 1405–1411.

Knapp, M., McCrone, P., Fombonne, E., *et al* (2002) The Maudsley long-term follow-up of child and adolescent depression: 3. Impact of comorbid conduct disorder on service use and costs in adulthood. *British Journal of Psychiatry*, **180**, 19–23.

Kolvin, I., Garside, R., Nicol, A., *et al* (1981) *Help Starts Here: The Maladjusted Child in the Ordinary School*. London: Tavistock.

Lahey, B., Loeber, R., Quay, H. C., *et al* (1998) Validity of DSM–IV subtypes of conduct disorder based on age of onset. *Journal of the American Academy of Child and Adolescent Psychiatry*, **37**, 435–442.

Langbehn, D., Cadoret, R., Yates, W., *et al* (1998) Distinct contributions of conduct and oppositional defiant symptoms to adult antisocial behavior: evidence from an adoption study. *Archives of General Psychiatry*, **55**, 821–829.

Liddle, H., Dakof, G., Parker, K., *et al* (2001) Multidimensional family therapy for adolescent drug abuse: results of a randomized clinical trial. *American Journal of Drug and Alcohol Abuse*, **27**, 651–688.

Lynam, D. & Henry, B. (2001) The role of neuro-psychological deficits in conduct disorders. In *Conduct Disorders in Childhood and Adolescence* (eds J. Hill & B. Maughan). Cambridge: Cambridge University Press.

Lynskey, M., Fergusson, D. & Horwood, L. (1998) The origins of correlations between tobacco, alcohol and cannabis use during adolescence. *Journal of Clinical Psychology and Psychiatry*, **39**, 995–1005.

Lyons-Ruth, K. (1996) Attachment relationships among children with aggressive behavior problems: the role of disorganised early attachment patterns. *Journal of Consulting and Clinical Psychology*, **64**, 64–73.

Mannuzza, S., Klein, R., Bessler, A., *et al* (1998) Adult psychiatric status of hyperactive boys grown up. *American Journal of Psychiatry*, **155**, 493–498.

Maughan, B., Pickles, A., Hagell, A., *et al* (1996) Reading problems and antisocial behaviour: developmental trends in comorbidity. *Journal of Child Psychology and Psychiatry*, **37**, 405–419.

McArdle, P., O'Brien, G. & Kolvin, I. (1995) Hyperactivity: prevalence and relationship with conduct disorder. *Journal of Child Psychology and Psychiatry*, **36**, 279–305.

McArdle, P., O'Brien, G. & Kolvin, I. (2000) The peer relations of children with hyperactivity and conduct disorder. *European Journal of Child and Adolescent Psychiatry*, **9**, 91–99.

McArdle, P., O'Brien, G. & Kolvin, I. (2002) Hyperactivity and conduct disorder: exploring origins. *Irish Journal of Psychological Medicine*, **19**, 42–47.

McArdle, P., Prosser, J. & Kolvin, I. (2004) Prevalence of psychiatric disorder: with and without psychosocial impairment. *European Child and Adolescent Psychiatry*, **13**, 347–353.

Meyer, J., Rutter, M., Silberg, J., et al (2000) Familial aggregation for conduct disorder symptomatology: the role of genes, marital discord and family adaptability. *Psychological Medicine*, **30**, 759–774.

Moffitt, T., Caspi, A., Harrington, H., et al (2002) Males on the life-course-persistent and adolescence-limited antisocial pathways: follow-up at age 26 years. *Development and Psychopathology*, **14**, 179–207.

Myers, W., Burton, P., Sanders, P., et al (2000) Project back-on-track at 1 year: a delinquency treatment program for early-career juvenile offenders. *Journal of the American Academy of Child and Adolescent Psychiatry*, **39**, 1127–1134.

O'Connor, T. & Rutter, M. (2000) Attachment disorder behavior following early severe deprivation: extension and longitudinal follow-up. English and Romanian Adoptees Study Team. *Journal of the American Academy of Child and Adolescent Psychiatry*, **39**, 703–712.

Peris, T. & Baker, B. (2000) Applications of the expressed emotion construct to young children with externalising disorder. *Journal of Child Psychology and Psychiatry*, **41**, 457–462.

Pickles, A., Starr, E., Kazak, S., et al (2000) Variable expression of the broader autism phenotype: findings from extended pedigrees. *Journal of Child Psychology and Psychiatry*, **41**, 491–502.

Rutter, M., Tizard, J. & Whitmore, K. (1970) *Education, Health and Behaviour*. London: Longman & Green.

Sampson, R. J., Raudenbush, S. W. & Earls, F. (1997) Neighbourhood and violent crime: a multilevel study of collective efficacy. *Science*, **277**, 918–924.

Schachar, R., Taylor, E., Wieselberg, M., et al (1987) Changes in family function and relationships in children who respond to methylphenidate. *Journal of the American Academy of Child and Adolescent Psychiatry*, **26**, 728–732.

Scott, S., Knapp, M., Henderson, J., et al (2001a) Financial cost of social exclusion: follow up study of antisocial children into adulthood. *BMJ*, **323**, 191.

Scott, S., Spender, Q., Doolan, M., et al (2001b) Multicentre controlled trial of parenting groups for childhood antisocial behaviour in clinical practice. *BMJ*, **323**, 194–198.

Smith, D. & Rutter, M. (1995) Time trends in psychosocial disorders of youth. In *Psychosocial Disorders in Young People* (eds M. Rutter & D. Smith). Chichester: John Wiley.

Snowling, M., Adams, J., Bowyer-Crane, C., et al (2000) Levels of literacy among juvenile offenders: the incidence of specific reading difficulties. *Criminal Behaviour and Mental Health*, **10**, 229–241.

Sroufe, L. A. (1995) *Emotional Development. The Organization of Emotional Development in the Early Years*. Cambridge: Cambridge University Press.

Still, G. F. (1902) The Coulstonian Lectures on some abnormal psychical conditions in children. *Lancet*, *i*, 1008–1012, 1077–1082, 1163–1168.

Swanson, J., Kraemer, H., Hinshaw, S., et al (2001) Clinical relevance of the primary findings of the MTA: success rates based on severity of ADHD and ODD symptoms at the end of treatment. *Journal of the American Academy of Child and Adolescent Psychiatry*, **40**, 168–179.

Target, M. & Fonagy, P. (1994) The efficacy of psychoanalysis for children: prediction of outcome in the developmental context. *Journal of the American Academy of Child and Adolescent Psychiatry*, **33**, 1134–1144.

Tomblin, B., Zhang, X. & Buckwalter, P. (2000) The association of reading disability, behavioural disorders and language impairment among second grade children. *Journal of Child Psychology and Psychiatry*, **41**, 473–482.

Weisz, J. R. (2000) Agenda for child and adolescent psychotherapy research: on the need to put science into practice. *Archives of General Psychiatry*, **57**, 837–838.

World Health Organization (1992) *Tenth Revision of the International Classification of Diseases and Related Health Problems* (ICD–10). Geneva: WHO.

CHAPTER 10

Disorders of attachment, anxiety and adjustment

Judith Trowell

There is a growing recognition that significant relationships and associated attachments play a large part in a child's resilience and vulnerability to difficulties. Disorders characterised by anxiety, fear and stress can be understood and interventions offered using an attachment framework. This chapter first reviews the role of attachment in the development of emotional disorders with onset specific to childhood (ICD–10 categories F93–F94; World Health Organization, 1992, 1995). The second half of the chapter outlines the presentation of anxiety and adjustment-related disorders (ICD–10 categories F40–F43).

Attachment

The population of children and their families who are seen in child and adolescent mental health services represent a group of children who are highly likely to have insecure attachments; this may also be true of their parents. These children's insecure attachments are anxious, avoidant or disorganised (see Chapter 2). Sadly, a very small number of children appear to have no attachment; they appear to be either indiscriminately attached to anyone and everyone they meet, or they are unresponsive and self-reliant in a quite inappropriate way. Bowlby (1973, 1980, 1982) suggested that separation from the primary caregiver leads to high levels of anxiety in the child. If the child experiences the loss of a carer by death, abandonment or lengthy separation, the risk of anxiety is increased, but it also becomes raised with insensitive, unresponsive or rejecting parenting; for all these children, insecure attachments are very likely (De Wolff & Van Izzendoorn, 1997). Depressed mothers have been studied extensively and their children frequently have insecure attachments (Murray, 1992). Disorganised attachments are of particular interest in the field of child protection, since they arise where there are unresolved losses and unresolved abuse and trauma.

Physical, emotional, psychological and sexual abuse may predispose to stress-related disorders as a result of unprocessed, undigested traumatic experiences and these have now been understood in attachment terms as strongly linked to fear (Main & Hesse, 1990). This may be fear on the part of the individual or it may result from witnessing fear in the behaviour, voice, facial expression and eyes of the parent or carer. The child is left confused and disoriented in relation to the secure base that should be provided by their attachment figure. The resultant disorganised attachment shows itself in the child's behaviour (such as odd movements, hand flapping, lying face down on the floor, backing away instead of approaching) or abnormalities of speech.

Many parents assessed in child and adolescent mental health services also have attachment difficulties and might have had childhood experiences that left them with an insecure attachment. These might be of the enmeshed kind, where they remain preoccupied by their early and current relationships that did not or do not meet their needs; or they might be dismissive, where they indicate that their early experiences are forgotten, irrelevant and of no current consequence. Adults too may have unresolved disorganised attachments arising from early separation, losses and trauma, or alternatively due to events in adolescence and adulthood such as rape, domestic violence or other traumatic experiences. Adult attachment difficulties are usually demonstrated in their conversation, particularly with reference to their autobiographical memory, i.e. their ability to give an account of their childhood and relationships within it. Their speech may be characterised by incoherent discourse, inconsistencies, lapses and failure of monitoring of reasoning. These have been most strikingly demonstrated using the Adult Attachment Interview (Main & Goldwyn, 1998). It has also been suggested (Main *et al*, 1985) that parents' attachment status influences their ability to attend to their children and hence contributes to the intergenerational transmission of attachment difficulties and subsequently anxiety disorders (Van Izzendoorn *et al*, 1995).

Assessment of attachment disorders

Assessing children

Many clinicians inevitably observe separations and reunions as part of their routine assessment of young children. The child is seen for a separate assessment session and so one can observe the way the separation is handled and the child's response to this (Ainsworth *et al*, 1978). One can also observe the reunion when the child returns to the waiting room. Can the carer facilitate the separation? Does the child, even when appropriately apprehensive, nevertheless manage to separate? How long can the child remain with the interviewer, and are there anxieties about being abandoned? On reunion, does the child make eye contact, perhaps have some physical contact and then settle, or does the child appear indifferent to any coming or going? Some children cannot separate and cling tearfully; this can be an indication of separation anxiety disorder. Attachment theory provides a basis to explain this.

Case example 1

A 6-year-old girl had been physically abused and neglected by her mother; she was currently in foster care and her mother was applying for rehabilitation. While in the room together, the young girl was able to play happily and passed Plasticine and small animals to mother, encouraging her to join in. It appeared a mutually warm, concerned relationship. When the separation was explained, the mother immediately stood up and walked out of the room. The young girl looked up but continued to play busily. Close observation, however, showed that the quality of the play changed. Instead of creative, pretend play involving the use of symbolic activity making use of the range of toys, the play changed to moving and replacing objects in a mechanical manner. When the mother returned, the young girl immediately found toys to give her and became very solicitous as to her welfare. Was mother all right, did she need or want anything? Mother, herself, sat without giving the child any explanation; there was no physical contact and no response to the child. Role reversal and parentified behaviour emerges in children with insecure attachment and this pattern was evident here (Toth *et al*, 2000).

Case example 2

Two small boys, 4 years and 2 years old, were referred for assessment, with suspicions of physical abuse or factitious illness induced by a parent. The two children and mother were seen together. Asked to separate, the mother walked out with no explanation. The 4-year-old watched, but the 2-year-old did not. Neither child followed or went to the door, neither child cried or appeared troubled. On the mother's return, the 2-year-old crawled under a chair and appeared stuck between a chair leg and the wall. The 4-year-old walked backwards away from his mother, hit the wall of the room, fell on to his face on the floor and lay there. The mother appeared not to notice the 2-year-old and a therapist had to extricate the child. The older child lay until encouraged to come and play. This older child was thought to have a disorganised attachment and the younger one to be avoidant. This aspect of the assessment was very significant. It was explained to the mother when she was seen individually. Over a series of interviews, it led to a partial disclosure of physical abuse and episodes of drowsiness and semi-consciousness in the older child due to nitrazepam, given by the mother.

Describing these examples, it is important to acknowledge that attachment is only one aspect of a full assessment and describes only one aspect of the child's functioning (Department of Health, 2000). It does, however, provide some indicators of future progress, relationships and school performance (Lyons-Ruth, 1992; Easterbrooks *et al*, 1993; Cicchetti &

Toth, 1995, 1998). The reactions to separations and reunions can be helpful in assessing children up to puberty and sometimes beyond.

Assessing adults

Assessing the parents, grandparents or substitute carers requires a range of skills, and may involve a multiprofessional team or network. Work is accumulating that indicates that the attachment status of the adult does provide quite a robust indicator of that person's capacity to provide an emotionally healthy environment for the child (Lyons-Ruth *et al*, 1992; Van Izzendoorn, 1992).

Meeting with such adults, one should take a history, assess physical and mental health and obtain a social history (see Chapter 7). Attachment theory provides a means of trying to understand the adult's state of mind during this account. Is there coherence and consistency, and – perhaps more importantly – have these individuals come to terms with and accepted the vicissitudes that life has thrown at them? Where these individuals have little or no recall of childhood, or where they are still engrossed in the wrongs and adversities they have experienced, then this is an indication of a need to explore in more depth, as there are likely to be attachment problems. The interview should enquire about early memories, and relationships with parents or caregivers. It can then move on to explore losses, separations and traumas. Questions about these may produce a flood of highly charged emotions. If there was a significant event in the past year (such as a bereavement), no conclusion can be drawn; but if the loss or trauma was some time ago, the response must be evaluated carefully. If the account shifts to the present tense or there are impossible elements included such as time sequences or place distortions, then the interviewer needs to be alerted; there may be unresolved issues. For example, a woman had already explained in her history about her period in care for 3 years as a child. In response to a question about any separations, there was a complete denial of any separation from her mother, who was described as loving and caring. This was seen as a lapse of reasoning and monitoring of the self, and led to further assessment. Where there is a history of abuse (physical, sexual or emotional) then there may be inconsistencies in the account of the trauma itself; but the experience may also intrude into the interview at other points in an inappropriate way. This indicates that the trauma is a preoccupying unresolved area, and this may well distort or change the adult's capacity to be available to the child (Main & Hesse, 1990).

Case example 3

Asked about any abuse in his own childhood, a father talked, in a distressed way, of being beaten by his father but was definite that this was in the past. Later in the interview, in the midst of another topic, he interjected in a very fearful way, using the present tense to describe a time he had been locked in the understairs cupboard for hours in the dark. Desperate to visit the toilet, he had feared a further beating if he messed himself. He needed to leave the room in the here and now to visit the toilet and on his return did not refer to this incident again.

These examples may be seen as extreme and have been chosen to emphasise the process, but lesser examples are surprisingly common.

Anxiety disorders

Fears and anxieties are common in childhood. To some extent anxiety is an appropriate emotional response, as children develop and new situations present, such as attending nursery or school, visiting friends or experiencing new events in the home. It is only of concern when it is persistent and becomes disabling. The presentation depends on the child's developmental stage. Young children may show separation anxiety or fears that are quite simple, such as of the dark. Older children may present with school-related fears or anxieties about monsters, television programmes or falling asleep. Adolescents become anxious about body image, their peer group's acceptance of them, school or society, and achievement relating to the opposite gender. There is increasing acknowledgement, however, of the extent to which anxiety may impair, limit and distort children's lives.

The anxious child or young person reacts with variable severity to external or internal events with sweating, shaking and internal changes. Fear is a normal response based on rational consideration of the source of concern. The responses of hyperarousal and tachycardia prepare the individual for 'fight or flight' – that is, assertive or aggressive approach or withdrawal. In anxiety the responses are similar, but anxiety arises because evaluation of the situation is irrational and unrealistic, often because of the emotional or mental state of the individual which makes it feel threatening. Adequate attachments mean the individual has a 'secure base' from which they feel confident with good self-esteem. Without this the individual is more vulnerable and more likely to feel threatened by a situation they perceive as aversive to themselves, and a likely response is anxiety in one form or another.

Anxiety disorders are more common than previously recognised (Anderson, 1994) and consist of a range of disorders with onset specific to childhood, and other disorders, commonly associated with stress and adjustment, which can occur at any age. The former category comprises a range of separation and phobic disorders. There are also some disorders of social functioning that include selective mutism and reactive attachment disorder. These disorders, which can be understood within an attachment framework, are discussed below. The more general emotional and adjustment disorders are reviewed later in this chapter.

Anxiety-related disorders with onset specific to childhood (ICD–10 categories F93–F94)

Separation anxiety disorder (F93.0)

Pre-school children all have some degree of separation anxiety when they are aware a significant other or attachment figure is leaving. They become anxious, clingy and vulnerable. In most children, this phase passes and there is enough confidence and trust to come to accept that others go but come back.

When this confidence is not there some children go on to show separation anxiety disorder. They are unable or very reluctant to attend school, and while away worry that something bad will happen to a close relative. They are unhappy in the home on their own and will not go away overnight to friends; if forced, they become very distressed. Separation anxiety underlies much of so-called 'school phobia'.

Phobic anxiety disorders (F93.1)

Minor fears of the dark, dogs, ghosts and monsters, for example, are extremely common in childhood. Most children suffer one or two such fears at some time. They become a phobic disorder when the fear becomes irrational and it leads to avoidance. Examples include a child who will not enter a shed for a fear of spiders, or cannot go down a street for fear of being bitten by a dog. For this to become a disorder, the avoidance should be of a degree that it leads to impairment of functioning.

Other phobias include claustrophobia or agoraphobia, in which the child is afraid in a small place such as a lift, where they feel trapped, or very anxious in wide-open spaces such as a park. This then leads to avoidance of these situations and subsequently to disruption of social functioning and age-appropriate independence. Social phobia describes a situation of extreme anxiety with new people or groups, or situations when the child is required to appear in front of others. School and out-of-school activities can present considerable difficulties for such a child. Behavioural therapies with a cognitive component for older children are the treatments of choice.

Elective mutism (F94.0) and selective mutism

This consists of a relative or absolute failure to speak in social situations, with interference with educational and social communication. It lasts for more than a month and is not accounted for by a communication disorder. For an excellent overview, see Standart & Le Couteur (2003).

The prevalence rate is about 0.4 per 1000 children and the differential diagnosis includes normal shyness, Asperger syndrome and incipient psychosis. In the family background, depression or social phobia may be present (Kolvin & Fundudis, 1981, 1993; Kolvin *et al*, 1997). The talking therapies are understandably challenged by these cases (Black & Uhde, 1995), but creative and cognitive–behavioural therapies are the treatments of choice. The use of psychopharmacological treatment is of uncertain benefit, but fluoxetine has been described as helpful in promoting communication (Black & Uhde, 1994).

Reactive attachment disorder (F94.1)

This refers to a pattern of insecure and disorganised attachment behaviours, specifying them as inhibited or indiscriminate.

Markedly disturbed and developmentally inappropriate social relatedness is seen in most contexts, beginning before the age of 5 years. The child shows either persistent failure to initiate or respond to social situations, or diffuse indiscriminate attachments. The disturbance cannot be accounted for by developmental delay. The cause is presumed to be due to poor care, with persistent disregard for the child's basic emotional or physical needs, or else to a repeated change of primary caregiver.

Stress-related disorders (F40–F48)

The word 'stress' is used frequently in lay media, and is defined in the *Oxford English Dictionary* as 'to subject a person to force, compulsion, constraint, restrain, confine, incarcerate, afflict, harass or oppress'. This indicates that stress or mental stress is inflicted by a situation or on a person by another. As with anxiety, to feel stressed can be an appropriate response to a situation or it can be an excessive response to a situation that is perceived to be less stressful by others.

Stress then is a broad term and is part of the individual's ordinary experience. It results in individual patterns of adaptation that are dependent on intelligence, affective state, previous experience, physical state and past/present relationships. When the stress cannot be managed, because of individual factors or because it is so great that it becomes overwhelming, then physical, cognitive or affective symptoms emerge.

Stress-related disorders are classified in ICD–10 as acute stress reaction, post-traumatic stress disorder and adjustment disorders.

Meade *et al* (2001) looked at stress, emotional skill and illness in children. They found that negative events (such as a new adult in the home, seeing serious violence) lead to stress and that the stress correlates positively with the children's poor health. They also found that where the children had the skills to communicate and identify their feelings, their health was better, but interestingly it was reported as worse by the parent.

Rutter (1979, 1994), writing on stress research, states that negative events and experiences are associated with psychopathology in childhood, such as bereavement, divorce and remarriage, chronic physical disorders, and man-made and natural disasters. However, it is the accumulation of events over time that contributes to psychological resilience or vulnerability of the individual, rather than the actual event itself. Major life changes may be desirable or undesirable and the cognitive appraisal of the events and the social context are important in considering the level of threat.

Stress is therefore mediated by mechanisms that lead to psychopathological disorder. Resilience factors such as social competence may protect the individual. There are sensitive periods in the developmental pathway when stress can have a more detrimental, longer-lasting effect. For example, maternal depression in the first year of life is associated with significant cognitive impairment, although later maternal depression does not have this effect (Murray, 1992).

Individual differences in vulnerability to stress may be mediated by genetic as well as environmental variables. Other factors include gender, the capacity to make active plans, and behaviour patterns of the individual such as aggression and racial discrimination. McMahon et al (2003) have undertaken an extensive review of the links between stress and psychopathology and found little specificity.

The ICD–10 classification system devotes a section to 'Reactions to Severe Stress and Adjustment Disorders'.

Phobic anxiety disorders (F40)

The ICD system includes in the general section those phobic disorders that may arise in childhood, but are not a part of psychosocial development, such as agoraphobia.

Panic disorder (F41.0)

The anxiety and fear is so overwhelming that the child has a massive psychological and autonomic reaction. The sweating and shaking can be unmanageable, and the child may become pale, feel faint or have a full vasovagal episode; the child may become terrified of losing consciousness or of dying.

Generalised over-anxious disorder (F41.1)

Generalised over-anxious disorder seems to arise from fear of a horrendous event occurring, such as a war, a bomb, an earthquake, a fire or a tornado. It is based on anxiety about the person's own survival or that of a loved one.

Obsessive–compulsive disorder (F42)

Obsessive–compulsive disorder is often a severe and disabling condition. In adolescents in the community prevalence rates range from 1% to 4% (Thompson, 1999; Zohar, 1999).

Obsessions are recurrent unwanted intrusive thoughts, ideas, images or impulses that the person experiences as distressing. Often they relate to contamination, harm and death or are somatic, religious or sexual. Compulsions are repetitive physical or mental acts that the person is driven to perform, such as checking, washing or touching. The course is often chronic and the onset peaks at puberty (Zohar, 1999), with slightly more boys than girls affected.

Cognitive–behavioural therapy is the treatment of choice for this disorder (March et al, 1997). Pharmacological treatments begin with selective serotonin reuptake inhibitors (SSRIs), of which only fluoxetine is now recommended for use with children and young people. For intractable obsessive–compulsive disorder a low dose of risperidone can often be very helpful, at a dosage of 0.5 mg or 1 mg (McDougle et al, 2000). There is a useful review of obsessive–compulsive disorder in children and adolescents by Shafran (2001).

Acute stress reaction (F43.0)

Acute stress reaction occurs when the individual has been subjected to a traumatic event that confronts the person with the possibility of death or serious injury, and the response involves intense fear or helplessness. The response lasts up to 4 weeks.

Post-traumatic stress disorder (F43.1)

Post-traumatic stress disorder (PTSD) is a form of anxiety disorder arising after a major traumatic event, the course of which has been established more clearly in recent years (Box 10.1) (Yule, 1991; Udwin, 1993). The DSM–IV criteria (American Psychiatric Association, 1994) are more inclusive than ICD–10, and are used more commonly in medico-legal claims.

A study reported by Udwin et al (2000) and Bolton et al (2000) explored the risk factors for long-term effects of trauma in adolescence in an attempt to predict PTSD. In this study individuals who were female, had had previous problems with learning or psychological problems and had experienced violence in the home were more likely to develop PTSD after a trauma. There was also a strong link with the perceived level of threat and the fear of being injured. These authors suggested that screening individuals for anxiety after a traumatic event with an account of their own appraisal of the experience could identify those most at risk.

Box 10.1 The course and diagnosis of post-traumatic stress disorder

A *Exposure to a traumatic event*

1. The person experienced, witnessed or was confronted by an event or events that involved actual or threatened death, serious injury or threat to their physical integrity
2. The person's response involved intense fear, helplessness or horror

B *The traumatic event is persistently re-experienced in one or more of the following ways*

1. Recurrent intrusive distressing recollections including images, thoughts or perceptions
2. Recurrent distressing dreams of the event
3. Acting or feeling as though the traumatic event was recurring
4. Intense psychological distress of exposure to internal or external cues of the event(s)
5. Physiological reactivity on such exposure

C *Avoidance is indicated by three or more of the following*

1. Efforts to avoid thoughts or feeling associated with the trauma
2. Efforts to avoid activity, places or people that arouse recollections
3. Inability to recall the important aspects of the trauma
4. Diminished interest in significant activities
5. Feelings of detachment
6. Restricted affect
7. Sense of foreshortened future

D *Symptoms of increased arousal (two or more)*

1. Difficulty in falling or staying asleep
2. Irritability or outbursts of anger
3. Difficulty concentrating
4. Hypervigilance
5. Exaggerated startle responses

E ***Duration is more than 1 month***

F ***Disturbance is clinically significant***

In a second study, this group of researchers looked at children and adolescents who had had traumatic experiences and developed PTSD, comparing them with a non-traumatised control group to see if there was any impact on their capacity to judge negative events. The PTSD sample stated that negative events were more likely to happen to others rather than themselves and this was true for physically and socially threatening events. The authors suggest that some form of inhibition is operating to limit their appraisal capacity (Dalgleish *et al*, 2000).

In a more recently reported study by Keppel-Benson *et al* (2002), post-traumatic stress was explored in children after motor vehicle accidents. They found that 7 children out of 50 developed PTSD, and that the degree of physical injury led to more PTSD symptoms, whereas

167

previous accident experience reduced them. Also, they found that the higher the level of social support, the fewer PTSD symptoms followed.

All these studies have looked at the response of children and young people to severe stressors and traumatic events. Another related field where stress, trauma and PTSD have been extensively explored is the aftermath of child abuse. Physical, emotional and sexual abuse is not generally a one-off event but involves a more prolonged exposure to stress and trauma. Post-traumatic stress disorder is now recognised as a significant problem for these children and young people (Beitchman *et al*, 1991; Deblinger *et al*, 1996; Trowell *et al*, 2002).

Abused children can be very troubled by PTSD. Trowell *et al* (2002) found that 76% of girls in their study had PTSD at assessment. Their symptoms consisted of flashbacks and re-experiencing phenomena, hyperarousal and dissociation. Perhaps because abuse can continue over many years, the PTSD can appear more 'chronic', with dissociation and the accommodation syndrome much in evidence. This consists of the child coming to experience the abuse as a normal part of life, and high level of distress, fear or other emotions become muted as the child dissociates more effectively. Their affective and cognitive functioning is limited, however, owing to the dissociation.

Adjustment disorders (F43.2)

Adjustment disorders comprise states of subjective distress and emotional disturbance usually interfering with social functioning and performance, arising in the period of adaptation to a significant life change or a stressful life event. The stress may involve the close relationships of the child, e.g. a bereavement, or the wider social environment, e.g. becoming a refugee or migrating.

Onset of symptoms occurs within a month and may be characterised by disturbance of emotions, conduct or both.

Epidemiology

Although childhood fears are common in middle childhood, Klein (1994), reviewing the rates of anxiety disorders, found the mean age of onset to be 16 years for generalised anxiety disorder. Twelve years of age is the mean for the onset of social or simple phobia (Bourdon *et al*, 1988). Anderson (1994) gave prevalence figures for any anxiety disorder of 2–9% of children and young people, the figure for each form of anxiety ranging from 1% to 9% of children (see Chapter 5). More girls than boys have anxiety disorders, and the coexistence of several forms of anxiety disorder is common. Comorbidity with other disorders such as conduct disorder or major depressive disorder is also frequently seen.

General treatment issues

Anxiety disorders can be disabling and merit energetic treatment. The first-line treatment is the psychological therapies. Behavioural or cognitive–behavioural therapy has been shown to be effective (Fonagy *et al*, 2002). Other psychological therapies such as family therapy and psychodynamic therapy are thought also to be helpful, but the evidence base for their use is limited to anecdote, clinical practice and small outcome studies.

Where these therapies fail, psychopharmacological treatment can play a part (Bramble, 2003) (see Chapter 18). Benzodiazepines are used rarely in children and young people and probably have little part to play. Buspirone is used in adult anxiety disorders, but research is lacking in children. The SSRIs are used most commonly, in particular fluoxetine, but fluvoxamine has a greater evidence base (Chapter 18). Where the physiological symptoms, such as sweating tremor, are severe in adolescents, beta-blockers such as propanolol or atenolol are sometimes used.

Cognitive–behavioural therapy, in which children and young people are encouraged and taught to develop relaxation strategies, coping strategies and planned exposure to the anxiety-provoking stressor, can be helpful. This may be individual or group therapy, usually given as a time-limited, focused course of 5–20 sessions.

Family therapy can be helpful in separation anxiety and some cases of generalised anxiety. Psychodynamic psychotherapy is favoured by its adherents for separation anxiety, generalised anxiety and panic attacks if the child or young person has had a traumatic, disrupted early childhood and the anxiety difficulties are part of an internalised confused sense of self, although the evidence base is not strong. Attachments are seen as insecure or disorganised, and the child or young person uses the therapist–patient relationship to develop and rebuild attachment patterns.

Carr (2000) and Fonagy *et al* (2002) have reviewed studies of outcome. An underrecognised part of the work is the need to work with and support the parents and carers (Rushton & Miles, 2000). This is not only to ensure children attend treatment, but also to work on helping parents and carers to allow the child or adolescent to change. They need to tolerate considerable anger that may now be expressed, particularly by the adolescent, and defiance, opposition and depression may emerge. Parents may also have considerable difficulties of their own and need a place to work on their issues to lift the burden from their child. Parents may suffer depression, with losses, separations and disruptions that have been hidden by the child's separation anxiety, generalised anxiety or panic attacks. Intergenerational issues are very common. Phobias are often more individual to the child, although social phobias, agoraphobia and claustrophobia may be linked to a depressed, phobic parent; often this is the mother.

Interventions

Most stress reactions that are excessive and lead to symptoms can be greatly helped by cognitive–behavioural therapy (Yule *et al*, 2000). Where there has been a shared experience of disaster, this could well be in a group situation, probably incorporating a psychoeducational emphasis, although critical incident debriefing on non-selected patients is not widely supported. Where the distress of PTSD is extreme, SSRI antidepressants may provide short-term relief for adolescents.

Some individuals with PTSD who have severe emotional difficulties after abuse where there have been many disruptions, losses and betrayals may benefit from psychodynamic psychotherapy. This individual child-led therapy allows the child or young person to work on the particular confusions, conflicts and issues at their own pace. Psychodynamic group work can also be beneficial post-abuse.

Conclusion

Many children and young people can become very distressed and troubled by anxiety and stress. Their attachment relationships are central to how these are managed. Securely attached children and young people are usually robust enough to manage, given support, whether the precipitating event is an internal or external stressor. The attachment relationship gives them resilience, particularly if constitutional factors are also robust.

Vulnerable individuals may have constitutional attachment relationship difficulties or other vulnerabilities and they may then develop symptoms or disorders. Interventions need to relieve distress and concentrate on reducing confusions, developing coping strategies and encouraging secure attachments.

References

Ainsworth, M. D. S., Blehar, M. C., Waters, E., *et al* (1978) *Patterns of Attachment: A Psychological Study of the Strange Situation*. Hillsdale, NJ: Erlbaum.

American Psychiatric Association (1994) *Quick Reference to the Diagnostic Criteria from DSM–IV* (4th edn). Washington, DC: American Psychiatric Association.

Anderson, J. (1994) Epidemiological Issues. In *International Handbook of Phobic and Anxiety Disorders in Children and Adolescents* (eds T. Ollendeck, N. King & W. Yule), pp. 43–46. New York: Plenum.

Beitchman, J. H., Zucker, K. J. & Wood, J. E. (1991) A review of the short-term effects of child sexual abuse. *Child Abuse and Neglect*, **15**, 537–556.

Black, B. & Uhde, T. (1994) Treatment of elective mutism with fluoxetine. A double-blind, placebo-controlled study. *Journal of the American Academy of Child and Adolescent Psychiatry*, **33**, 1000–1006.

Black, B. & Uhde, T. (1995) Psychiatric characteristics of children with selective mutism: a pilot study. *Journal of the American Academy of Child and Adolescent Psychiatry*, **34**, 847–856.

Bolton, D., O'Ryan, D., Udwin, O., *et al* (2000) The long-term psychological effects of a disaster experience in adolescence. II: General psychopathology. *Journal of Child Psychiatry and Psychology*, **41**, 513–523.

Bourdon, K., Boyd, J., Rae, D., *et al* (1988) Gender differences in phobias: results of the ECA community survey. *Journal of Anxiety Disorders*, **2**, 227–241.

Bowlby, J. (1973) *Attachment and Loss, vol. 2. Separation*. New York: Basic Books.

Bowlby, J. (1980) *Attachment and Loss, vol. 3. Loss: Sadness and Depression*. New York: Basic Books.

Bowlby, J. (1982) *Attachment and Loss, vol.1. Attachment* (2nd edn). New York: Basic Books.

Bramble, D. (2003) Annotation: the use of psychotropic medications in children: a British view. *Journal of Child Psychiatry and Psychology*, **4**, 169–179.

Carr, A. (ed.) (2000) *What Works with Children and Adolescents? A Critical Review of Psychological Interventions with Children, Adolescents and Their Families*. London: Routledge.

Cichetti, D. & Toth, S. (1995) Developmental psychopathology and disorders of affect. In *Developmental Psychopathology*, vol. 2: *Risk Disorder and Adaptations* (eds D. Cichetti & D. Cohen), pp. 369–420. New York: Wiley.

Cicchetti, D. & Toth, S. (1998) The development of depression in children and adolescents. *American Psychologist*, **53**, 221–241.

Dalgleish, T., Moradi, A., Taghavi, R., *et al* (2000) Judgements about emotional events in children and adolescents with post-traumatic stress disorder and controls. *Journal of Child Psychology and Psychiatry and Allied Disciplines*, **41**, 981–988.

Deblinger, E., Lippermann, J. & Stern, R. (1996) Sexually abused children suffering post-traumatic stress symptoms: initial treatment outcome findings. *Child Maltreatment*, **1**, 310–321.

Department of Health (2000) *Framework for the Assessment of Children in Need and Their Families*. London: Stationery Office.

De Wolff, M. & Van Izzendoorn, M. (1997) Sensitivity and attachment: a meta-analysis on parental antecedent of infant attachment. *Child Development*, **68**, 571–591.

Easterbrooks, M., Davidson, C. & Chazan, R. (1993) Psychosocial risk, attachment and behaviour problems among school aged children. *Development and Psychopathology*, **5**, 389–402.

Fonagy, P., Target, M., Cottrell, D., *et al* (2002) *What Works for Whom? A Critical Review of Treatments for Children and Adolescents*. New York: Guilford Press.

Keppel-Benson, J., Ollendick, T. & Benson, M. (2002) Post-traumatic stress in children following motor vehicle accidents. *Journal of Child Psychology and Psychiatry*, **43**, 203–212.

Klein, R. (1994) *Anxiety Disorders in Child and Adolescent Psychiatry*. Oxford: Blackwell.

Kolvin, I. & Fundudis, T. (1981) Elective mute children: psychological development and background factors. *Journal of Child Psychology and Psychiatry*, **22**, 219–232.

Kolvin, I. & Fundudis, T. (1993) Communicative behaviour with neurotic developmental disorder: elective mutism. In *Linguistic Disorders and Pathologies* (eds G. Blanken, J. Dittman, H. Grimm, *et al*). New York: Walter de Gruyter.

Kolvin, I., Trowell, J., Le Couteur, A., *et al* (1997) *The Origins of Selective Mutism: Some Strategies for Attachment and Bonding Research*. ACPP Occasional Paper 14, pp. 17–25. London: Association for Child Psychology and Psychiatry.

Lyons-Ruth, K. (1992) Maternal depressive symptoms, disorganized infant–mother attachment relationships and hostile aggressive behaviour in the pre-school classroom. A prospective longitudinal view from infancy to age five. In *Rochester Symposium on Developmental Psychopathology*, vol. 4: *Developmental Perspectives in Depression* (eds D. Cichetti & S. Toth), pp. 131–171. Rochester, NY: University of Rochester Press.

Lyons-Ruth, K., Repacholi, B., McLeod, S., *et al* (1992) Disorganised attachment behaviour in infancy: short-term stability, maternal and infant correlates and risk related subtypes. *Development and Psychopathology*, **3**, 377–396.

Main, M. & Goldwyn, R. (1998) *Adult Attachment Scoring and Classification System*. Berkeley, CA: University of California at Berkeley, Department of Psychology.

Main, M. & Hesse, E. (1990) Parents' unresolved traumatic experiences are related to infant disorganized attachment status. Is frightened and/or frightening parental behaviour the linking mechanism? In *Attachment in the Pre-school Years* (eds M. T. Greenberg, D. Cicchetti & E. M. Cummings), pp. 161–182. Chicago, IL: University of Chicago.

Main, M., Kaplan, N. & Cassidy, J. (1985) Security in infancy, childhood and adulthood: a move to the level of representation. In *Growing Points of Attachment Theory and Research* (eds I. Bretherton & E. Waters), pp. 66–104. Chicago, IL: University of Chicago Press.

March, J. S., Frances, A., Kahn, D., *et al* (1997) Consensus guidelines treatment of obsessive–compulsive disorder. *Journal of Clinical Psychiatry*, **58**, 1–72.

McDougle, C. J., Epperson, C. N., Pelton, G. H., *et al* (2000) A double-blind placebo-controlled study of risperidone addition in serotonin reuptake inhibitor in refractory obsessive compulsive disorder. *Archives of General Psychiatry*, **57**, 794–801.

McMahon, S., Grant, K., Compas, B., *et al* (2003) Stress and psychopathology in children and adolescents: is there evidence of specificity? *Journal of Child Psychiatry and Psychology*, **44**, 107–133.

Meade, J., Lumley, M. & Casey, R. (2001) Stress, emotional skill and illness reports. *Journal of Child Psychiatry and Psychology*, **42**, 405–412.

Murray, L. (1992) The impact of post-natal depression in infant development. *Journal of Child Psychology and Psychiatry*, **33**, 543–561.

Rushton, A. & Miles, G. (2000) Study of support service for current carers of sexually abused girls. *Journal of Clinical Child Psychology and Psychiatry*, **5**, 411–426.

Rutter, M. (1979) Protective factors in children's responses to stress and disadvantage. In *Primary Preventions of Psychopathology*, vol. 3: *Social Competence in Children* (eds M. W. Kent & J. E. Rolt), pp. 49–74. Hanover, NH: University Press of New England.

Rutter, M. (1994) Stress research: accomplishment and tasks ahead. In *Stress Risk and Resilience in Children and Adolescents* (eds R. Heggerty, L. Sherrod, Y. N. Garmez, *et al*). Cambridge: Cambridge University Press.

Shafran, R. (2001) Obsessive–compulsive disorder in children and adolescents. *Child Psychology and Psychiatry Review*, **6**, 50–58.

Standart, S. & Le Couteur, A. L. (2003) The quiet child: a literature review of selective mutism. *Child and Adolescent Mental Health*, **8**, 154–160.

Thompson, P. H. (1999) *From Thoughts to Obsessions: Obsessive–Compulsive Disorder in Children and Adolescents*. London: Jessica Kingsley.

Toth, S., Cicchetti, D., Macfie, J., *et al* (2000) Narrative representation of caregivers and self in maltreated preschoolers. *Attachment and Human Development*, **2**, 271–305.

Trowell, J., Kolvin, I., Weeramanthri, T., *et al* (2002) Psychotherapy for sexually abused girls: psychopathological outcome findings and patterns of change. *British Journal of Psychiatry*, **180**, 234–247.

Udwin, O. (1993) Annotation: children's reactions to traumatic events. *Journal of Child Psychology and Psychiatry*, **34**, 115–127.

Udwin, O., Boyle, S., Yule, W., *et al* (2000) Risk factors for long-term psychological effects of a disaster experienced in adolescence: predictors of post traumatic stress disorder. *Journal of Child Psychology and Psychiatry*, **41**, 969–979.

Van Izzendoorn, M. H. (1992) Intergenerational transmission of parenting: a review of studies in non-clinical populations. *Developmental Review*, **12**, 76–99.

Van Izzendoorn, M. H., Juffer, F. & Duyresteyn, M. (1995) Breaking the intergenerational cycle of insecure attachment: a review of the effects of attachment based interventions on maternal sensitivity and infant security. *Journal of Child Psychology and Psychiatry*, **36**, 225–248.

World Health Organization (1992) *The ICD-10 Classification of Mental and Behavioural Disorders: Clinical Descriptions and Diagnostic Guidelines*. Geneva: WHO.

World Health Organization (1995) *Multi-Axial Version of ICD–10: Prepared for Use by Clinicians Dealing with Children and Adolescent Psychiatric Disorders*. Cambridge: Cambridge University Press.

Yule, W. (1991) Working with children following disasters. In *Clinical Child Psychology: Social Learning, Development and Behaviour* (ed. M. Herbert), pp. 349–633. Chichester: John Wiley.

Yule, W., Bolton, D., Udwin, O., *et al* (2000) The long-term psychological effects of a disaster experience in adolescence: I. The evidence and course of post-traumatic stress disorder. *Journal of Child Psychology and Psychiatry*, **41**, 503–511.

Zohar, A. H. (1999) The epidemiology of obsessive compulsive disorder in children and adolescents. *Child and Adolescent Psychiatric Clinics of North America*, **8**, 445–460.

CHAPTER 11

Depression and self-harm

Andrew J. Cotgrove

Depression is a widely used and commonly understood term. In lay language, it is often used synonymously with sadness or unhappiness. However, in psychiatry, depression refers to a syndrome consisting of more than just an isolated symptom. Self-harm, on the other hand, is a behaviour that may or may not be associated with a psychiatric disorder. The two are linked, in that both can be associated with feelings of despair or hopelessness, and in addition both are commonly associated with a range of comorbid psychiatric disorders that can affect their course and outcome.

This chapter systematically reviews the epidemiology, clinical features, aetiology, management and prognosis for both depression and self-harm.

Depression

Epidemiology

Community prevalence rates for depressive disorder increase during childhood and adolescence from approximately 0.5–2.5% in pre-adolescence to between 2% and 8% during adolescence (Harrington, 1994). In mental health settings, prevalence rates rise dramatically, with as many as 60% of referred children having depressive symptoms (Carlson & Cantwell, 1980) and one in four being diagnosable with a major depressive disorder (Kolvin et al, 1991). This serves to illustrate further the high levels of comorbid disorder, as most of these children were referred to mental health services for other difficulties (Harrington et al, 1990).

Gender ratios also change with age. At the age of 11 years there is no difference between the rates of depression for boys and girls. Prevalence rates for both sexes then increase steadily through adolescence, most markedly in girls. By the mid-teens, the rates resemble those of the adult disorder, with depression being twice as likely in females as in males (Angold & Rutter, 1992).

Diagnosis and clinical features

The presentation of a depressive disorder varies according to the developmental stage of the child or adolescent. Children's cognitive experiences, for example feelings of guilt, and their abilities to communicate their feelings and experiences accurately are different from adults. However, despite these differences it is generally accepted that depressive disorders akin to those seen in adults occur in children and adolescents (Harrington & Wood, 1995). Indeed, in DSM–IV (American Psychiatric Association, 1994), the criteria for pre-pubertal, adolescent and adult depression are almost identical.

The typical symptoms of a depressive episode (ICD–10, World Health Organization, 1992) or major depressive episode (DSM–IV) are listed in Table 11.1.

Both ICD–10 and DSM–IV require that symptoms be present for at least 2 weeks in order for a diagnosis to be made; DSM–IV, which operationalises its criteria for major depressive episodes by requiring five or more symptoms, also requires that the symptoms result in significant distress or impairment in social, occupational or other important areas of functioning. Thus, there is an attempt to exclude those with mild or transient symptoms.

In younger children, low mood may manifest itself in frustration or temper outbursts, and there may be additional psychosomatic symptoms such as headaches or stomach aches. Loss of interest, poor concentration and poor attention may also be prominent, as well as separation anxiety, school refusal or failure to progress academically. In older children and adolescents, irritability, anxiety (or motor agitation) and social withdrawal tend to feature more than in adults with depressive disorder.

Table 11.1 Typical symptoms of depression

Symptom	Included in	
Depressed mood	DSM–IV	ICD–10
Loss of interest and enjoyment	DSM–IV	ICD–10
Reduced energy leading to increased tiredness and diminished activity	DSM–IV	ICD–10
Psychomotor agitation or retardation	DSM–IV	
Reduced concentration and attention	DSM–IV	ICD–10
Reduced self-esteem and self-confidence		ICD–10
Ideas of guilt and unworthiness	DSM–IV	ICD–10
Bleak and pessimistic views of the future, including thoughts of death	DSM–IV	ICD–10
Ideas or acts of self-harm or suicide	DSM–IV	ICD–10
Disturbed sleep, diminished appetite and weight loss	DSM–IV	ICD–10

There are high rates of comorbid disorder in children and adolescents with depression. In one study, 93% of cases of depression presenting to child and adolescent mental health services were found to have a comorbid diagnosis (Goodyer *et al*, 1997). The most common of these were separation anxiety disorder (65%), oppositional defiant disorder (44%), conduct disorder (37%), social phobia disorder (37%), panic disorder (25%), generalised anxiety disorder (25%) and dysthymia (25%). Other studies have also reported high rates of comorbid attention-deficit disorder and anorexia nervosa. High levels of alcohol consumption may be an additional association. Children and adolescents with a depressive disorder are therefore likely to have multiple problems. In addition to the 'endogenous symptoms' listed in Table 11.1, they often experience difficulties with school work and social withdrawal, and they are likely to have significant problems relating to peers.

Classification

A range of approaches have been used in the classification of depressive disorders in children and adolescents (Harrington & Wood, 1995).

The subdivision of affective disorders into bipolar disorder (episodes of depression and mania) and unipolar disorder (depression only) is well accepted in adults and there is increasing evidence of its validity in younger people. Juvenile probands with bipolar disorder are more likely to have relatives with bipolar disorder than probands with unipolar depression (Kutcher & Marton, 1991). Further evidence is available: first, in the prognostic implications of this diagnosis; second, in the response of bipolar disorder to lithium prophylaxis; and third, evidence that an episode of mania may be induced by a tricyclic antidepressant in children with a family history of bipolar disorder.

Another sub-classification with validity in adults distinguishes between those with and without somatic symptoms (e.g. appetite disturbance, early morning wakening and psychomotor retardation). Studies in younger people have been less conclusive, and the distinction between somatic and non-somatic depression appears to be more one of severity rather than representing qualitatively different disorders.

The DSM–IV classification makes the distinction between acute depression (major depressive disorder) and chronic depression (dysthymia), which lasts for more than 1 year but has fewer symptoms. This has resulted in some confusion, in that some investigators have included both dysthymia and chronic major depressive disorder in the same group. Young people with dysthymia tend to have an earlier age of onset, a slower rate of improvement, higher rates of social impairment and comorbidity with behavioural disorders. However, on long-term follow-up, the two disorders have similar outcomes and the distinction may just be one of severity and duration.

Many researchers have classified depression according to whether its onset comes before or after puberty. The rapid rise in the incidence of this disorder after puberty suggests there may be a biological explanation for this, but social or cognitive changes may be just as significant.

Finally, it is also possible to sub-classify depressive disorders according to comorbidity. In particular, children with comorbid depression and conduct disorder have been found to have lower rates of depression among relatives and greater variability of mood when compared with depressed children with no conduct problems. The ICD–10 recognises the significance of this association with a classification of mixed disorder of conduct and emotion: 'depressive conduct disorder' (F92.0). Just as with conduct disorder, it would seem likely that a significant proportion of this group will go on to develop personality disorders with an affective component such as emotionally unstable personality disorder, borderline type F60.31 (ICD–10).

Those with comorbid anxiety disorder and depressive disorder tend to have increased severity and duration of depressive symptoms, particularly suicidality, increased risk of substance misuse, poor response to psychotherapy and increased psychosocial problems.

Aetiology

There are clear familial links in child and adolescent depression. Children of depressed parents have greater than expected rates of depression (Radke-Yarrow et al, 1992). Harrington et al (1993) demonstrated that lifetime prevalence rates of depression in relatives of depressed children were twice that of relatives of non-depressed controls. Although these and other studies show a strong familial component, there has to date been no conclusive twin or molecular genetic study supporting a genetic aetiology of depressive symptoms in childhood (Rice et al, 2002), with the exception of a small group who have bipolar affective disorder.

A link between adverse events and depressive symptoms has been demonstrated. Specific events including loss, parental divorce and exposure to suicide have been associated with the onset of depression. Friendship difficulties may also be relevant, as well as schooling difficulties and bullying. These links are non-specific and those experiencing an event are as likely to develop anxiety as depression.

The role of biological mechanisms in the aetiology of depression remains unclear. As with adults, the monoamine hypothesis proposes that depression can result from hypoactivity of monoamine neurotransmitter systems in the brain (Deakin & Crow, 1986). Support for this hypothesis comes from observations that drugs that deplete monoamines can cause depression and drugs that inhibit monoamine reuptake have an antidepressant effect. However, there is no direct evidence to support this as an aetiological factor in depression. Abnormalities in basal cortisol levels have been found in some young people with depression (Goodyer et al, 1991) and some have abnormal sleep electroencephalograms (EEGs), usually relating to abnormal rapid eye movement sleep (Kutcher et al, 1992). However, these are not homogeneous findings and their significance is unclear.

Management

Assessment

The management of all suspected cases of depressive disorder should start with a thorough assessment. Indeed, from the evidence presented earlier it may be appropriate to screen others presenting to child and adolescent mental health services for evidence of depressive disorder. Multiple sources of information should be sought, including information taken individually from the child, the family and the school. The young person should be seen individually to assess his or her mental state, including an assessment of suicidal thoughts. Studies have consistently shown that family members underestimate the presence of depressive symptoms, many of which are purely subjective (Barrett et al, 1991). Children are often reticent about discussing how they are feeling with their parents for fear of upsetting them, and this may be exacerbated by feelings of guilt and low self-worth. In addition, children seen alone may feel able to disclose a precipitant such as bullying or abuse, which they would not reveal in front of their parents.

The diagnosis may be aided by the use of questionnaires or standardised interviews. These can provide both an aid to diagnosis and an objective measure of response to treatment. However, although several of these instruments show good interrater reliability, their test–retest reliability has not been as good because affective symptoms seem to be particularly unstable in this age group (Birmaher et al, 1996).

A full medical history and examination to exclude a physical cause for the symptoms should be included, with further investigations if appropriate. Additional psychobiological measures such as the dexamethasone suppression test, nocturnal growth hormone levels and sleep EEGs probably add nothing to the diagnosis or management of the individual.

As depressed children often have multiple problems such as educational failure, impaired psychosocial functioning and other comorbid disorders, exploring these issues needs to be included in the assessment.

Treatment

Treatment depends on the nature of the problems identified at assessment. If the disorder is mild, it may respond to supportive therapy and an amelioration of any maintaining factors. More severe disorder will need a more focused approach and therapy needs to be individually tailored to the needs of the patient. Specific and realistic goals should be agreed with the child and the family. An aim of reducing depression should go hand in hand with strategies designed to address related problems such as academic difficulties or peer relationship difficulties that may be serving to maintain the disorder.

Many different psychosocial interventions have been used to treat young people with depression. These include cognitive–behavioural therapy (CBT), interpersonal therapy, play therapy, psychodynamic psychotherapy, family therapy, psychodrama, art therapy and social skills training programmes. In the adult literature most evidence exists to support the efficacy of CBT or interpersonal therapy. Studies of these therapies have also shown promise with young people, and a meta-analysis of six randomised trials by Harrington et al (1998a) found CBT to be significantly superior to comparisons such as remaining on a waiting list or having relaxation training. Cognitive–behavioural therapy aims to treat the cognitive distortions identified in the depressed youngster. Sessions usually run for 8–12 weeks on a weekly basis, during which time the young person is encouraged to monitor his or her feelings and thoughts by means of a diary, and cognitive distortions can then be challenged (Harrington et al, 1998b). This style of therapy can also be effective as part of relapse prevention work.

Most families would benefit from attending sessions intended to educate them about the disorder and to provide general support. In cases where family pathology seems to be contributing to the disorder, it is sensible to offer family therapy, although studies have yet to demonstrate its effectiveness.

Psychosocial problems related to depressive disorders can be addressed by social skills training. This may be offered in a group setting or as a component of cognitive–behavioural or supportive therapy.

Medication has been a mainstay of treatment for many years, particularly with moderate to severe depressive disorders. Until the 1990s this was mostly with tricyclic antidepressants, despite numerous studies failing to demonstrate the effectiveness of such treatment (Hazell et al, 1995). Tricyclic antidepressants have a problematic side-effect profile and are cardiotoxic in overdose. In view of this the selective serotonin reuptake inhibitors (SSRIs) and the newer serotonergic and noradrenergic antidepressants have become popular over recent years. Drug company-sponsored randomised controlled trials have shown some benefits from fluoxetine, paroxetine and sertraline over placebo in the treatment of depressive symptoms (Emslie et al, 1997, 2002; Keller et al, 2001; Wagner et al, 2003). Although these drugs show some efficacy and are generally well tolerated, a question has arisen over their safety. All SSRIs (with the exception of fluoxetine) and venlafaxine have been contraindicated in the UK because of an increased risk of suicidality. The mechanism for this is as yet unclear; for example, it could be a side-effect or partial treatment effect. At the time of writing, the UK National Institute for Clinical Excellence (NICE) Depression in Children Guideline Development Group and an Expert Working Group of the Committee on Safety of Medicines are reviewing the use of antidepressants in children. Until clear guidance is given, this group of drugs should be prescribed only with caution.

If antidepressant medication is used, and there is a good response, it is wise to continue it for 6 months after the resolution of symptoms, before a gradual withdrawal is considered. During the stage of withdrawal the patient will need to be seen regularly to monitor for 'rebound effects' or for a recurrence of symptoms. If there is a failure to respond to medication, a review of diagnosis may be necessary as well as a check for compliance. Kutcher (1997) advises that medication should not be discounted until it has been tried at the maximum dosage without undue side-effects. At this point an alternative antidepressant could be considered.

In severe cases lithium augmentation may be useful, and studies suggest that lithium reduces the risk of further episodes of illness in children and adolescents with bipolar disorder (Strober *et al*, 1990). Carbamazepine and valproate are also used for bipolar disorder, and may be more effective than lithium in the younger age group and in those with rapid cycling or mixed affective symptoms. If there are psychotic symptoms, the use of antipsychotic medication should be considered.

In cases of severe, persistent disorder, cases with comorbid difficulties or those in which there is a significant suicide risk, in-patient treatment may be an option. In addition, where environmental factors appear to be maintaining or exacerbating the disorder, an admission could be useful both diagnostically and therapeutically. If a dramatic improvement follows this intervention, further consideration should be given to how to bring about change in aspects of the youngster's environment, such as the home or the school.

If all other treatments fail and severe symptoms persist, particularly if they are life-threatening, electroconvulsive therapy (ECT) can be considered. There is no randomised controlled trial to support the use of ECT, but case series of adolescents treated in this way, especially when there are also psychotic symptoms, suggest good outcomes in 60–70% of cases (Walter *et al*, 1999).

Prognosis

The vast majority of adolescents with a depressive disorder will recover from the index episode. Strober *et al* (1993), in a study of adolescents with severe depression requiring in-patient treatment, found that 90% had recovered in 2 years. However, recurrence rates are high, and in long-term follow-up, Fombonne *et al* (2001*a*) found that over 60% of children diagnosed with major depressive disorder had a recurrence of this disorder later in life. Previous suggestions that the presence of comorbid conduct disorder reduced the likely recurrence of depression in adult life were not borne out by this study. A small but significant number of cases will go on to develop a bipolar affective disorder. At 20-year follow-up, the rate of attempted suicide was 44% and completed suicide 2.5% (Fombonne *et al*, 2001*b*).

Self-harm and suicide

Epidemiology

Self-harm is extremely commonplace, with approximately 19 000 young people in England and Wales aged 10–19 years referred to hospital each year (Hawton & Fagg, 1992). It is far less common in children, rising in incidence through the teenage years. In comparison, the number of recorded deaths from suicide is small: 73 males and 19 females aged 15–19 years in England and Wales in 1997 (Office of Population Censuses and Surveys, 1998), with fewer still for children and adolescents under the age of 15 years. However, these figures are probably an under-estimate because of uncertainties around intent in younger children and because coroners are reluctant to burden bereaved parents with a stigmatising label. Despite this, suicide still represents the fourth most common cause of death in the adolescent age group in the UK and the suicide rate for young males continues to increase (Hawton, 1992; Fombonne, 1998).

The gender ratio for self-harm is approximately 1:6 male to female (Cotgrove *et al*, 1995), but this ratio is reversed for completed suicides with a male to female ratio of about 4:1 (Office of Population Censuses and Surveys, 1998).

Methods of self-harm

The most common form of self-harm is probably cutting or scratching. This is characteristically seen in young females and is not usually associated with suicidal ideation. Cutting behaviour rarely presents at hospital for treatment and so does not feature in most medical statistics of self-harm such as those quoted above. The most frequently recorded form of self-harm in the UK is self-poisoning (Hawton *et al*, 1996) and the majority of this in the adolescent age group is from paracetamol overdose. High levels of alcohol intake are commonly associated with overdosing, taken before, with or after the overdose.

In the UK, self-poisoning also represents the most common means of completed suicide among females, whereas for males it is hanging. In the USA, guns are used in over 50% of adolescent suicides, reflecting their easy availability.

Characteristics of those who self-harm

Adolescents who self-harm are a heterogeneous group. They form a spectrum ranging from those who scratch or cut themselves to relieve a sense of inner tension to those who have a clear intent to kill themselves. Although those who have an unequivocal wish to die are rare, there are many who are ambivalent and express suicidal ideation (27% in a community sample of 14- to 17-year-olds; Centre for Disease Control, 1991). Very few actually go on to complete suicide, but accurate predictions in this group are difficult. Clinicians are, therefore, left with relying on what is known of the main characteristic features associated with completed suicide. These features are summarised in Table 11.2.

The role of major mental illness (particularly major depressive disorder, conduct disorder and substance misuse) as an associated or predisposing factor to self-harm is still unclear. Some studies based on routine clinical practice suggest that a relatively small proportion of adolescents who self-harm have a psychiatric disorder – for example, Hawton & Fagg (1992) found a rate of only 3.5% and Cotgrove *et al* (1995) 6%. Others, however, using detailed research evaluations, have reported higher rates – for example, Kerfoot *et al* (1996) and Burgess *et al* (1998) respectively diagnosed 75% and 100% of adolescents as having a psychiatric disorder at, or soon after, the time of self-harm.

Immediate precipitants to self-harm and suicide include inter-personal conflicts with a boy- or girlfriend (50%) and arguments with parents (25%) (Hawton *et al*, 1982*a*). Additional precipitants include losses through bereavement and external stressors such as bullying, disciplinary problems, legal difficulties, unemployment (in the older age group), abuse/neglect and exposure to self-harm or suicide.

Table 11.2 Characteristic features associated with completed suicide

Circumstances of attempt	Individual factors	Family and environment

• High degree of isolation
• High level of premeditation
• Potential lethality of means used
• Precautions to avoid detection
• Leaving a suicide note
• High degree of expressed suicidal intent
	• Psychiatric disorder:
	  depression
	  psychosis
	  substance misuse
	  conduct disorder
	• Social isolation
	• Low self-esteem
	• Hopelessness
	• Male gender
	• Physical illness
		• Loss of parent in childhood
		• Family dysfunction
		• Abuse/neglect
		• Family history of psychiatric illness or suicide

The meaning of self-harm

The act of self-harm can have a range of meanings. It may be a serious attempt to die in order to escape from unbearable feelings or an unbearable situation. However, rather than death an overwhelming wish to escape may be the main intention, the adolescent knowing that they want things to change but feeling powerless to bring this about without taking dramatic action. Most adolescents who take overdoses (as opposed to cutting) express a wish to die, but when the circumstances of their self-harm are examined most ensure that it is likely they will receive help. In these cases, it can be helpful to view the act of self-harm as a communication. This communication may include a 'cry for help', but may also involve feelings of guilt or hostility and anger with others (Kingsbury, 1993).

Alternatively, there may be no expressed suicidal intent (more commonly with cutting than overdosing), the act helping to release feelings of inner tension. There may be an associated sense of low self-worth and guilt, with the self-harm being seen as a means of self-punishment.

Management

The immediate management of an act of self-poisoning should generally include admission to a paediatric or medical ward overnight, even if there is no medical indication for this, to facilitate a considered assessment (Royal College of Psychiatrists, 1998). Further management is strongly influenced by the clinical assessment and risk assessment, there being a need for more proactive management with an emphasis on safety if the risk of repetition or completed suicide is considered high. The clinical and risk assessment should include exploration of the factors listed in Table 11.2. Rating scales such as the Pierce Suicide Intent Score (Pierce, 1981) can help with such an assessment, although it is important that this is not used as a substitute for a full clinical assessment, particularly if significant risk factors are identified.

Practical methods such as reducing the availability of the means of self-harm can be helpful at both an individual and a societal level. In the UK, the switch from coal gas to natural gas reduced suicide rates significantly in the 1960s, and more recently repackaging of paracetamol into smaller 'blister' packs is an attempt to reduce the quantities easily available for overdosing. Other social measures, such as attempting to reduce the availability and consumption of drugs and alcohol, have been shown to have an impact on suicide rates in adults.

Underlying psychiatric disorder needs to be identified and treated, for example with cognitive–behavioural therapy for depression and feelings of hopelessness. Other precipitating or predisposing factors

183

should be addressed wherever possible, although little can be done about some of these, e.g. relationship break-ups, except through the offer of support. Evidence of abuse or neglect should be addressed, and if there is a suggestion that this is ongoing, a multi-agency approach including social services should ensure the child's safety.

Adolescents who attempt suicide and their families are often not compliant with follow-up treatment, so interventions need to address this issue in order to have any likelihood of success. Interventions need to be both convenient and acceptable to adolescents and their families. On reviewing a range of treatments, both with adults and with adolescents, Brent (1997) concluded that interventions are most likely to be achieved through aggressive outreach. Suggested treatment goals include improved social adjustment, reduced suicidal ideation and attempts, reduction in dysfunctional cognitions, and improved problem solving and interpersonal skills.

To date, there have only been three randomised controlled trials evaluating specific interventions with young people to reduce repetition. Cotgrove et al (1995) used a 'green card' to allow youngsters immediate access to a paediatric bed should they feel suicidal; although the results looked promising, a lack of power produced inconclusive results. Harrington et al (1998c) evaluated a home-based family intervention: although this achieved a greater compliance with treatment, good parental satisfaction and a reduction of children received into care, there was no reduction in repetition. Wood et al (2001) compared group therapy with routine care in a group of adolescents who had already repeatedly harmed themselves; these authors found the group therapy, specifically designed for adolescents who self-harm, to be effective in reducing further self-harm.

There is not a large role for in-patient psychiatric treatment, but occasionally, when there is an underlying psychiatric disorder and an immediate risk from repetition is judged to be high, admission may be indicated. Despite uncertainty regarding efficacy, in one study referrals to an adolescent unit following self-harm made up the largest pro- portion of emergency referrals (Cotgrove, 1997). Often such referrals reflect concerns about the environment, which need addressing through social care, with or without involvement of mental health services.

Prognosis

Following an episode of self-harm, approximately 10% will go on to repeat it within a year (Goldacre & Hawton, 1985; Spirito et al, 1989; Cotgrove et al, 1995). Repetition rates appear much higher than average (50%) among those whose self-harm is comorbid with conduct disorder (Hawton et al, 1982b). A small but significant proportion of those who self-harm will go on to kill themselves. Estimates of this group vary, partly depending on duration of follow-up, but Goldacre & Hawton (1985) found that at 3-year follow-up of a group of 16- to 20-year-olds who had self-harmed, 0.7% of males and 0.1% of females had completed suicide.

Conclusion

Those who self-harm are a heterogeneous group who harm themselves for a range of reasons and intent. Measures to predict repetition of self-harm or completed suicide remain crude and unreliable, but nevertheless are worth attempting in order to focus resources where they are most needed.

An absence of evidence supporting particular interventions makes management difficult, but systematically attending to predisposing psychosocial factors and treating any underlying psychiatric disorder offer an appropriate way of managing such cases.

References

American Psychiatric Association (1994) *Diagnostic and Statistical Manual of Mental Disorders* (4th edn) (DSM–IV). Washington, DC: American Psychiatric Association.

Angold, A. & Rutter, M. (1992) Effects of age and pubertal status on depression in a large clinical sample. *Development and Psychopathology*, **4**, 5–28.

Barrett, M. L., Berney, T. P., Bhate, S., *et al* (1991) Diagnosing childhood depression: who should be interviewed – parent or child? The Newcastle Child Depression Project. *British Journal of Psychiatry*, **159** (suppl. 11), 22–27.

Birmaher, B., Ryan, N. D., Williamson, D. E., *et al* (1996) Childhood and adolescent depression: a review of the last ten years. Part 1. *Journal of the American Academy of Child and Adolescent Psychiatry*, **35**, 1427–1439.

Brent, D. A. (1997) Practitioner review: the aftercare of adolescents with deliberate self-harm. *Journal of Child Psychology and Psychiatry*, **38**, 277–286.

Burgess, S., Hawton, K. & Loveday, G. (1998) Adolescents who take overdoses: outcome in terms of changes in psychopathology and the adolescent's attitudes to care and to their overdose. *Journal of Adolescence*, **21**, 209–218.

Carlson, G. A. & Cantwell, D. P. (1980) A survey of depressive symptoms, syndrome and disorder in a child psychiatric population. *Journal of Child Psychology and Psychiatry*, **21**, 19–25.

Centre for Disease Control (1991) Attempted suicides among high school students – United States 1990. *Morbidity and Mortality Weekly Report*, **40**, 633–635.

Cotgrove, A. J. (1997) Emergency admissions to a regional adolescent unit: piloting a new service. *Psychiatric Bulletin*, **21**, 604–608.

Cotgrove, A. J., Zirinsky, L., Black, D., *et al* (1995) Secondary prevention of attempted suicide in adolescence. *Journal of Adolescence*, **18**, 569–577.

Deakin, J. F. W. & Crow, T. J. (1986) Monamine, rewards and punishments – the anatomy and physiology of the affective disorders. In *The Biology of Depression* (ed. J. F. W. Deakin), pp. 1–25. London: Gaskell.

Emslie, G., Rush, A., Weinberg, W., *et al* (1997) A double-blind, randomised placebo-controlled trial of fluoxetine in depressed children and adolescents. *Archives of General Psychiatry*, **54**, 1031–1037.

Emslie, G., Heiligenstein, J. H., Wagner, K., *et al* (2002) Fluoxetine for acute treatment of depression in children and adolescents: a placebo controlled, randomized clinical trial. *Journal of the American Academy of Child and Adolescent Psychiatry*, **41**, 1205–1215.

Fombonne, E. (1998) Suicidal behaviours in vulnerable adolescents: time trends and their correlates. *British Journal of Psychiatry*, **173**, 154–159.

Fombonne, E., Wostear, G., Cooper, V., *et al* (2001*a*) The Maudsley long-term follow-up of child and adolescent depression: 1. Psychiatric outcomes in adulthood. *British Journal of Psychiatry*, **179**, 210–217.

Fombonne, E., Wostear, G., Cooper, V., *et al* (2001*b*) The Maudsley long-term follow-up of child and adolescent depression: 2. Suicidality, criminality and social dysfunction in adulthood. *British Journal of Psychiatry*, **179**, 218–223.

Goldacre, M. & Hawton, K. (1985) Repetition of self-poisoning and subsequent death in adolescents who take overdoses. *British Journal of Psychiatry*, **146**, 395–398.

Goodyer, I., Herbert, J., Moor, S., *et al* (1991) Cortisol hypersecretion in depressed school-aged children and adolescents. *Psychiatry Research*, **37**, 237–234.

Goodyer, I., Herbert, J., Secher, S. M., *et al* (1997) Short-term outcome of major depression: I. comorbidity and severity at presentation as predictors of persistent disorder. *Journal of the American Academy of Child and Adolescent Psychiatry*, **36**, 179–187.

Harrington, R. (1994) Affective disorders. In *Child and Adolescent Psychiatry* (eds M. Rutter, E. Taylor, & L. Hersolv), pp. 330–374. London: Blackwell Science.

Harrington, R. C. & Wood, A. J. (1995) Validity and classification of child and adolescent depressive disorders. Review of the field circa 1995. In *Childhood Depression: ACPP Occasional Paper 11* (ed. G. Forrest), pp. 3–22. London: Association for Child Psychology and Psychiatry.

Harrington, R., Fudge, H., Rutter, M., *et al* (1990) Adult outcomes of child and adolescent depression: I. Psychiatric status. *Archives of General Psychiatry*, **47**, 465–473.

Harrington, R. C., Fudge, H., Rutter, M., *et al* (1993) Child and adult depression: a test of continuities with data from a family study. *British Journal of Psychiatry*, **162**, 627–633.

Harrington, R., Whittaker, J., Shoebridge, P., *et al* (1998*a*) Systematic review of efficacy of cognitive behaviour therapies in child and adolescent depressive disorder. *BMJ*, **316**, 1559–1563.

Harrington, R., Whittaker, J. & Shoebridge, P. (1998*b*) Psychological treatment of depression in children and adolescents: a review of treatment research. *British Journal of Psychiatry*, **173**, 291–298.

Harrington, R. C., Kerfoot, M., Dyer, E., *et al* (1998*c*) Randomised trial of home-based family intervention for children who have deliberately poisoned themselves. *Journal of the American Academy of Child and Adolescent Psychiatry*, **37**, 512–518.

Hawton, K. (1992) By their own young hand. *BMJ*, **304**, 1000.

Hawton, K. & Fagg, J. (1992) Deliberate self-poisoning and self-injury in adolescents: a study of characteristics and trends in Oxford, 1976–89. *British Journal of Psychiatry*, **161**, 816–823.

Hawton, K., Osborn, M., O'Grady, J., *et al* (1982*a*) Adolescents who take overdoses: their characteristics, problems and contacts with helping agencies. *British Journal of Psychiatry*, **140**, 118–123.

Hawton, K., Osborn, M., O'Grady, J., *et al* (1982*b*) Classification of adolescents who take overdoses. *British Journal of Psychiatry*, **140**, 124–131.

Hawton, K., Fagg, J. & Simkin, S. (1996) Deliberate self-poisoning and self-injury in children and adolescents under 16 years of age in Oxford, 1976–1993. *British Journal of Psychiatry*, **169**, 202–208.

Hazell, P., O'Connell, D., Heathcoat, D., *et al* (1995) Efficacy of tricyclic drugs in treating child and adolescent depression, *BMJ*, **310**, 897–890.

Keller, M. B., Ryan, N. D., Stober, M., *et al* (2001) Efficacy of paroxetine in the treatment of adolescent major depression: a randomised, controlled trial. *Journal of the American Academy of Child Psychiatry*, **40**, 762–772.

Kerfoot, M., Dyer, E., Harrington, V., et al (1996) Correlates and short-term course of self-poisoning in adolescents. British Journal of Psychiatry, 168, 38–42.

Kingsbury, S. (1993) Parasuicide in adolescents: a message in a bottle. Association of Child Psychology and Psychiatry Review and Newsletter, 15, 253–259.

Kolvin, I., Barrett, M. L. & Bhate, S. R. (1991) The Newcastle Child Depression Project: diagnosis and classification of depression. British Journal of Psychiatry, 159 (suppl. 11), 9–21.

Kutcher, S. (1997) Practitioner review; the pharmacotherapy of adolescent depression. Journal of Child Psychology and Psychiatry, 32, 755–767.

Kutcher, S. P. & Marton, P. (1991) Affective disorders in first-degree relatives of adolescent onset bipolar, unipolar and normal controls. Journal of the American Academy of Child Psychiatry, 30, 75–78.

Kutcher, S., Williamson, P., Marton, P., et al (1992) REM latency in endogenously depressed adolescents. British Journal of Psychiatry, 161, 399–402.

Office of Population Censuses and Surveys (1998) 1997 Mortality Statistics. Cause: England and Wales. London: HMSO.

Pierce, D. W. (1981) The predictive validation of a suicide intent scale: a 5-year follow-up. British Journal of Psychiatry, 139, 391–396.

Radke-Yarrow, M., Nottelmann, E., Martinez, P., et al (1992) Young children of affectively ill parents: a longitudinal study of psychosocial development. Journal of the American Academy of Child Psychiatry, 31, 68–77.

Rice, F., Harold, G. & Thapar, A. (2002) The genetic aetiology of childhood depression: a review. Journal of Child Psychology and Psychiatry, 43, 65–79.

Royal College of Psychiatrists (1998) Managing Deliberate Self-Harm in Young People. London: Royal College of Psychiatrists.

Spirito, A., Brown, L., Overholser, J., et al (1989) Attempted suicide in adolescence: a review and critique of the literature. Clinical Psychology Review, 9, 335–363.

Strober, M., Morrell, W., Lampert, C., et al (1990) Relapse following discontinuation of lithium maintenance therapy in adolescents with bipolar I illness: a naturalistic study. American Journal of Psychiatry, 147, 457–461.

Strober, M., Lampert, C., Schmidt, S., et al (1993) The course of major depressive disorder in adolescents: recovery and risk of manic switching in a follow-up of psychotic and non-psychotic subtypes. Journal of the American Academy of Child and Adolescent Psychiatry, 32, 34–42.

Wagner, K., Ambrosinin, P., Rynn, M., et al (2003) Efficacy of Sertraline in the treatment of children and adolescents with a major depressive disorder: two randomized controlled trials. JAMA, 290, 1033–1041.

Walter, G., Rey, J. M. & Mitchell, P. B. (1999) Practitioner review: electroconvulsive therapy in adolescents. Journal of Child Psychology and Psychiatry, 40, 325–334.

Wood, A., Trainor, G., Rothwell, J., et al (2001) Randomized trial of group therapy for repeated deliberate self-harm in adolescents. Journal of the Academy of Child and Adolescent Psychiatry, 40, 1246–1253.

World Health Organization (1992) The ICD–10 Classification of Mental and Behavioural Disorders. Geneva: WHO.

187

CHAPTER 12

Psychosis

Clare Lamb

Psychotic disorders cause significant distress and disruption to young people and their families and have a major impact on adolescent development. They are rare before puberty, but the incidence increases with age during adolescence. In a Swedish population-based study, Gillberg *et al* (1986) showed a prevalence of 0.54% during the teenage years, increasing from 0.9% per 10 000 at 13 years to 17.6% per 10 000 at 18 years. Most episodes of psychotic disorder in adolescents will be the first episode. Presentations vary and there is likely to be significant diagnostic uncertainty. Where definite psychotic symptoms occur, as opposed to fleeting or 'pseudo-psychotic' experiences, the clinical picture may reflect an underlying schizophrenic, mixed affective, bipolar or affective disorder. It may be a single, brief psychotic episode followed by full recovery. It may be as a result of substance misuse. In rare cases, it may be secondary to a medical cause such as epilepsy, other central nervous system disorders, or an endocrine or metabolic disorder. For these reasons, a full diagnostic assessment is essential.

Adolescents suffering a first episode of psychosis frequently present with mixed symptomatology, and the presence of non-specific hallucinations, particularly in younger adolescents, does not necessarily imply the development of a psychotic disorder. However, the early course of psychosis is often characterised by changing symptoms, and where there are clear signs and symptoms of psychosis but significant diagnostic uncertainty, the most appropriate and clinically useful diagnosis is of a psychotic disorder.

The embracing of diagnostic uncertainty is crucial in work with first-episode psychosis. Provided that organic causes are excluded, a symptom-based approach to treatment has been advocated (McGorry, 1995), but thorough assess-ment is essential before treatment is commenced (Werry *et al*, 1994).

Over recent years, a number of studies have linked a long duration of psychosis prior to treatment with a poor treatment outcome (Larsen *et al*, 1996; Scully *et al*, 1997). Intensive and sophisticated interventions in the early phase of illness could more effectively promote recovery (McGorry *et al*, 1996). Evidence is also emerging that the early phase following the onset of a first psychotic illness can be conceived of as a critical period, influencing the long-term course of illness (Birchwood *et al*, 1998). This is a period when individuals and their families may develop adverse psychological reactions to the psychosis and how it is managed. These factors have resulted in the establishment of specialised services for the management of first-episode psychosis, notably in Australia and Scandinavia. Similar services are now developing in the UK. These early-intervention services share a common set of aims:

- to shorten the duration of untreated psychosis and produce rapid, expert multidisciplinary assessment;
- to achieve remission through the implementation of prompt, effective biological and psychosocial interventions;
- to provide an acceptable, developmentally appropriate service to the individuals and carers/family, which aims to maximise social functioning and education, training and work opportunities;
- to prevent relapse and treatment resistance.

The particular diagnostic complexities of adolescent psychosis combined with the developmental issues and transition from adolescence to adulthood imply a need for special attention to the assessment and management of psychosis presenting in adolescence.

Presentation and assessment of the first psychotic episode

Emotional, social and cognitive developmental processes that are still ongoing in adolescents influence the presentation of psychosis. However, the core signs and symptoms of a psychotic disorder with onset in adolescence are similar to those of adult onset (Clark, 2001*a*).

Adolescent schizophrenia frequently presents with an insidious onset. Non-specific behavioural change, e.g. social withdrawal, declining school performance, and uncharacteristic and odd behaviour, can begin more than a year before the onset of positive symptoms such as hallucinations and delusions. In some cases, positive psychotic symptoms are preceded by other psychiatric symptoms such as anxiety, depression or obsessive–compulsive symptoms.

In younger adolescents, social and intellectual deterioration may present itself as a failure to make progress and gain new skills. Some young people, including those with symptoms suggestive of schizotypal disorder, show social awkwardness, anxiety and unusual ways of thinking but no evidence of active symptoms of psychosis. It is not currently possible to predict which of these young people may be in the prodromal phase of a psychotic illness. However, they could be considered as a vulnerable group with an enhanced risk of schizophrenia, particularly where there is a strong family history. A suggested course of action in these cases is to offer practical and psychotherapeutic support, and attempt to facilitate early recognition of those who may eventually develop psychosis (Roberts *et al*, 2001).

Many young people present to the family doctor. However, a number will present to youth services, social services, voluntary agencies, or school or college staff. It is important that child and adolescent mental health services have good working links with the range of agencies involved with young people.

An adolescent with psychosis may also present through the youth justice system. A study from the Office of National Statistics (Lader, 2000) shows significantly higher rates of functional psychosis in male young offenders compared with the same-age general population. Hence, close links with the youth justice system and youth offending teams are vital in ensuring prompt assessment of young people at risk of psychosis. There is little evidence to date exploring the relationship between psychosis and criminal violence in adolescence. A case-note study reported that criminally violent behaviour in psychosis was associated more closely with developmental and social factors than with recorded psychopathology. The majority of first-episode psychoses do not present with criminally violent behaviour (Clare *et al*, 2000).

Assessment

History

An accurate and detailed history of recent events and changes in the young person's mental state and behaviour must be recorded, and should include an account of the developmental history and premorbid personality and functioning. The developmental history should pay particular attention to cognitive, social and emotional factors. Cognitive impairment and early developmental delays (particularly with respect to language development, reading and bladder control) are more common in adolescent-onset schizophrenia than in adult-onset schizophrenia (Hollis, 2000).

It is important to elicit as much information as possible about any family history of psychiatric disorder. A detailed history of substance misuse should be sought. The details of any offending behaviour and any contact with the youth justice system should be recorded. It is also essential to record any behaviour that poses a risk to the young person or other people, including family members.

Histories should be obtained from the young person and from parents or carers. It is important to seek consent from the young person and any adult holding parental responsibility, before contacting other people. In the case of a young person over 16 years, it is important to seek his or her consent before speaking to parents or carers. Family involvement is crucial and most young people expect and accept it. It is helpful to seek consent to contact school or college in order to obtain further information on changes in social or cognitive functioning.

Mental state examination

The key to a detailed assessment of the mental state of a young person is effective engagement. Engagement or the formation of a therapeutic alliance is an independent predictor of treatment retention rates and a range of symptomatic and functional outcomes in psychosis. Spencer *et al* (2001) suggest it is fostered by a search for common ground with the young person, an avoidance of premature confrontation of their own explanatory model of illness, and a delivery of treatment in as flexible a manner as possible. Every reasonable effort should be made to be as flexible as possible and to see the young person in an age-appropriate and non-stigmatising setting. Special attention should be paid to the needs and expectations of different ethnic and cultural groups. In some cases, and taking levels of risk into account, several shorter assessment meetings may prove more useful than one long one. It is particularly important in the case of children and adolescents that the clinician does not express shock or disbelief at ideas or experiences related by the young person.

Specific questions should be asked to elicit symptoms such as mood disturbance, obsessions and compulsions, persecutory ideation, abnormal perceptual experiences, and cognitive and social impairment. Particular attention should be given to the assessment of suicidal ideas or ideas of harm to self or others. This information is vital to the risk assessment, which is an important part of the diagnostic assessment. It is important to have a detailed record of the symptoms and signs elicited, including samples of speech verbatim. Such details can be the key to establishing diagnosis and developing knowledge of the symptoms to watch for in monitoring recovery and preventing future relapse.

The use of a semi-structured interview such as the Schedule for Affective Disorders and Schizophrenia for School-Age Children – Epidemiologic version (K–SADS–E; Orvaschel & Puig-Antich, 1987) may be helpful in ensuring detailed diagnostic assessment.

Physical examination

Psychotic disorder secondary to underlying physical disorder is rare, but a formal physical examination, including a full neurological assessment, is essential.

Investigations

These should include blood investigations for full blood count, urea and electrolytes, thyroid function and liver function; in addition, most authors recommend that an electroencephalogram and a computed tomographic or magnetic resonance imaging scan should be arranged (Clark & Lewis, 1998). Urinary or hair drug screening is frequently indicated. Second-line investigations to exclude rare neurodegenerative and metabolic disorders should be considered only when there are specific abnormalities or indications from the history and physical examination.

Differential diagnosis of a psychotic disorder

Developmental disorders (atypical autism, Asperger syndrome, language disorders)

Autistic-spectrum disorders are clearly distinguished as separate and different disorders from a schizophrenic disorder. Children on the autistic spectrum can develop psychotic symptoms in adolescence. Some of these show a clear progression into schizophrenia. However, comorbidity is rare and the risk is not increased.

Schizotypal and schizoid disorder

Schizoid disorder is characterised by egocentricity and aloofness from human relationships. Schizophrenic-like positive symptoms are absent.

Schizotypal disorder is characterised by eccentricity and oddness of ideation, short of frank thought disorder or delusions. There is no active psychotic phase and schizophrenic positive symptoms are mild, localised and/or inconspicuous. There is some evidence to suggest that schizotypal disorder might be linked to schizophrenia by familial distribution as a risk factor, and symptomatologically as a milder version (Werry & Taylor, 1994). In doubtful cases where it is clinically difficult to separate schizotypal disorder and schizophrenia, it is suggested that a trial of antipsychotic medication is considered, remembering that schizotypal disorder may also respond to medication in much lower dosage (Andrews, 1990).

Schizophrenia

Criteria for a diagnosis of schizophrenia have been progressively changed since the first descriptions. The ICD–10 (World Health Organization, 1992) requires specific symptoms to have been present for at least 1 month with no evidence of major affective symptoms or organic brain disease. Major symptoms include thought echo, insertion, withdrawal and broadcast; control or passivity delusions or delusional perception; running commentary, auditory hallucinations from a third person or from some part of the body; and other persistent delusions. Minor symptoms include persistent hallucinations associated with fleeting or half-formed delusions; disruption of train of thought causing incoherence, irrelevance or neologism; catatonic symptoms; and 'negative symptoms'.

The DSM–IV (American Psychiatric Association, 1994) requires symptoms to have been present for at least 6 months and reflects an alternative grouping of the core symptoms as positive (active) and negative (deficit) symptoms. Positive symptoms include delusions, hallucinations, thought disorder, excitement and suspiciousness. Negative symptoms include flattening of affect, alogia, apathy, an-hedonia and asociality.

Delusions and hallucinations are not unique to schizophrenia. Delusions in adolescent-onset schizophrenia may be fleeting or half-formed and are mostly paranoid in nature. The presence of hallucinations in children does not necessarily predict later development of psychosis (Garralda, 1984). Non-specific auditory hallucinations in combination with a mistrust of others may occur in a number of non-psychotic conditions, such as conduct or emotional disorders, dissociative states, borderline personality disorders and post-traumatic stress disorder. However, hallucinations are the most consistently reported symptoms in early-onset schizophrenia. They are usually auditory but may be visual, tactile, olfactory or somatic. Children and adolescents in the early stages of psychosis will frequently describe feeling perplexed, confused or unable to think properly. Flattened or inappropriate affect and social withdrawal are common in adolescent schizophrenia. Depressive symptoms are also frequent. Catatonic behaviour is uncommon in adolescent schizophrenia.

Schizoaffective disorder

According to ICD–10, schizoaffective disorder requires the coexistence of prominent mood and schizophrenic symptoms. Some children and adolescents first diagnosed with schizophrenia will receive a diagnosis of schizoaffective disorder at longer-term follow-up. The stability of diagnostic status of schizoaffective psychosis in childhood and adolescence is much less certain than in adults.

Bipolar affective disorder

The diagnostic criteria for bipolar affective disorder are broadly the same irrespective of age of onset. The core feature is at least two episodes of elevated and depressed mood; ICD–10 discriminates between lesser degrees of mood elevation (hypomania) and more severe degrees (mania with or without psychotic symptoms). Manic disorder is characterised by elevated mood, overactivity, grandiosity and flight of ideas. Psychotic symptoms of grandiose or persecutory delusions may occur, as well as auditory or visual hallucinations. Irritability and challenge of authority is a common feature and can result in verbal and physical aggression. Sexual disinhibition and risk-taking behaviour can occur. Performance in school or college is likely to deteriorate.

Mixed affective states are not uncommon in adolescence and contain symptoms of severe depression and mania present over a period of at least 2 weeks, e.g. coexistence of low mood with overactivity and pressure of speech, or of elevated mood and grandiosity with agitation and loss of energy and drive.

Between episodes of disturbed mood, most adolescents will be asymptomatic. Embarrassment about behaviour when unwell may be a major focus of work during recovery, especially where it results in resistance to reintegration with peers in school, college or work.

Borderline personality disorder

The development of this disorder has not been well studied in children and adolescents. The characteristic symptoms are intense, demanding interpersonal relationships, emotional instability, impulsiveness, self-harm and hallucinations. Background factors frequently associated include grossly inappropriate parental behaviour, expulsion or removal from the family home and sexual abuse (Ludolph *et al*, 1990).

Organic psychoses

Psychotic symptoms, in particular schizophrenic-type positive symptoms, can be produced in adolescents by acute drug-induced psychoses, complex partial seizures and some rare neurodegenerative disorders. The neurodegenerative disorders usually involve significant extrapyramidal and other motor abnormalities and progressive loss of skills (dementia). Short-lived psychotic episodes of a few hours are highly suggestive of drug-induced states. However, in some cases of drug-induced episodes the psychosis endures. There is some evidence to suggest that there is a group of young people in whom drug or alcohol misuse may represent self-medication of symptoms of psychosis.

Aetiology

There are a number of theories relating to the aetiology of schizophrenia and bipolar affective disorder. Intrinsic and extrinsic factors are believed to interact to play a part in a multifactorial process. Biological factors are primary, but the disorder is shaped and influenced by psychosocial factors.

Genetic inheritance

Twin and adoption studies provide evidence for a substantial genetic component (Gottesman & Shields, 1982; Kendler, 1998). The elevated risk applies chiefly to schizophrenic and schizotypal disorders. However, bipolar affective disorder is twice as common among relatives of people with schizophrenia (McGuffin et al, 1987). A positive family history is more commonly found in early-onset schizophrenia and early-onset bipolar disorder than in cases with onset in adult life (Werry, 1992; Hollis, 1995). It has been proposed that a multifactorial polygenic model of inheritance could coexist with a single gene of large effect (McGue et al, 1985).

Environmental factors

Possible causes in early development that have been implicated in schizophrenia research include birth and perinatal trauma, foetal exposure to pathogenic agents, seasonality and viral infections, postnatal brain damage and genetic factors affecting early brain damage. Temporal lobe epilepsy can give rise to a psychiatric syndrome resembling schizophrenia, as can drug intoxication, notably with amphetamines. There is increasing evidence for the role of cannabis as a risk factor for schizophrenia (Arseneault et al, 2002; Patton et al, 2002; Zammit et al, 2002).

Developmental theories

There is increasing evidence of abnormal neurodevelopment and poor premorbid function in people with schizophrenia and the affective psychoses, in particular delayed language development, reading, bladder control and premorbid social impairment. There are particular neuropsychological deficits associated with adolescent-onset schizophrenia (Hollis, 1999; Kumra et al, 2000); however, the pattern is not specific to schizophrenia and is present in other neurodevelopmental disorders such as attention-deficit hyperactivity disorder. Research findings show greater impairments in early-onset schizophrenia (onset before 18th birthday) compared with adult schizophrenia (Hollis, 2003; Vourdas et al, 2003). In the case of early-onset schizophrenia, there appears to be developmental continuity from premorbid impairment to negative symptoms (Hollis, 2003).

Debate continues as to whether schizophrenia is a neurodevelopmental or neurodegenerative disorder. In the 1980s, several research groups began to speculate that schizophrenia might have a significant developmental component (Murray & Lewis, 1987). The 'neurodevelopmental hypothesis' received support from neuropathological studies implicating anomalies in early brain development, for example aberrant migration of neurons. Evidence in the 1990s provided information on cerebral ventricular enlargement and reduction in volume of certain brain structures in subgroups of people with schizophrenia. Studies in adolescent schizophrenia have confirmed a broadly similar pattern to that in adult schizophrenia (Jacobsen & Rappoport, 1998). Increasing evidence demonstrates that the complex symptoms of schizophrenia are paralleled by complex functional and structural abnormalities in the temporal lobe, prefrontal cortex and thalamus. Research suggests that abnormal development of dopamine innervation of the prefrontal cortex may have a role in the cognitive deficits of schizophrenia (Finlay, 2001).

The neurodevelopmental hypothesis postulates that deviations in early development establish a neuronal phenotype that predisposes to, or in some versions determines, the later onset of schizophrenia. The second theory proposes that schizophrenic symptoms arise from abnormalities in neuronal connectivity. Bullmore *et al* (1997) suggested an integration of findings from these two separate lines of inquiry into a unitary framework: the dysplastic net hypothesis. This proposes that anatomical and physical disconnectivity of the adult schizophrenic brain is determined by dysplastic foetal brain development.

Arguments continue as to whether schizophrenia is the final consequence of a cascade of increasing developmental deviance or whether there is additional brain degeneration following onset of psychosis which is superimposed on the developmental impairment. It has been postulated that the onset of psychotic symptoms may reflect the maturationally mediated triggering of an active disease process that is associated with progressive deterioration unless attenuated by antipsychotic medication. Waddington *et al* (1997) proposed a developmental trajectory to link first or early second trimester dysplasia to the chronic course of the illness. They argue that schizophrenia is inherently a progressive disorder, but that antipsychotic drugs may act to ameliorate the progressive component and thus confer on the disease course some of the characteristics of a 'static encephalopathy'.

Cotter & Pariante (2002) discuss the evidence for a common neuropathology in major depression, bipolar disorder and schizophrenia and the role of glucocorticoids. They conclude that evidence is accumulating to support the theory that changes in macroscopic and microscopic brain structure occur during and possibly after the period of first acute psychosis. These changes are present in people with schizophrenia and to a milder degree in people with mood disorder and are in keeping with glucocorticoid-related brain changes.

Management

The management of a young person presenting with an acute psychotic disorder is complex and challenging. It must address biological, psychological and social factors. Management of psychosis requires a multidisciplinary, multimodal approach that includes pharmacotherapy, individual psychological treatments, family-based interventions and educational or vocational strategies (Clark & Lewis, 1998; Spencer *et al*, 2001; Clark, 2001c). The impact of psychosis on adolescent development and the high risk of suicide in the early years of psychotic illness is of particular importance.

Early detection and assessment

The emphasis in the initial phase is on early detection and assessment. In the UK, clear care pathways from the primary care setting should be established, and general practitioners and other agencies routinely involved with young people should be made aware of the warning signs and indicators of possible psychosis.

Once the diagnosis is suspected, the first task is the engagement of the young person, and family or carers. In most cases, attempts at engagement succeed with a flexible approach within an age-appropriate, non-stigmatising setting. However, in some cases of increased severity of illness, engagement may prove more problematic. Admission to hospital may be required. This should be into an age-appropriate adolescent psychiatric unit. The National Service Framework (NSF) (Department of Health, 1999) for the NHS in England and Wales requires NHS Trusts to make explicit plans for provision of services for teenagers requiring acute psychiatric admission. In rare, particularly severe and extreme cases, it may be necessary, in order to ensure safety, to consider compulsory admission against the wishes of the adolescent (Clark, 2001a). This may be achieved either through the use of the mental health legislation, or through consent on behalf of the minor, by the parent or person with parental responsibility under the Children Act 1989. A helpful current overview of the complex issue of competence and consent to treatment in children and adolescents is given by Shaw (2001). Compulsory admission should be rare.

In most cases where admission is indicated, this will be informal and in many cases treatment can be given at home. Home treatment requires careful expert assessment, including risk assessment and intensive support by the clinical team. Consideration must be given to the environment and daily structure and access to education. Home treatment may be supported by attendance at an age-appropriate day care unit. The decision on the treatment setting needs careful discussion with the individual and with the carers.

Psychopharmacology

There is a paucity of robust research evidence on the treatment of psychosis in children and adolescents, most evidence being extrapolated from adult research. However, antipsychotic medication is the mainstay of treatment in schizophrenia spectrum disorders and is also useful in affective psychosis (Clark, 2001a,b). The majority of antipsychotic drugs that are effective in adults are not licensed for use in children and adolescents. This must be explained to the families involved.

If possible, there should be an antipsychotic-free observation period during which diagnosis can be confirmed and organic causes excluded. If sedation is needed during this time, benzodiazepines may be used as an alternative to antipsychotic medication.

The newer 'atypical' antipsychotic drugs (risperidone, olanzapine, quetiapine and amisulpride) have been found to cause fewer side-effects in general and tardive dyskinesias in particular, while having equal efficacy compared with the more conventional drugs. Children and adolescents are particularly sensitive to the side-effects of antipsychotic medication. Reduced side-effects are likely to be associated with better compliance. The atypical antipsychotics are now the drug of first choice in the treatment of first-episode psychoses in adults (National Institute for Clinical Excellence, 2002). A small number of clinical trials have investigated the use of antipsychotic medications in adolescents. Care-ful use can be justified in this population, but more research is needed.

The positive symptoms of most young people with psychosis will respond to the equivalent of 2–4 mg risperidone daily. It is, however, important to start at the lowest dosage and build up slowly. In some cases, adolescents will show significant improvement on risperidone 0.5 mg or 1 mg daily. The equivalent lowest effective dosage of quetiapine is 150 mg daily, olanzapine 5 mg daily, and amisulpride 50 mg daily. In the case of younger adolescents, it is often advisable to start lower than this and titrate the dose to the response. It is advisable to carry out haematological screening and to monitor liver function and serum prolactin levels in young people on long-term medication.

When sedation is needed it is recommended to use benzodiazepines in conjunction with a low dosage of an atypical antipsychotic, e.g. lorazepam 2–4 mg daily or diazepam 5–10 mg daily for a limited period (Clark & Lewis, 1998).

The antipsychotic medication chosen should be continued for 6–8 weeks at a therapeutic dose before being considered ineffective. In cases where remission is not being achieved, despite adequate doses of two different antipsychotics and appropriate psychosocial input, it is important to review for unsuspected organic factors, mood disorder, substance misuse or non-compliance with medication. Consideration should then be given to clozapine, which is of proven benefit in treatment-resistant schizophrenia. This must be instituted on an in-patient basis. It is only available in the UK on an off-label and named patient basis for young people under 16 years old and needs specific discussion with pharmaceutical companies in addition to the usual routine blood monitoring arrangement of the Clozapine Patient Monitoring Service (National Institute for Clinical Excellence, 2002).

In the rare case of a young person who does not comply with oral medication despite all attempts to encourage and support, it may be necessary to prescribe a depot preparation. Atypical antipsychotic agents are now available in this form.

Management of acute manic disorder follows the same approach as other acute psychotic presentations. The use of antipsychotic medication may be indicated. However, the preferred first line of treatment is a mood stabiliser (Clark, 2001b).

In the past, lithium preparations were the only choice of mood stabiliser. Now, carbamazepine and sodium valproate are increasingly being considered as first-line treatment. There is a lack of robust research evidence but they appear to be as least as effective as lithium and better tolerated. There is, however, a significant risk of hepatotoxicity and blood dyscrasias, and routine monitoring should be carried out. In addition, prescribers must be aware that their usage is beyond the product licence for both drugs in adulthood and childhood, with the exception of carbamazepine in rapid-cycling mood disorders. This should be explained to the young person and family (Clark, 2001b). There is no established agreement on therapeutic dosages, but recommended doses and levels tend to be similar to those governing their use as anticonvulsants: for valproate, between 1000 mg and 3000 mg daily, and for carbamazepine, up to 1200 mg daily. In both carbamazepine and valproate, doses should be built up slowly and be accompanied by monitoring of serum levels.

Adjunctive treatment with an atypical antipsychotic or, for preference, a benzodiazepine may be useful in the acute phase if additional sedation is required. A study by Kafantaris et al (2001) concluded that where a combination of antipsychotic and mood stabiliser is used in the initial treatment of adolescents with acute psychotic mania, the antipsychotic medication needs to be maintained for longer than 4 weeks in the vast majority. In young people who remain ill despite adequate doses of a mood stabiliser, combination therapy may be necessary. In the very rare cases of severe, non-responsive, life-threatening manic disorder, electroconvulsive treatment may be considered.

In addition to pharmacotherapy, all young people with psychosis must have access to a multimodal treatment package that includes family and individual counselling and education about the illness, and assessment of social, educational and vocational needs (Hollis, 2000; Clark, 2001a; Spencer et al, 2001).

The establishment of a supportive psychotherapeutic relationship with the young person is vital. The key seems to be to provide the opportunity for the patient to develop a positive, trusting relationship with a single mental health worker who is part of the multidisciplinary team and available for the 'critical period'. Special attention must be paid to providing developmentally and culturally appropriate interventions and environment. The initial focus will be on coming to terms with the illness, and its effect on the young person and family.

Adverse reactions to the experience of psychosis and its treatment, including depression, post-traumatic stress disorder and suicide are well established in the adult literature. Spencer *et al* (2001) provide a review of work in this area. They recommend the focus of work is on blame-free acceptance of the illness, together with encouragement of a sense of mastery over it.

Family interventions focusing on providing information and support, clarifying expectation and improving communication have been shown to be associated with improvements in the course of disorder by reducing relapse rates and improving social functioning (Birchwood *et al*, 1998; Clark, 2001*a*). It is important to provide education on relapse prevention, and to aim to help the family in achieving a balance between support, supervision and overprotection of the young person. Parents of children and adolescents with schizophrenia express lower levels of criticism and hostility than parents of adult-onset patients (Asarnow *et al*, 1994); however, strategies aimed at reduction of 'expressed emotion' may still be beneficial in some cases.

Individual psychological therapies have been shown to be of use in adult-onset psychosis. Problem-solving skills, social skills training, coping strategy enhancements and cognitive–behavioural approaches have been advocated (Birchwood *et al*, 2000). These have not as yet been formally evaluated in adolescents.

Most individual therapy can be provided in the context of an ongoing therapeutic relationship with a key mental health worker. In some cases, effective therapeutic work is facilitated by using a range of settings, for example a local snooker club or café. The focus is on adjustment and the maintenance of social roles. Gradual return to education or vocational training is undertaken within the therapeutic programme. Close links with school or college are vital. In the UK, the 'Connexions' organisation can have a key role in working with professionals and families to link a young person back into education, training or work.

Relapse prevention

Current consensus guidelines suggest continual use of antipsychotic medication for 1–2 years following remission of a first episode of non-affective psychosis, although there is little age-specific information on this. Many young people wish to stop medication sooner than recommended. If persuasion to continue medication fails, it is important to try to negotiate gradual reduction and to retain engagement with ongoing individual, family, social and educational interventions. With a thoughtful approach from professionals, it is possible to engage the majority of young people and their families or carers in ongoing work.

The basis of relapse prevention is the modification of stress and vulnerability factors by means of the best practice interventions discussed above. Young people and their families should be informed about risk factors. A shared and documented relapse prevention plan is recommended for each individual, and this can be developed with the young person and his or her social network (Birchwood *et al*, 1998). This plan should aim to identify the young person's unique and early-warning signs of psychotic relapse and to prepare and rehearse a response to these. The recommended response draws on cognitive therapy of emerging delusions and the use of coping mechanisms, drug intervention and family resources.

In essence, the work of the team involved with the young person and family should focus on maintaining treatment engagement and compliance and providing support and strategies to enable the young person to achieve, as far as possible, the developmental tasks of adolescence.

A few young people will have a single psychotic episode and make a full recovery. However, in most cases, long-term management is required and transition from child and adolescent to adult mental health services will be necessary. The transition must be managed with care and discussed with the young person, the family and the other agencies involved. In the UK, transfer of care from child and adolescent mental health services to adult mental health services should be implemented with the use of the care programme approach. This ensures the appointment of a case manager and facilitates engagement with the new team, and helps to ensure clear plans for future care. A period of joint working with the adult team is often helpful. In cases where specialist follow-up is not indicated, the young person's care should be discussed with the general practitioner and follow-up in primary care agreed. In these cases, it is important to highlight the early-warning signs of potential relapse and to clarify rapid access to psychiatric help.

Outcomes

There is a paucity of longitudinal studies of outcome in adolescent-onset psychosis. Adolescent-onset psychosis appears to be in continuity with adult-onset psychosis, but there is no statistically significant prediction of diagnosis or outcome. Long-term follow-up studies of adolescent in-patients in Sweden, Oxford and the Maudsley Hospital, London, have been carried out (Gillberg *et al*, 1993; Cawthron *et al*, 1994; Hollis, 2000). These report a majority of cases with poor prognosis, i.e. recurrent illness and impaired social functioning. Individuals with lower IQ scores did less well. Individuals with affective symptoms did better. Younger age of onset correlates with greater diagnostic instability. Symptoms often change and evolve over time. Substance misuse is an important confounding variable, with impact on diagnosis, presentation and evolution of psychotic disorder. In the adult literature, substance misuse is correlated with younger age of onset of psychosis, lower premorbid functioning and increased risk of suicide. The degree of recovery after the first episode of psychosis is a substantial predictor for outcome in schizophrenia (Werry *et al*, 1994).

It may be that the introduction of atypical antipsychotics and a multimodal treatment package may improve prognosis of adolescent-onset psychosis through a possible direct effect of medication, better early compliance and improved social functioning (Clark, 2001*a*).

Service provision

There are examples of services that provide excellent treatment for adolescents with psychosis, but the national picture in the UK is of patchy provision. A solution put forward by the UK government NHS Plan under the National Service Framework for Adults of Working Age is the development of early intervention services for 14- to 35-year-olds; the National Service Framework for Children will also address psychosis. Outside the UK, services such as the Early Psychosis Prevention and Intervention Centre (EPPIC) in Melbourne, Australia (McGorry, 1993) provide innovative models of intensive first-episode interventions for psychosis spanning adolescent and early adult life.

It is important that child and adolescent and adult mental health professionals work together to provide developmentally appropriate, integrated and effective models of service for intervention in early-onset psychosis.

References

American Psychiatric Association (1994) *Diagnostic and Statistical Manual of Mental Disorders* (4th edn) (DSM–IV). Washington, DC: American Psychiatric Association.
Andrews, G. (1990) Treatment outlines for paranoid, schizotypal and schizoid personality disorders: the quality assurance project. *Australia and New Zealand Journal of Psychiatry*, **24**, 339–350.
Arseneault, L., Cannon, M., Poulton, R., *et al* (2002) Cannabis use in adolescence and risk for adult psychosis: longitudinal prospective study. *BMJ*, **325**, 1212–1213.
Asarnow, J. R.,Tompson, M., Hamilton, E. B., *et al* (1994) Family expressed emotion, childhood onset depression and childhood onset schizophrenia spectrum disorders. Is expressed emotion a non-specific correlate of psychopathology or a specific risk factor for depression? *Journal of Abnormal Psychology*, **22**, 129–146.
Birchwood, M., Todd, P. & Jackson, C. (1998) Early intervention in psychosis. The critical period hypothesis. *British Journal of Psychiatry*, **172** (suppl. 33), 53–59.

Birchwood, M., Jackson, C. & Fowler, D. (2000) *Early Intervention in Psychosis*. Chichester: John Wiley.

Bullmore, E. T., Woodruff, P. W., Wright, I. C., *et al* (1997) The dysplastic net hypothesis; an integration of developmental and dysconnectivity theories of schizophrenia. *Schizophrenia Research*, **28**, 143–156.

Cawthron, P., James, A., Dell, J., *et al* (1994) Adolescent onset psychosis. A clinical and outcome study. *Journal of Child and Adolescent Psychology and Psychiatry*, **35**, 1321–1322.

Clare, P., Bailey, S. & Clark, A. (2000) Relationship between psychotic disorders in adolescence and criminally violent behaviour. A retrospective examination. *British Journal of Psychiatry*, **177**, 275–279.

Clark, A. F. (2001*a*) Proposed treatment for adolescent psychosis: schizophrenia and schizophrenia-like psychoses. *Advances in Psychiatric Treatment*, **7**, 16–23.

Clark, A. F. (2001*b*) Proposed treatment for adolescent psychosis. 2: Bipolar illness. *Advances in Psychiatric Treatment*, **7**, 143–149.

Clark, A. F. (2001*c*) Psychotic disorders. In *Adolescent Psychiatry in Clinical Practice* (ed. S. Gowers). London: Arnold.

Clark, A. & Lewis, S. (1998) Practitioner review: the treatment of schizophrenia in childhood and adolescence. *Journal of Clinical Psychology and Psychiatry*, **39**, 1071–1081.

Cotter, D. & Pariante, C. M. (2002) Stress and the progression of the developmental hypothesis of schizophrenia. *British Journal of Psychiatry*, **181**, 363–365.

Department of Health (1999) *National Service Framework for Mental Health*. London: Department of Health.

Finlay, J. M. (2001) Mesoprefrontal dopamine neurones and schizophrenia: role of developmental abnormalities. *Schizophrenia Bulletin*, **27**, 431–442.

Garralda, M. E. (1984) Hallucinations in children with conduct and emotional disorders. II. The follow-up study. *Psychological Medicine*, **14**, 597–604.

Gillberg, C., Wahlstrom, J., Forsman, A., *et al* (1986) Teenage psychoses – epidemiology, classification and reduced optimality in the pre-, peri- and neonatal periods. *Journal of Child Psychology and Psychiatry*, **27**, 87–98.

Gillberg, I. C., Hellgren, L. & Gillberg, C. (1993) Psychotic disorders diagnosed in adolescence. Outcome at 30 years. *Journal of Child Psychology and Psychiatry*, **34**, 1173–1186.

Gottesman, I. & Shields, J. (1982) *Schizophrenia: The Epigenic Puzzle*. Cambridge: Cambridge University Press.

Hollis, C. (1995) Child and adolescent (juvenile onset) schizophrenia. A case–control study of premorbid developmental impairment. *British Journal of Psychiatry*, **166**, 489–495.

Hollis, C. (1999) *A Study of the Course and Adult Outcomes of Child and Adolescent Psychosis* (PhD thesis). London: University of London.

Hollis, C. (2000) Adolescent schizophrenia. *Advances in Psychiatric Treatment*, **6**, 83–92.

Hollis, C. (2003) Developmental precursors of child and adolescent schizophrenia and affective psychoses: diagnostic specificity and continuity with symptom dimensions. *British Journal of Psychiatry*, **182**, 37–44.

Jacobsen, L. & Rapoport, J. L. (1998) Research update: childhood onset schizophrenia. *Journal of Child Psychology and Psychiatry and Allied Disciplines*, **39**, 101–113.

Kafantaris, V., Coletti, D. J., Dicker, R., *et al* (2001) Adjunctive antipsychotic treatment of adolescents with bipolar psychosis. *Journal of the American Academy of Child and Adolescent Psychiatry*, **40**, 1448–1455.

Kendler, A. S. (1998) The genetics of schizophrenia: an overview. In *Handbook of Schizophrenia* (eds M. Tsuang & P. Simpson), vol. 3, pp. 437–462. New York: Elsevier.

Kumra, S., Wiggs, E., Bedwell, J., *et al* (2000) Neuropsychological deficits in pediatric patients with childhood-onset schizophrenia and psychotic disorder not otherwise specified. *Schizophrenia Research*, **42**, 135–144.

Lader, D. (2000) *Psychiatric Morbidity Among Young Offenders in England and Wales*. London: Stationery Office.

Larsen, T. K., McGlashan, T. H. & Moe, L. C. (1996) First episode schizophrenia I. Early course parameters. *Schizophrenia Bulletin*, **22**, 241–256.

Ludolph, P. S., Westen, D., Misle, B., *et al* (1990) The borderline diagnosis in adolescents: symptoms and developmental history. *Archives of General Psychiatry*, **147**, 470–476.

McGorry, P. (1993) Early Psychosis Prevention and Intervention Center (EPPIC). *Australasian Psychiatry*, **1**, 32–34.

McGorry, P. D. (1995) Psychoeducation in first-episode psychosis: a therapeutic process. *Psychiatry*, **58**, 313–328.

McGorry, P. D., Edwards, J., Mihalopoulos, C., *et al* (1996) EPPIC: an evolving system of early detection and optimal management. *Schizophrenia Bulletin*, **22**, 305–229.

McGuffin, P., Murray, R. M. & Reveley, A. M. (1987) Genetic influence on the psychoses. *British Medical Bulletin*, **43**, 531–556.

McGue, M., Gottesman, I. & Rao, D. C. (1985) Resolving genetic models for the transmission of schizophrenia. *Genetic Epidemiology*, **2**, 99–110.

Murray, R. M. & Lewis, S. W. (1987) Is schizophrenia a neurodevelopmental disorder? *BMJ*, **295**, 681–682.

National Institute for Clinical Excellence (2002) *Guidance on the Use of Newer (Atypical) Antipsychotic Drugs for the Treatment of Schizophrenia* (Technical Appraisal no. 43). London: NICE.

Orvaschel, H. & Puig-Antich, J. (1987) *Schedule for Affective Disorders and Schizophrenia for School-Age Children - Epidemiologic Version (K–SADS–E)*. Philadelphia: Medical College of Pennsylvania.

Patton, G. C., Coffey, C., Carlin, J. B., *et al* (2002) Cannabis use and mental health in young people: cohort study. *BMJ*, **325**, 1195–1198.

Roberts, S., Garralda, E. & Renfrew, D. (2001) Schizotypal disorder among child and adolescent mental health service users. *Journal of the American Academy of Child and Adolescent Psychiatry*, **40**, 12.

Scully, P. J., Coakley, G., Kinsella, A., *et al* (1997) Psychopathology, executive (frontal) and general cognitive impairment in relation to duration of initially untreated versus subsequently treated psychosis in chronic schizophrenia. *Psychological Medicine*, **27**, 1303–1310.

Shaw, M. (2001) Competence and consent to treatment in children and adolescents. *Advances in Psychiatric Treatment*, **7**, 150–159.

Spencer, E., Birchwood, M. & McGovern, D. (2001) Management of first episode psychosis. *Advances in Psychiatric Treatment*, **7**, 133–140.

Vourdas, A., Pipe, R., Corrigall, R., *et al* (2003) Increased developmental deviance and premorbid dysfunction in early onset schizophrenia. *Schizophrenia Research*, **62**, 13–22.

Waddington, J. L., Scully, P. J. & Youssef, H. A. (1997) Developmental trajectory and disease progression in schizophrenia: the conundrum, and insights from a 12-year prospective study in the Monaghan 101. *Schizophrenia Research*, **23**, 107–118.

Werry, J. S. (1992) Child and adolescent (early onset) schizophrenia: a review in light of DSM–III–R. *Journal of Autism and Developmental Disorders*, **22**, 601–624.

Werry, J. S. & Taylor, E. (1994) Schizophrenic and allied disorders. In *Child and Adolescent Psychiatry: Modern Approaches* (eds M. Rutter, E. Taylor & L. Hersov), p. 606. Oxford: Blackwell.

Werry, J. S., McClellan, J. M., Andrews, L. K., *et al* (1994) Clinical features and outcome of child and adolescent schizophrenia. *Schizophrenia Bulletin*, **20**, 619–630.

World Health Organization (1992) *The ICD–10 Classification of Mental and Behavioural Disorders*. Geneva: WHO.

Zammit, S., Allebeck, P., Andreasson, S., *et al* (2002) Self reported cannabis use as a risk factor for schizophrenia in Swedish conscripts of 1969: historical cohort study. *BMJ*, **325**, 1199–1201.

CHAPTER 13

Substance misuse

Clare Lamb

Substance use or misuse is generally accepted to mean the non-medical use of chemical substances in order to achieve alterations in psychological functioning.

Adolescents who misuse substances are different from adults with drug and alcohol problems in number of ways. Reported differences include shorter drug histories, less involvement with opiates, more involvement with alcohol and cannabis, more binge drinking and more poly-drug use. There are significant differences relating to the developmental and social aspects of adolescents, including rapid social and physical changes and the relatively normative nature of high-risk behaviours.

For a comprehensive and detailed overview of different substances, their use and adverse effects, refer to Merrill & Peters (2001).

Substances commonly used include:

- nicotine, alcohol and illegal drugs, e.g. cannabis, lysergic acid diethylamide (LSD), ecstasy (methylenedioxymethamphetamine, MDMA), amphetamines, cocaine and heroin;
- prescription drugs when not used for medical purposes, e.g. benzodiazepines;
- volatile substances or solvents, e.g. aerosols, bottled gas, lighter fuel.

The usefulness of the ICD–10 (World Health Organization, 1992) and DSM–IV (American Psychiatric Association, 1994) diagnostic criteria of dependence syndromes in adolescents has been questioned by some experts working in substance misuse.

There has been a move towards a dimensional model of substance misuse disorder, in which substance misuse may be categorised as:

- **Experimental use**   Initial use, prompted by curiosity.
- **Recreational use**   Infrequent or regular use to fit in with peer group.
- **Instrumental use**   Frequent drug use, active drug-seeking where the primary motive may be hedonistic or compensatory to help cope with negative emotions.

- **Problem use** The primary means of recreation or way to cope with stress, or both. There is a change in peer group and lifestyle. Drug use is regular and continues despite negative consequences.
- **Dependent use** Compulsive use and loss of control over use. There is development of tolerance, and physical and psychological complications. Physiological withdrawal symptoms occur and there is rapid reinstatement after abstinence. There are significant impairments in almost all areas of life.

Prevalence

There is a significant amount of data on the prevalence of substance misuse. Most data covers the three major areas of concern: cigarette smoking, the use of alcohol and the use of illegal drugs. Studies producing data on prevalence are not always comparable because of different methods used. However a good source of summary data is to be found in *Key Data on Adolescence* (Coleman & Schofield, 2001).

Smoking

In community studies in the UK, 31% of boys and 41% of girls describe themselves as current smokers by 15 years of age. In addition, 37% of boys at aged 15 smoked more than 40 cigarettes weekly (Haselden *et al*, 1999; Goddard & Higgins, 2000).

Alcohol

By the age of 16 years, 94% of British school children had drunk alcohol and 78% had been intoxicated in the previous month (Miller & Plant, 1996). There is evidence that young people drink more frequently and get drunk more often than they did a decade ago (Royal College of Physicians and British Paediatric Association, 1995).

Illegal drugs

By the age of 16 years, 40% of UK school children have taken an illegal drug. By the late teens, 50% have used an illegal drug and 25% use an illegal drug on a regular basis (Miller & Plant, 1996). Another study reports that 30% of UK 15-year-olds have used cannabis and 6% have used psychedelic drugs (Goddard & Higgins, 2000). A similar picture was found in a Health Advisory Service study (Haselden *et al*, 1999). However, illegal drug use among teenagers and young adults varies markedly according to region, and in a large prevalence study among 14- to 18-year-olds in the north-west of England, rates were higher; in this study, 41% of 15-year-olds reported cannabis use, 13% had used solvents, 4% had used cocaine and 2.5% heroin (Parker *et al*, 1998). Adolescent drug use is higher in the UK than in the rest of Europe.

Aetiology

A number of studies are available on the predisposing and protective factors for substance misuse (Tsuang *et al*, 1998).

Predisposing factors

These include environmental risk factors such as widespread drug availability, poverty, acceptance of drug use in the community, parental substance misuse, peers who use drugs, family conflict and failure at school. Individual risk factors include low self-esteem, high risk-taking behaviour, early and persistent behaviour problems and mental health problems.

Harmful substance misuse in young adolescents usually occurs in the context of behaviour disorder, and most of the risk factors are also predictive of problem behaviour.

Protective factors

Protective factors include positive temperament, intellectual ability, supportive family environment and a social support system that encourages positive values. Reducing risk factors and enhancing protective factors is important to both preventing and managing substance misuse.

Psychological and psychiatric problems associated with substance misuse

The relationship between substance misuse and psychiatric disorder is complex, the presence of one predisposing to the development of the other. There is some evidence that substance misuse may develop as a form of self-medication for some young people with pre-existing mental illness (Wilens *et al*, 1999).

Psychiatric comorbidity is especially common in young adolescents. Studies confirm that young people with alcohol and other drug use problems frequently suffer from concomitant psychiatric disorders (Lewinsohn *et al*, 1995; Zeitlin, 1999). Significant rates of comorbid psychiatric disorder are found in community samples of adolescents who misuse substances, as well as clinic and in-patient samples. A study in the USA of a community sample of 1285 children and adolescents aged 9–18 years found that 66% of weekly drinkers met diagnostic criteria for a psychiatric disorder. Of those who reported use of illicit drugs three or more times in the past year, 85% of females and 56% of males met criteria for a least one psychiatric disorder (Kandel *et al*, 1997). The rates of comorbid substance misuse disorder and psychiatric disorder in a study of juvenile offenders referred for psychiatric evaluation were higher than for a community sample (Neighbors *et al*, 1992).

The psychiatric disorders that are most often reported concomitant with substance misuse among adolescents include mood disorders, anxiety disorders, conduct disorder and attention-deficit hyperactivity disorder. Comorbidity of drug use with a psychotic disorder is a significant and particular problem.

Recent studies have provided more research evidence on the link between cannabis use and psychiatric illness (Hall & Degenhardt, 2000; McKay & Tennant, 2000). In a historical cohort study of 50 000 Swedish conscripts, Zammit *et al* (2002) reported that cannabis use in adolescence was a risk factor for schizophrenia, independent of the effects of other drugs or social personality traits. In a New Zealand cohort, Arseneault *et al* (2002) found that adolescent cannabis use was a risk factor for schizophrenia even after adjustment for pre-existing childhood psychosis. This study shows that cannabis use by age 15 is of greater risk than later use at 18. Risk was specific to cannabis rather than other drugs.

Frequent use of cannabis has been linked to high rates of depression and anxiety in a number of cross-sectional surveys and studies of long-term users. However, the reason for the high rates is uncertain. Patton *et al* (2002) followed a cohort of 1600 Australian adolescents for 7 years. Results showed that rates of depression and anxiety increased with greater frequency of cannabis use: weekly use significantly increased later risk. There was a strong association between daily use of cannabis and depression and anxiety in girls. In contrast, depression and anxiety did not predict later cannabis use; self-medication was therefore unlikely to be the reason for the association. This study supports the link between frequent cannabis use and mental health problems in young people.

Substance misuse has been shown to be a significant factor in suicide attempts, repeated attempts and completed suicide (Hawton *et al*, 1993; Williams & Morgan, 1994).

Physical problems associated with substance misuse

Physical problems associated with substance misuse include those resulting from intoxication, such as accidents and overdose, and those related to a drug lifestyle, such as poor nutrition, increased vulnerability to infection and the consequences of risk-taking behaviour. Young injectors of opiates will be at particular risk of the consequences of unclean equipment and the transmission of hepatitis B and C and HIV.

Young people who binge drink are more likely to experience negative consequences, including involvement in damaging property, trouble with the police, sustaining injuries, driving after drinking, engaging in unplanned and unprotected sexual activity, and impaired academic performance (Wechsler *et al*, 2000).

Interventions

There is a relative dearth of systematic research-generated information about the kind of clinical interventions and services that are effective with adolescents who have substance misuse problems. However, many of the agencies routinely involved with young people, such as education, youth services, youth offending teams, accident and emergency staff, social services, family doctors and child mental health services, are likely to have an important role in the treatment of substance misuse. Effective interventions usually entail addressing multiple targets through a coordinated multi-agency approach with statutory, non-statutory and generic services, e.g. multisystemic therapy (Henggeler et al, 1996). There are risks in providing adolescent substance misuse services in adult-orientated services. The Health Advisory Service outlines the recommended criteria for substance misuse services for young people (Health Advisory Service, 1995).

Harm reduction

This is a pragmatic response to substance misuse which often uses a series of intermediate goals. The principles are applied to individual behaviour and also community interventions such as improved education on substance misuse and easier access to treatment (Miller et al, 2001).

Motivational interviewing

Strategies for change assume the client is motivated to cooperate with treatment. Motivation is a state of readiness to change. Motivational interviewing is a directive, client-centred counselling style that is designed to assist in exploring and resolving ambivalence to increase motivation for change. Motivation is a factor that changes over time and has the potential to be influenced by the therapist. Motivational interviewing assists client movement through the stages of change (Prochaska & DiClemente, 1992).

The process of change is described as a number of phases. The assumption is that the client is likely to pass through these phases several times, each time coming closer to recovery. The phases described consist of pre-contemplation, contemplation, determination, action and maintenance. Relapse is seen as inevitable and to be expected. The client is encouraged to accept the situation and start again. Motivational interviewing is distinguished from other approaches by its empathic, non-confrontational style and the stage-specific strategies it utilises. These stages consist of giving advice; removing barriers; providing choice, decreasing desirability, practising empathy, providing feedback, clarifying goals and active helping (Miller & Rollnick, 1992).

A number of studies support motivational interviewing as a useful clinical intervention. Further work is needed on applying this technique to the younger age group (Monti *et al*, 2001).

Family therapy

Several theory-based therapies have been shown to be effective in improving family relationships and reducing substance use, including systems-based, strategic and behavioural models (Weinberg *et al*, 1998). In most cases, family interventions should take place in conjunction with other interventions in a multimodal treatment approach.

Treatment of comorbidity

The treatment of comorbid mental illness is vital and must begin with diagnosis. Thorough mental state and physical examination and assessment of psychosocial circumstances is key to the identification of the range of difficulties to be addressed.

The most challenging diagnostic dilemma is that of comorbid psychosis and substance misuse. The primary aim of intervention is meaningful engagement of the young person and alleviation of mental distress, while undertaking further assessment and risk management. The case for the pharmacological treatment of psychoses and other psychiatric disorders in substance-misusing adolescents is accepted. However, more intense treatment may be required and special vigilance is needed when using pharmacotherapy in this group (Myles & Willner, 1999).

Treatment of withdrawal syndromes

Substance misuse withdrawal syndromes are rare in adolescents (Chung *et al*, 2000), hence pharmacotherapy to treat them should also be rare. Pharmacotherapy to relieve withdrawal in adolescents should proceed only when the quantity and frequency of substance use is sufficient to produce a withdrawal syndrome, e.g. daily use for a month or longer. In the case of alcohol or heroin withdrawal, treatment of adolescents should usually be undertaken by or under the supervision of a specialist trained in substance misuse.

Service provision

Every opportunity should be taken to identify and engage young people with problematic substance misuse. Studies of substance misuse services suggest that aspects of service delivery processes such as home visits, short waiting lists and frequent short contacts with a single worker can maximise engagement.

In many areas of the UK, primary care professionals, youth offending teams, child and adolescent mental health services, paediatricians, social services, youth services and education are working together with outreach substance misuse workers to meet the need of this vulnerable group of young people. Strategies for developing models of service for young people who misuse substances must include a needs-led, evidence-based service design in which multi-agency, multidisciplinary planning and implementation are central (Williams *et al*, 2004).

References

American Psychiatric Association (1994) *Diagnostic and Statistical Manual of Mental Disorders* (4th edn) (DSM–IV). Washington, DC: American Psychiatric Association.

Arseneault, L., Cannon, M., Poulton, R., *et al* (2002) Cannabis use in adolescence and risk for adult psychosis: longitudinal prospective study. *BMJ*, **325**, 1212–1213.

Chung, T., Colby, S. M., Barnett, N. P., *et al* (2000) Screening adolescents for problem drinking. *Journal of Studies on Alcohol*, **61**, 579–587.

Coleman, J. & Schofield, J. (2001) *Key Data on Adolescence*. Brighton: TSA Publications.

Goddard, E. & Higgins, V. (2000) *Smoking, Drinking and Drug Use Among Young Teenagers in 1998. Volume 1: England*. London: Office of National Statistics.

Hall, W. & Degenhardt, L. (2000) Cannabis and psychosis. *Australia and New Zealand Journal of Psychiatry*, **34**, 26–34.

Haselden, L., Angle, H. & Hickman, M. (1999) *Young People and Health: Health Behaviour in School-aged Children. A Report of the 1997 Findings*. London: Health Education Authority.

Hawton, K., Fagg, J., Platt, S., *et al* (1993) Factors associated with suicide after parasuicide in young people. *BMJ*, **306**, 1641–1644.

Health Advisory Service (1995) *Child and Adolescent Mental Health Services: Together We Stand*. London: HMSO.

Henggeler, S. W., Pickrel, S. G., Brondino, M. J., *et al* (1996) Eliminating (almost) treatment dropout of substance abusing or dependent delinquents through home-based multi-systemic therapy. *American Journal of Psychiatry*, **153**, 427–428.

Kandel *et al* (1997) Psychiatric disorders associated with substance use among children and adolescents: findings from the MECA study. *Journal of Abnormal Psychology*, **25**, 121–132.

Lewinsohn, P. M., Rohde, P. & Seeley, J. R. (1995) Adolescent psychopathology: III. The clinical consequences of comorbidity. *Journal of the American Academy of Child and Adolescent Psychiatry*, **34**, 510–519.

McKay, D. R. & Tennant, C. C. (2000) Is the grass greener? The link between cannabis and psychosis. *Medical Journal of Australia*, **172**, 284–286.

Merrill, J. & Peters, L. (2001) Substance misuse. In *Adolescent Psychiatry in Clinical Practice* (ed. S. Gowers), pp. 150–176. London: Arnold.

Miller, P. M. & Plant, M. (1996) Drinking, smoking and illicit drug use among 15 and 16-year-olds in the UK. *BMJ*, **313**, 394–397.

Miller, W. R. & Rollnick, S. (1992) *Motivational Interviewing. Preparing People to Change Addictive Behaviour*. London: Guilford.

Miller, E. T., Turner, A. P. & Marlatt, G. A. (2001) The harm reduction approach in adolescents. In *Adolescents, Alcohol and Substance Abuse: Reaching Teens Through*

Brief Interventions (eds P. M. Monti, S. M. Colby & T. O'Leary), pp. 58–79. London: Guilford.

Monti, P., Colby, S., O'Leary, T., *et al* (2001) Motivational enhancement for alcohol-involved adolescents. In *Adolescents, Alcohol and Substance Abuse: Reaching Teens through Brief Interventions* (eds P. M. Monti. S. M. Colby & T. O'Leary), pp. 145–182. London: Guilford.

Myles, J. & Willner, P. (1999) Substance misuse and psychiatry co-morbidity in children and adolescents. *Current Opinion in Psychiatry*, **12**, 287–290.

Neighbors, B., Kempton, T. & Forehand, R. (1992) Co-occurrence of substance abuse with conduct, anxiety and depression disorders in juvenile delinquents. *Addictive Behaviours*, **17**, 379–386.

Parker, H., Bury, C. & Egginton, R. (1998) *New Heroin Outbreaks Amongst Young People in England and Wales*. London: Home Office.

Patton, G. C., Coffey, C., Carlin, J. B., *et al* (2002) Cannabis use and mental health in young people: cohort study. *BMJ*, **325**, 1195–1198.

Prochaska, J. O. & DiClemente, C. C. (1992) Stages of change in the modification of problem behaviours. *Program of Behaviour Modifications*, **28**, 183–218.

Royal College of Physicians & British Paediatric Association (1995) *Report of a Joint Working Party: Alcohol and the Young*. London: Royal College of Physicians.

Tsuang, M. T., Lyons, M. J., Meyer, J. M., *et al* (1998) Co-occurrence of abuse of different drugs in men: the role of drug-specific and shared vulnerabilities. *Archives of General Psychiatry*, **55**, 967–972.

Wechsler, H., Lee, J. E., Kuo, M., *et al* (2000) College binge drinking in the 1990s. A continuing problem – results of the Harvard School of Public Health 1999 College Alcohol Study. *Journal of American College Health*, **48**, 199–210.

Williams, R. & Morgan, H. G. (1994) *Suicide Prevention – The Challenge Confronted*. London: NHS Health Advisory Service.

Williams, R., Gilvarry, E. & Christian, J. (2004) Developing an evidence-based model for services. In *Young People and Substance Misuse* (eds I. Crome, H. Ghodse, E. Gilvarry, *et al*), pp. 195–222. London: Gaskell.

Weinberg, N. Z., Rahdert, E., Colliver, J. D., *et al* (1998) Adolescent substance abuse. A review of the past 10 years. *Journal of the American Academy of Child and Adolescent Psychiatry*, **37**, 252–261.

Wilens, T., Biederman, J., Millstein, R., *et al* (1999) Risk of substance use disorders in youths with child and adolescent onset bipolar disease. *Journal of the American Academy of Child and Adolescent Psychiatry*, **38**, 680–685.

World Health Organization (1992) *The ICD-10 Classification of Mental and Behavioural Disorders. Clinical Descriptions and Diagnostic Guidelines*. Geneva: WHO.

Zammit, S., Allebeck, P., Andreasson, S., *et al* (2002) Self reported cannabis use as a risk factor for schizophrenia in Swedish conscripts of 1969: historical cohort study. *BMJ*, **325**, 1199–1201.

Zeitlin, H. (1999) Psychiatric comorbidity with substance misuse in children and teenagers. *Drug and Alcohol Dependence*, **55**, 225–234.

CHAPTER 14

Eating disorders

Simon G. Gowers

Concern about a child's eating or weight is a common cause of parental
contact with primary care services. Health visitors in particular are
consulted about difficulties with feeding and sleeping more than any
other problem. In childhood, responsibility for maintaining an adequate
food intake is seen to rest primarily with parents or other carers, but in
the course of development it transfers to the young person. Thus,
teenagers may make the decision to diet for the first time. The ICD–10
(World Health Organization, 1992) and DSM–IV (American Psychiatric
Association, 1994) psychiatric classification systems reflect this
developmental shift in responsibility in distinguishing between 'feeding
disorders of childhood' and 'eating disorders', which generally arise in
adolescence and which are similar to those seen in early adulthood. The
transitional nature of adolescence, however, suggests that different
approaches to the assessment and treatment of these disorders are
required.

Feeding disorders of childhood
and eating disorders of adolescence

Feeding disorders arise in the first 6 years of life, and involve food
refusal or extreme faddiness in the presence of adequate food and the
absence of organic disease. They are extremely common; faddy eating
occurs in over 20% of pre-school children, rumination and regurgitation
of food more rarely. In contrast to adolescent eating disorders, there is
usually an absence of concern with appearance, or other psychological
or behavioural abnormality. These disorders tend to be treated by
interventions focused on parental management. In practice there is
some overlap between feeding disorders and early-onset eating disorders,
as some of the latter present with prior histories of feeding problems. In
addition, early-onset eating disorders tend not to conform readily to
strict ICD–10 or DSM–IV criteria, and are thus often considered atypical

(Lask & Bryant-Waugh, 2000). The terms 'selective eating', 'pervasive refusal' and 'food avoidance emotional disorder' have been coined to describe some of the atypical eating disorders that occur in older childhood and puberty.

This chapter focuses on the related syndromes of anorexia nervosa and bulimia nervosa, which involve profound disturbances of physical, psychological, behavioural and social functioning. Obesity will be mentioned briefly, as attention is increasingly being directed to the problems of overweight adolescents, both because of the rapid increase in prevalence and their relationship with other eating disorders.

Epidemiology

Prevalence

Anorexia nervosa

The point prevalence of anorexia nervosa in the UK determined by a screening questionnaire followed by semi-structured interview for girls aged 14–19 years has been reported as 0.2% in state schools and 0.8% in private schools (Szmukler, 1983). The condition is rare at age 12 years, but reaches about 1 in 200 girls at age 16 years. The figure for teenage boys is about 1 in 2000, with a more equal gender ratio at the younger end, where eating disorders are in general less typical. In boys, less fear of fatness and more obsessive–compulsive symptoms may be seen.

There are suggestions of an increasing incidence of anorexia nervosa over the past 50 years, calculated at 36% every 5 years from 1950 to 1984 in adolescent American girls (Lucas *et al*, 1991). It is also thought that anorexia nervosa may have changed over time, becoming more evenly distributed among the social classes and occurring in younger and younger children. The purging form (with vomiting and laxative use) is believed to have become more common.

Bulimia nervosa

Since 1980, there have been reports of a growing epidemic of bulimia nervosa: 19% of Dutch female students report bulimic symptoms, with a point prevalence of 1500 definite cases per 100 000 young females, a rate approximately five times that for anorexia nervosa (Hoek, 1995). As the mean age of onset of bulimia nervosa is 18–19, it remains a relatively rare disorder in early adolescence. Bulimia nervosa is a common outcome of anorexia nervosa. More rarely, young people may progress from normal weight bulimia into anorexia nervosa.

Cultural influences

Anorexia nervosa was formerly seen as a middle-class disorder of the White, Western world. This is no longer the case, although it is not clear whether this is due to a change in identification of cases in different cultures or a spread to immigrants and developing nations as they have taken on Western culture and aspirations. Becker *et al* (2002) reported an interesting study suggesting that rates of disordered eating rose in Fijian adolescents after the introduction of television. Second-generation migrants may be at higher risk than the indigenous population of developed countries, owing to conflict between parental and peer aspirations.

Diagnosis

Anorexia nervosa

The diagnosis of anorexia nervosa is based on the maintenance of low weight as a result of the over-evaluation of the self in terms of weight and shape. This may be manifested as concern about fatness and distorted body image. Weight must be low enough that sex hormone levels regress to or are maintained at pre-pubertal levels. The diagnosis is more difficult to make in younger adolescents, for whom growth has not been completed, than in adults. The ICD–10 (Box 14.1) and DSM–IV criteria address the diagnostic difficulty in younger children by allowing for failure to gain weight and delay in the process of puberty, rather than specifying the presence of secondary amenorrhoea.

Malnutrition stunts linear growth and consequently the degree of underweight can be underestimated if based solely on weight for current height. Body mass index (BMI; weight in kg/height in m²) is a less useful guide to degree of thinness under the age of 16 years, when the normal range of BMI is lower. Reference to the BMI centiles for age may be useful, although these are also based on current (possibly stunted) height.

Although not part of the core diagnosis, social withdrawal, regressive behaviour, rigid self-control, obsessionality and perfectionism are

---

Box 14.1 Summary of diagnostic criteria for anorexia nervosa, ICD–10 code F50.0 (World Health Organization, 1992)

- Body weight is maintained at least 15% below that expected (lost or never achieved) or body mass index is below 17.5 kg/m².
- Weight loss is self-induced by avoidance of fattening foods, exercise, vomiting or purgation.
- There is a body image distortion, manifested as a dread of fatness.
- A widespread endocrine disorder involving the hypothalamic–pituitary–gonadal axis is present. In the female this is manifest as amenorrhoea and in the male as impotence and loss of sexual interest.

> **Box 14.2** Three examples of entry into anorexia nervosa
>
> Patient A shows premorbid normal growth followed by marked weight loss. Her height chart shows a slowing of growth with dietary abstinence.
>
> Patient B, having followed a similar premorbid course, has not lost weight but maintained a pre-pubertal weight when the normal pubertal trajectory started steeply upwards. She has also ended up underweight with a similar effect on her height to patient A.
>
> Patient C has always been small and indeed thin for her age. With the onset of adolescence, however, despite slow growth, she has crossed centile lines and become more underweight, taking into account her 'expected' weight and height.

common in adolescents with anorexia. The striving for control often extends to others and the family will often report feeling controlled by their son or daughter. Classical restricting anorexia nervosa often seems to represent an excess rather than a loss of control. Box 14.2 illustrates the route into anorexia nervosa for three 13-year-old girls.

Bulimia nervosa

The ICD–10 criteria apply across the age range (Box 14.3). Typically, the young person falls into a daily cycle of dietary restriction early in the day, which cannot be sustained for both physiological and psychological reasons in the evening. The resultant binge is followed by vomiting, associated feelings of guilt and a resolve to redress the situation the following day.

The alternating cycle of control and catastrophic loss of control is often mirrored in other areas of the young person's life; thus, they may have difficulties with drug and alcohol use, delinquency or promiscuous sexual behaviour. This may render girls vulnerable to sexual exploitation and unwanted pregnancy.

> **Box 14.3** Summary of diagnostic criteria for bulimia nervosa, ICD–10 code F50.2 (World Health Organization, 1992)
>
> - Persistent preoccupation with eating, with irresistible craving that results in episodes of binge eating (DSM–IV requires subjective feeling of loss of control while bingeing).
> - Vomiting, purging or drug use (amphetamines, diet pills or diuretics) in an attempt to counteract the effect of a binge.
> - Dread of fatness.

Table 14.1 Grading of obesity by body mass index

Grade of obesity	BMI (kg/m²)
0	<25
1	25–29.9
2	30–40
3	>40

Obesity

Although obesity is not classified as a psychiatric syndrome (it is coded E66 in Section E), a number of teenagers will identify emotional factors that contribute to their overeating and volunteer adverse psychosocial consequences of their condition. Difficulties with self-esteem and in peer relationships predominate. Desirable body weight is usually considered to be between 90% and 120% of ideal weight. Obesity can be graded according to BMI as shown in Table 14.1.

Investigations

Pre-pubertal children are at greater risk than adults of physical complications of starvation, because of their relative deficiency of body fat and tendency to dehydrate more quickly. Routine blood count, electrolyte levels, and liver and thyroid function should be measured. Serum calcium, phosphate, vitamin B$_{12}$ and folate levels should be monitored in severe starvation or during re-feeding.

Height and weight should be plotted on centile charts and if possible related to premorbid values. Stunting of growth, interruption of the process of puberty and failure of bone mineralisation provide extra dimensions to the physical risks of the condition, which may only be partially reversible if recovery is significantly delayed.

Heart rate and blood pressure should be measured and an electro-cardiogram (ECG) performed if cardiac function is compromised or antidepressant treatment proposed. Pubertal status can be assessed by Tanner staging, which provides mean ages and ranges for the development of secondary sexual characteristics. Concerns arise if this staging is more than two standard deviations behind the mean. Ultrasonography can confirm (and enable monitoring of) ovarian function.

Differential diagnosis

The diagnosis is usually straightforward, if the young person's defensiveness can be overcome by engagement and a corroborative parental history. It is usually possible to ascertain dietary restriction in the face of normal or increased appetite. Depression in adolescence rarely leads to selective dietary restriction or the degree of weight loss seen in older adults, although it occurs comorbidly with anorexia nervosa in nearly 50% of cases.

Unusual physical differential diagnoses include intracranial tumours, thyrotoxicosis (in which there is raised metabolic rate), Addison's disease and growth hormone deficiency.

Aetiology

In many ways, eating disorders typify adolescent mental health problems. Their origins are multifactorial, sociocultural factors and life events tending to have an impact on a vulnerable personality, possibly shaped by family environment against a background of genetic and biological predisposition. It is often possible to identify difficulties in the areas of identity formation, independence, behavioural control and physical growth, which are the essence of the teenage years. As the illness develops, it is just these areas of development that are adversely affected by anorexia nervosa. The condition can therefore be seen to be maintained by difficulties meeting the challenges of adolescence which originally predisposed to the condition.

Case example 1

Emma was 15 and studying hard for her GCSE exams. At the New Year she was invited to a party at which she was shocked by a friend's sexual precocity. She noticed the disappointment in her parents' eyes when she returned home slightly intoxicated. Over the next few days they reminded her that she would now have to buckle down and study hard if she were to achieve her required exam grades. When up in her bedroom attempting to study, however, she found difficulty concentrating and would regularly interrupt her work to slip downstairs for a couple of biscuits. When term restarted, she was shocked to find her school uniform was uncomfortably tight. She really had let herself go over the Christmas holidays! As anorexia nervosa developed, she found her willpower increase and she became more single-minded. Her partying days were over – at least until her exams had passed. In any case, she wouldn't want anyone to watch her eat, so invitations had to be declined. As April came, Emma became quite unwell with a persistent virus, which resulted in further weight loss and time off from school. She feared that she would not do as well in her exams as she should, because only the top grades would satisfy her. Maybe, her parents suggested, it would be better if they got a letter from the doctor explaining her illness and took the pressure off her by postponing her exams. She could take them next year when she was fully recovered and really do justice to her abilities.

Biological factors

A number of risk factors for the development of eating disorders have been postulated, from premorbid obesity to excessive tallness. Biological vulnerability may be present as genetic predisposition to early pubertal development. In general, early pubertal development is experienced negatively by girls, who may suffer high levels of body dissatisfaction extending into adulthood. It is likely that once starvation has become established, the condition may be maintained by a distortion of the hunger drive.

Personality

Many children who develop eating disorders in adolescence are described as having been compliant, ideal children. A strong sense of morality, concern about the welfare of others, conscientiousness and perfectionism are common. These features apply in the main to restricting anorexia, the purging form being more associated with periodic loss of control and impulsivity.

Family factors

Structure

Anorexia nervosa more commonly arises in intact families than do other adolescent mental health problems, although parental marital breakdown can act as a life event precipitant. It has been shown to occur equally in any position in the sibship.

Functioning

There are dangers in extrapolating from a situation of crisis and presuming aetiological significance. The notion of the psychosomatic family described by Minuchin *et al* (1978) has now largely been rejected owing to lack of supportive evidence. Families themselves report no greater difficulties in functioning than community controls and somewhat fewer than families with other adolescent psychiatric disorders. Adolescents with anorexia nervosa themselves are more critical of their families, and their views and those of clinicians have been shown to predict the outcome of anorexia nervosa at 1 year (North *et al*, 1997). An inverse relationship between family difficulties and severity of anorexia has supported the notion of anorexia nervosa as an adaptive strategy to reduce family distress.

Precipitants and life events

Crisp (1994) has provided a compelling case for an adolescent maturational crisis underlying anorexia nervosa. A controlled study into the role of life event precipitants suggested that severe negative life events occurred in the year before onset in about one-quarter of cases, somewhat fewer than in those with other psychiatric conditions, but more than in a community control group (Gowers *et al*, 1996).

219

Sociocultural factors

The uneven distribution of eating disorders across populations and possibly time has led many to postulate the role of family eating patterns, prevailing attitudes to female fatness in different societies, gender roles and television (Becker *et al*, 2002) in the aetiology of eating disorders. The power of advertising to promote the desirability of foods and lifestyles, particularly for women, has come under recent scrutiny.

Management

Anorexia nervosa

Evidence is growing to suggest that complete recovery is dependent on the patient owning changes to their diet and weight. Thus engagement is important in ensuring an effective treatment alliance, aiming for restoration of normal weight and eating, with appropriate psychological adjustment. Most advocate a target weight of around 95% average body weight and certainly above the menarcheal threshold for post-pubertal cases. Whereas in adults, treatment usually aims to return the patient to a state of premorbid health, in adolescents the task frequently involves achieving a healthy post-pubertal weight for the first time. This is usually accompanied by a new experience of engagement with adolescence in all its aspects, which can be as challenging as the adjustment to increased weight, for patients and parents alike.

Setting

Pragmatic guidelines suggest that admission may be the logical step for those in whom physical concerns are greatest and for those who fail to make progress on an out-patient basis. In case series, however, hospital in-patients often lose weight after discharge before subsequently recovering, raising the question of the part played by in-patient treatment in recovery (Gowers *et al*, 2000). On the one hand, ensuring completion of puberty and avoiding stunting of growth may be extremely important. On the other, disruption of education and normal social development may especially harm a younger person. An individual decision about admission may rest on such issues as the wishes of the patient and family, the expertise available and the degree of physical concern.

Day programmes have the advantage of combining the benefits of intensive treatment, peer support and behavioural therapies (particularly around meal-times) without the disadvantages (and costs) of admission.

Therapeutic style

There are advocates of family systemic, cognitive–behavioural and cognitive–analytic approaches, but as yet empirical evidence fails to favour one approach over another. All young people are likely to require parental counselling to address practical issues such as dietary planning, education and return to physical activities. Where family communication is poor, family therapy may be helpful. A trial of two forms of family intervention suggested that separated family therapy might be more effective than conjoint therapy, particularly in families with high expressed emotion (Eisler *et al*, 2000).

Pharmacotherapy

Pharmacological interventions have been disappointing in the treatment of both anorexia nervosa and accompanying mood disorder. Suspicion of medication (in terms of its calorific value and potential for taking away control) may affect compliance. Fluoxetine may help prevent relapse in weight-restored patients.

Bulimia nervosa

Most treatment research is based on adult series. Numerous trials have confirmed the efficacy of psychotherapy and pharmacotherapy, generally delivered on an out-patient basis. Both cognitive–behavioural therapy and interpersonal therapy have been shown to decrease binge eating, purging and related attitudes and behaviours in women with bulimia nervosa. With appropriate modification to allow for the young person's age, it seems appropriate to use a similar approach.

Teenagers have strong beliefs about the morality of eating and purging behaviours, which they will assume the interviewer shares. It is helpful to establish a non-judgemental approach to recording rates of bingeing and vomiting, in order to establish an accurate baseline against which to measure recovery. This helps when cognitive distortions make it hard for young people to acknowledge progress and cause them to lose heart during treatment. Antidepressants – in particular fluoxetine and desipramine – appear to be an effective adjunct to treatment in combination with cognitive–behavioural therapy, although less effective alone.

Case example 2

Michelle was 17 when she developed bulimia nervosa. The traumatic break-up of her relationship with her boyfriend had left her feeling used and physically unattractive. Her friends had never liked Steve and now their predictions had been confirmed; she was beginning to doubt her own judgement. She was left somewhat bruised by the experience and with a police caution for possession of drugs. Each day she woke with a resolution to start afresh, with a new commitment to getting her life back on track. When she restricted her eating, at least that gave her a sense of achievement; she did have some willpower after all. No breakfast then and no lunch. By evening she was starving, her blood sugar was so low, it demanded she eat and high-calorie food too. Once she started, she found it difficult to stop. She was home much of the time now, so it was easy to indulge herself. At the back of her mind she knew she would easily be able to vomit back the excess, so what the heck. As she flushed the lavatory later, she reflected on the fact that her parents still didn't seem to have noticed her distress. How many signals did she have to give before they gave her any time these days? As she retired to bed she chastised herself again. What a fool! She dare not think about the weight she must have put on. Tomorrow she must turn over a new leaf – no breakfast for sure. At least that would be a start and in any case all she deserved.

Involving parents

The role of parents alongside cognitive–behavioural therapy programmes is unclear, but parents will need to be kept informed of the treatment plan and progress, particularly for younger patients, ideally in their presence. Family therapy may usefully be employed where the patient identifies family relationship difficulties alongside her eating disorder.

Obesity

Some will be helped by psychotherapeutic measures, with or without behavioural intervention aimed at weight loss. Obesity treatment programmes rarely achieve consistently maintained weight loss greater than 10% and many now aim for weight stabilisation rather than weight loss. Although this might seem a limited aim, where adult height has not been attained, weight maintenance will result in reduction in fatness (and therefore BMI) over time.

Prognosis

Anorexia nervosa

Predictors of good outcome include healthy family functioning and a severe negative life event precipitant (North *et al*, 1997). A weight below 65% of that expected is a negative prognostic feature. Admission to hospital for extensive psychiatric treatment is often associated with a poor outcome. Cases with a number of adverse physical and psychological features are likely to be selected for admission, but it is probable that the negative effects of loss of schooling on peer relationships and self-esteem are underestimated. A long-term adolescent follow-up study (Herpertz-Dahlmann *et al*, 2001) suggested that two-thirds were free of an eating disorder by 10 years (slightly better than adult series), but that 51% had an Axis I psychiatric disorder.

Bulimia nervosa

Bulimia nervosa generally has a better outcome than anorexia nervosa and complete remission is more likely. Poor prognostic indicators include borderline personality functioning and multi-impulsivity. Long-term follow-up suggests that 71% of patients receiving intensive treatment maintain gains over 6 years. As the mean age of onset for bulimia is 19, there are few reports specifically focusing on adolescents.

Prevention

Primary prevention programmes aim to target at-risk populations (e.g. girls in secondary school) and deliver interventions aimed at preventing the development of eating disorders in those who are asymptomatic. A number of educational programmes have been tried, based on the uncertain assumption that knowledge changes attitudes, which in turn modify behaviour. Such interventions aimed at reducing dieting may clash with those aimed at reducing obesity. Programmes focusing on self-esteem might be more fruitful.

Secondary prevention programmes aim to detect cases and provide early intervention. Education of health workers in primary care is vital, while de-stigmatising child mental health services should reduce patient resistance. There is good evidence that early intervention reduces long-term morbidity.

References

American Psychiatric Association (1994) *Diagnostic and Statistical Manual of Mental Disorders* (4th edn) (DSM–IV). Washington, DC: American Psychiatric Association.

Becker, A. E., Burwell, R. A., Gilman, S. E., *et al* (2002) Eating behaviours and attitudes following prolonged exposure to television among ethnic Fijian adolescent girls. *British Journal of Psychiatry*, **180**, 509–514.

Crisp, A. H. (1994) *Anorexia Nervosa: Let Me Be* (2nd edn). London: Academic Press.

Eisler, I., Dare, C., Hodes, M., *et al* (2000) Family therapy for adolescent anorexia nervosa: the results of a controlled comparison of two family interventions. *Journal of Child Psychology and Psychiatry*, **41**, 727–736.

Gowers, S. G., North, C., Byram, V., *et al* (1996) Life event precipitants of adolescent anorexia nervosa. *Journal of Child Psychology and Psychiatry*, **37**, 469–478.

Gowers, S. G., Weetman, J., Shore, A., *et al* (2000) Impact of hospitalisation on the outcome of adolescent anorexia nervosa. *British Journal of Psychiatry*, **176**, 138–141.

Herpertz-Dahlmannn, B., Muller, B., Herpertz, S., *et al* (2001) Prospective 10 year follow up in adolescent anorexia nervosa – course, outcome, psychiatric comorbidity and psychosocial adaptation. *Journal of Child Psychology and Psychiatry*, **42**, 603–612.

Hoek, H. W. (1995) The distribution of eating disorders. In *Eating Disorders and Obesity* (eds K. D. Brownell & C. G. Fairburn), pp. 207–211. New York: Guilford.

Lask, B. & Bryant-Waugh, R. (2000) Childhood onset anorexia nervosa and related disorders (2nd edn). Hove: Psychology Press.

Lucas, A. R., Beard, C. M., O'Fallen, W. M., *et al* (1991) Fifty year trends in the incidence of anorexia nervosa in Rochester, Minnesota. A population study. *American Journal of Psychiatry*, **148**, 917–922.

Minuchin, S., Rosman, B. & Baker, L. (1978) *Psychosomatic Families; Anorexia Nervosa in Context*. Cambridge, MA: Harvard University Press.

North, C. D., Gowers, S. G. & Byram, V. (1997) Family functioning and life events in the outcome of adolescent anorexia nervosa. *British Journal of Psychiatry*, **171**, 545–549.

223

Szmukler, G. (1983) Weight and food preoccupation in a population of English schoolgirls. In *Understanding Anorexia Nervosa and Bulimia* (ed. G. I. Bargman), pp. 21–27. Report of the Fourth Ross Conference on Medical Research. Columbus, Ohio: Ross Laboratories.

World Health Organization (1992) *The ICD–10 Classification of Diseases: Clinical Descriptions and Diagnostic Guidelines.* Geneva: WHO.

CHAPTER 15

Biological factors

Lindsey Kent

The past decade has seen a rapidly expanding interest in biological markers and risk factors for childhood psychiatric disorders. Technological advances in molecular genetics and functional neuroimaging techniques have fuelled this growing interest and have provided new insights into aetiological factors underlying common diseases. Identification of susceptibility genes for a number of childhood psychiatric disorders has the potential to transform future clinical management. As the biological mechanisms responsible for disease are unravelled, new approaches to diagnosis and classification, as well as an improved understanding of the course of disorders, may emerge. Ultimately, future therapeutic interventions can be developed rationally based on a clear understanding of pathogenesis. In addition, biological approaches may identify individuals who are most likely to respond to certain pharmacological interventions or develop particular side-effects. Understanding the biological basis of disorders provides an opportunity to investigate the contribution that environmental factors may make to disease processes, and how biology and environment interact and influence each other in the development of disorders. This chapter discusses the evidence for the involvement of biological risk factors and underlying biological markers relevant to a number of childhood psychiatric disorders, and in particular discusses pertinent findings from the research literature on genetics, neurophysiology, neuropsychology and neuroimaging.

Before discussing the different disorders, it is useful to discuss some general issues that have a bearing on the interpretation of findings in the literature. It is often not clear whether many of the biological factors associated with various disorders represent primary causative factors, and as such are true risk factors for illness, or whether the associated factor has occurred as a consequence of having the disorder. For example, is the disturbed hypothalamic function seen in patients with anorexia nervosa a risk factor for anorexia or does it arise as a consequence of having the condition? Although for many biological markers, examining unaffected first-degree relatives and performing twin studies will help clarify this, a 'cause or effect' model is oversimplistic. The development of disorders is a constantly evolving process, with biological and environmental factors influencing each other in ways that we currently have little understanding of. A particularly demonstrative example of this is seen with depression. Genes have only a small role in the susceptibility to childhood depression, but genetic liability to depression increases considerably throughout adolescence and into adulthood, although this increase is seen predominantly in females. In parallel with this is the finding that childhood depression is more common in boys, whereas by adolescence this gender bias has reversed, with a greater prevalence evident in girls. Although genes do not change, their relative influence on the development and expression of a phenotype may change over time as environmental influences change and interplay with genetic factors. It is useful, therefore, to consider when reading this chapter that even quite apparently obvious biological risk factors are operating within a broader context, and rarely alone.

Autism

Both family and twin studies demonstrate a significant genetic influence in infantile autism. The rate of autism among siblings of affected individuals is around 3% (e.g. Smalley *et al*, 1988), which is 75–150 times greater than the rate of autism within the general population. Within families of autistic individuals, a much broader range of cognitive disabilities, particularly speech and language problems and social deficits, are also seen, providing support for the existence of a spectrum of autistic disorders. A number of studies have demonstrated higher concordance rates in monozygotic twin pairs with autism (36–91%) compared with dizygotic pairs (0–10%) (Folstein & Rutter, 1977; Bailey *et al*, 1995). The heritability of autism is of the order of 80–90%. Molecular genetic research in autism has recently attracted considerable interest with the publication of several whole-genome linkage scans identifying some overlapping regions of interest (International Molecular Genetics Study of Autism Consortium, 2001; see summary in Liu *et al*, 2001). Of particular interest are regions of chromosome 15q, which contains the region where several imprinted genes lie, including the Prader–Willi/Angelman critical region. All of the chromosome 15q duplications associated with autism have been derived from the mother (Cook *et al*, 1997), further raising the possibility of imprinting effects. Although no genes have yet been identified for autism, the most promising areas from the genome scans also include a region on 7q and another region on 2q, which have been replicated by several groups.

Approximately 10–15% of cases of autism are associated with an underlying medical disorder (Barton & Volkmar, 1998). For instance, a wide range of chromosomal abnormalities are associated with autistic-spectrum disorders, but these are only found in around 5% of autistic individuals. Autism has also been associated with other genetic disorders such as fragile-X syndrome, Rett's syndrome and tuberous sclerosis.

A number of studies have identified possible biological markers for autism, most notably increased levels of platelet serotonin (5-HT) and monoamine oxidase activity, and low dopamine beta-hydroxylase activity. However, these findings have not proved particularly useful in furthering our understanding of these disorders. Elevated levels of whole blood serotonin have been observed in around 30% of individuals with autism (Anderson *et al*, 1987), but have also been noted in individuals with severe mental retardation as well as unaffected family members. Support for the involvement of 5-HT in autism also comes from functional neuroimaging studies which have suggested that 5-HT synthesis may be disrupted in children with autism, although these results are preliminary (Chugani *et al*, 1999). Although not of widespread benefit in autism, selective serotonin reuptake inhibitors (SSRIs) may be helpful in a subset of children with autism and may especially help anxiety and obsessional symptoms. Findings from structural and functional neuro-imaging studies have been largely contradictory. Several studies have reported increased brain volume and hippocampal and amygdala changes, although these changes differ between studies.

Attention-deficit hyperactivity disorder

Family, twin and adoption studies all support the role of genes in attention-deficit hyperactivity disorder (ADHD). Siblings of children with ADHD are at up to 5 times greater risk of ADHD than siblings of normal controls. Twin studies report higher concordance in monozygotic (70–80%) than in dizygotic twin pairs (30%). Heritability estimates range from 70% to 90% (Faraone & Biederman, 1998). Methylphenidate, the stimulant most commonly used in treatment, has blockade of the dopamine transporter and release of dopamine as two of its actions, and low-dose methylphenidate preferentially releases noradrenaline. In addition, decreased central serotonin has been implicated in poor impulse control, and nicotine is known, like methylphenidate, to stimulate the release of dopamine, improving attention in smokers, non-smokers and adults with ADHD. Maternal smoking during pregnancy is associated with an increased risk of ADHD in offspring and ADHD is a risk factor for early initiation of smoking (Milberger *et al*, 1997), further suggesting a role for the cholinergic nicotinic system in ADHD. Evidence from animal studies also supports the potential role of these neurotransmitter systems in the pathogenesis of ADHD. For example, a dopamine transporter gene knockout mouse is hyperactive and demonstrates a number of spatial cognitive deficits.

To date, molecular genetic studies of ADHD have mainly focused on the candidate gene association study approach. A variety of candidate genes have been examined, largely selected from genes involved in the neurotransmitter system pathways discussed above. Despite a number of contradictory findings, the most interesting results to date suggest a possible role for the dopamine receptor gene *DRD4* and the dopamine transporter gene *DAT1* (Thapar & Scourfield, 2002).

Neuropsychology studies have repeatedly demonstrated deficits in response inhibition, verbal and non-verbal working memory and other 'executive' functions, but these deficits are also seen in other conditions and as such do not represent specific underlying biological markers for ADHD. Structural and functional imaging techniques have provided supportive evidence for the involvement of fronto-striatal pathways, the corpus callosum, caudate nuclei, globus pallidum and cerebellum in ADHD, with preferential reduction in volume in these areas in addition to decreased total brain volume (Tannock, 1998; Eliez & Reiss, 2000). More recent functional neuroimaging studies conducted during neuro-psychological and motor control testing have also suggested the importance of prefrontal, basal ganglia and anterior cingulate dys-function in this disorder (Rubia *et al*, 1999; Teicher *et al*, 2000), with task performance on a number of neuropsychological tests being shown to correlate with functional deficits. The common finding in event-related potential (ERP) studies employing continuous performance tests of children with ADHD is impaired target processing, shown by attenuated P300 amplitudes in response to targets. Several ERP abnormalities in children with ADHD are ameliorated by methyl-phenidate (Jonkman *et al*, 1997).

Reading disorders

Although it has been recognised for many years that reading difficulties (dyslexia) run in families, twin studies have confirmed that several components of reading have a significant genetic contribution, e.g. reading recognition and spelling. Molecular genetic studies in reading disability have predominantly focused on linkage strategies, and several whole-genome linkage scans for reading disability have reported regions of interest on chromosomes 15q and 6p (Grigorenko, 2001). In addition, several twin studies have suggested that the phenotypic association between reading disability and attention-deficit hyperactivity disorder, particularly inattention symptoms, is largely attributable to common genetic influences (Willcutt *et al*, 2000). Children at risk of developing dyslexia demonstrate a characteristic pattern of poor phonological awareness and limited letter knowledge that presages reading difficulties. Moreover, structural neuroimaging studies have demonstrated symmetry of the planum temporale in the brain of dyslexic readers, and evidence from functional neuroimaging studies suggests that differences in left-hemisphere brain functioning may underlie phonological processing deficits seen in dyslexia (Filipeck, 1999).

Tourette syndrome and tic disorders

Family and twin studies have provided evidence that genetic factors are involved in Tourette syndrome and related tic disorders (Pauls & Leckman, 1986). Family studies have indicated that first-degree relatives of those with this syndrome are at a higher risk of developing not only Tourette syndrome but also chronic motor tic disorders and obsessive–compulsive disorder, compared with unrelated individuals. Twin studies for Tourette syndrome alone demonstrate monozygotic concordance rates of around 50% and dizygotic concordance rates of around 10%. However, when this phenotype is broadened to include co-twins with chronic motor tic disorders as well, the concordance figure for mono-zygotic twins rises to nearly 80% and the dizygotic rate is around 30%. Despite initial studies suggesting autosomal dominant transmission in Tourette families, subsequent linkage studies failed to identify a susceptibility gene using traditional linkage approaches. Sib-pair linkage approaches have suggested possible linkages to regions on chromosomes 4q and 8p (Tourette Syndrome International Consortium for Genetics, 1999) and 11q (Simonic et al, 2001).

In terms of which neurotransmitter pathways may be involved in Tourette syndrome, the dopaminergic system is the most implicated, with D_2 receptors receiving attention given the preferential blockade of these receptors by a number of neuroleptics that ameliorate tics, such as haloperidol and tiapride (Chappell et al, 1997). Some functional neuroimaging studies also support the role of D_2 receptors in Tourette syndrome (Wong et al, 1997). A number of other neurotransmitters and pathways have been implicated in Tourette syndrome, including the glutamate, gamma-aminobutyric acid (GABA), cholinergic, serotonergic and noradrenergic systems, but results from studies are contradictory and preliminary. Neuroimaging studies have also lent support to the role of prefrontal cortex/basal ganglia circuits in the aetiology of Tourette syndrome and obsessive–compulsive disorder (Peterson et al, 1998).

There has been recent interest in the possibility that paediatric autoimmune neuropsychiatric disorder associated with streptococcal infection (PANDAS) may underlie some cases of Tourette syndrome and obsessive–compulsive disorder (Swedo et al, 1998). This is based on the finding that many patients with childhood-onset Tourette syndrome or obsessive–compulsive disorder have elevated expression of a marker that identifies nearly 100% of rheumatic fever patients (a delayed sequela of group A beta-haemolytic streptococcus infection), but is present at very low levels of expression in healthy control populations. Patients with rheumatic fever may develop Sydenham's chorea, a movement disorder which also involves the basal ganglia, and may include motor and vocal tics and obsessive–compulsive symptoms as part of its presentation. Although these findings are preliminary, they have attracted considerable interest.

Obsessive–compulsive disorder

Family and twin studies implicate a role for genetics in obsessive–compulsive disorder (OCD). Several studies have demonstrated that both OCD and tic disorders run through the same families. In fact, some researchers have proposed that OCD and Tourette syndrome are in fact alternate expressions of the same underlying genetic susceptibility. Given the effectiveness of SSRIs in the treatment of OCD, it is likely that serotonin has a role in this disorder. In addition, functional neuro-imaging studies have provided evidence for decreased serotonin synthesis in the prefrontal cortex and caudate nucleus in children with OCD (Rosenburg *et al*, 1998). This study also supports the role of the involvement of frontal-basal ganglia pathways in OCD, in keeping with the knowledge that areas within the basal ganglia are thought to be involved in Tourette syndrome. It is likely that both disorders involve a balance between the dopaminergic and serotonergic systems. Further evidence for the involvement of the basal ganglia in OCD is provided by the improvements seen in patients who have undergone psychosurgical procedures that involve separating the basal ganglia from the frontal cortex. In addition, orbital frontal cortex and caudate nuclei regional glucose metabolism has been demonstrated to be elevated in OCD.

Conduct disorders

Genetic factors appear to be of less importance in childhood conduct disorder, in contrast to studies of adult criminality, but they are still present. McGuffin & Gottesman (1985) reported pooled concordance rates from five twin studies of juvenile delinquency of 87% for mono-zygotic twins and 72% for dizygotic twins. Children with conduct disorder and delinquency are more likely to come from families with a criminal parent, but twin and adoption studies suggest that a complex interaction between both genetic and environmental factors underlies susceptibility to conduct problems. Gene–environment correlation is thought to be of particular importance in the development of conduct disorder, i.e. genes influence our behaviour, and our behaviour influences how we interact with our environment and how others interact with us.

In terms of possible underlying biological markers, children with conduct disorder have demonstrated lower levels of electrodermal activity, lower heart rate reactivity and resting heart rate, and lower heart rate variability (Mezzacappa *et al*, 1997; Pine *et al*, 1998). These characteristics have been noted to be most marked in individuals who have an earlier onset of conduct disorder and whose disorder involves poor socialisation and predatory aggression. In addition to these autonomic indices, a number of neuro-endocrinological and neurohumoral indices have been studied. Diminished levels of salivary cortisol and elevated levels of salivary testosterone in patients with aggressive and impulsive behaviour have been replicated in some studies. Conduct disorder is known to be associated with lower IQ scores and also some executive function deficits, which are independent of IQ.

Affective disorders

Family studies clearly demonstrate increased rates of depression among the offspring of depressed parents. It is known from twin studies in adults that affective disorders have significant genetic contributions. Heritability for bipolar disorder is high at around 80% and unipolar depression also has a significant genetic component at around 40–50% (Jones *et al*, 2002).

Twin studies suggest a moderate genetic influence on depressive symptoms in adolescents. However, it appears that shared environmental factors are more important contributors to depression in younger children (Thapar & McGuffin, 1994). A number of researchers have reported that early-onset bipolar disorder is associated with a greater genetic loading than bipolar disorder occurring in adulthood, with higher rates of affective disorder occurring in first-degree relatives of early-onset probands compared with later-onset probands.

The underlying biochemical hypothesis of depression proposes that depression arises from underactivity in monoamine systems. There is evidence to implicate the role of 5-HT in childhood-onset depression, partly coming from the treatment response of some – particularly adolescents – to SSRIs. In addition, the finding of reduced levels of 5-HT transporter protein in the platelets from the blood of some children and adolescents with major depression is also supportive (Salee *et al*, 1998). In adolescents, however, endocrine studies have attracted the most attention in terms of attempting to elucidate the underlying biological processes involved. A number of studies have demonstrated that depressed young people are more likely to demonstrate non-suppression of cortical secretion following administration of dexamethasone. In addition, several studies have demonstrated a relationship between the cortisol level and course of depression in adolescents (Goodyer *et al*,

1998). However, raised cortisol is a normal physiological response to stress, and it remains unclear what role cortisol has in mediating links between stress and subsequent depression.

Although it was generally assumed that patients with bipolar disorder did not have underlying neuropsychological deficits, evidence has now emerged that this may not be the case. Frontal executive difficulties have been reported by a number of groups, particularly deficits in verbal working memory (Ferrier *et al*, 1999). Some neuroimaging studies of adults with bipolar disorder have demonstrated frontal, temporal, corpus callosal and basal ganglia differences, but other studies have failed to support these findings, partly as a result of different diagnostic and neuroimaging methods (Videbech, 1997). Adolescent bipolar imaging studies have reported decreased cerebral volume, with increased frontal and temporal sulcal size (Friedman *et al*, 1999), as well as subcortical focal signal hyperintensities (Botteron *et al*, 1995). However, findings from neuroimaging studies are not specific enough to be of value in identifying children at risk.

Schizophrenia

From a neurobehavioural point of view, schizophrenia has been one of the most extensively studied psychiatric disorders, although studies have predominantly investigated adult patients. Most individuals with schizophrenia have some underlying central nervous system dysfunction, but the nature of this dysfunction is not well understood. Biochemical theories of schizophrenia, predominantly derived from the mechanism of action of antipsychotic drugs, have focused on the role of dopamine and more recently serotonin and the excitatory neurotransmitter glutamate. Preliminary work using magnetic resonance spectroscopy demonstrates that there are indeed decreased levels of cerebral glutamate in the frontal lobes of children with schizophrenia (Thomas *et al*, 1998).

Neuroimaging findings in children are similar to those observed in adults and provide evidence for the neurobiological continuity between childhood-onset and adult-onset schizophrenia. These findings include a smaller total cerebral volume and larger caudate, putamen, globus pallidus and lateral ventricles in children with schizophrenia compared with controls. Functional neuroimaging studies have also consistently demonstrated relative hypometabolism in several brain structures, particularly in the frontal lobes. In addition, histological studies have demonstrated loss or disorganisation of hippocampal tissue.

Increasingly, schizophrenia is considered to be a neurodevelopmental condition. Both retrospective studies of children with schizophrenia and studies of high-risk offspring of patients with schizophrenia demonstrate that these children manifest certain neurobehavioural impairments during childhood well before the onset of psychotic symptoms; these include delayed language acquisition and motor impairments in infancy (Watkins *et al*, 1988) and also a preference for solitary play. Children with schizophrenia typically have a mild intellectual deficit with below-average IQ scores. In addition, more specific deficits in various aspects of cognition are also apparent. Slow reaction times and deficits in verbal and spatial working memory and in sustained attention have been demonstrated. In a group of children diagnosed with schizophrenia, Gordon *et al* (1994) demonstrated impaired smooth pursuit eye movements and high baseline levels of autonomic activity with slow habituation and adaptation.

Psychophysiological studies of the processes involved in information processing have demonstrated some reasonably consistent findings that may reflect underlying biological markers in children with schizophrenia. Event-related potentials possess extremely high temporal resolution (milliseconds) and have the potential to identify processing stages involved in a variety of neurocognitive test paradigms. Studies of event-related potentials in children (and adults) with schizophrenia have demonstrated reduced P300 amplitude and smaller Np components. The Np and P300 components provide an index of allocation of attentional and perceptual resources during cognitive task performance.

Although several reasonably consistent findings emerge from the literature with respect to possible underlying biological vulnerability markers for childhood schizophrenia, many of these are not necessarily specific to schizophrenia. They may also be associated with other conditions, for example reduced P300 amplitude is also a consistent finding in patients with alcoholism. As yet, they cannot be used reliably to identify children who will later develop schizophrenia.

Family, twin and adoption studies have all consistently demonstrated the involvement of genes in schizophrenia (Scourfield & McGuffin, 2001), although most genetic research has involved adults. There is some evidence that early-onset schizophrenia may represent a more heritable form with a greater genetic loading. Many groups have been involved in molecular genetic studies of schizophrenia, although few have had adequate numbers of childhood-onset patients to examine. Despite numerous linkage and association studies, however, there has been only a modest amount of replication across studies, and current interest is focusing on chromosomes 15, 10 and 5. In addition the velo-cardio-facial syndrome, caused by a microdeletion on chromosome 22q11, is associated with learning difficulties, cardiac abnormalities, short stature and parkinsonism. Individuals with this syndrome are around a hundred times more likely to have schizophrenia compared with the general population. This chromosomal region may, therefore, harbour a susceptibility gene for schizophrenia.

Eating disorders

Anorexia nervosa

Family studies provide evidence that anorexia nervosa may have a genetic component, with around 5–10% of first-degree relatives of a proband also affected. There is also an increased risk of major affective disorder, alcoholism and drug misuse in the first-degree relatives of people with anorexia. Twin studies have demonstrated a significant genetic liability for anorexia. For any eating disorder, monozygotic concordance rates are around 50%, compared with around 25% for dizygotes, whereas a more narrowly defined phenotype such as restricting anorexia nervosa demonstrates higher monozygotic rates of around 60%, with dizygotic rates of around 8%. Heritability for anorexia has been estimated at around 70–80%. No gene has as yet been identified as definitely having a role in anorexia, but many investigators have focused on the serotonergic system. Physiologically, there is evidence for disturbed hypothalamic/pituitary function in anorexia. However, this may be secondary to weight loss, carbohydrate starvation and stress, and may represent an effect of having anorexia nervosa rather than an underlying biological cause. However, given that amenorrhoea occurs before the weight loss in around 20% of cases, there remains the possibility that disturbed hormonal function may underlie susceptibility to anorexia.

Bulimia nervosa

In contrast, although patients with bulimia often demonstrate similar endocrine changes to those seen in patients with anorexia as a result of low weight and depressed mood, there is little evidence for any genetic susceptibility to bulimia. In fact, twin studies demonstrate a very small genetic contribution and a very large environmental influence (Wade *et al*, 1998). Quantitative genetic studies of both anorexia and bulimia nervosa have been contradictory, however, with a couple of studies failing to find much of a genetic influence for anorexia and other studies reporting evidence of significant genetic influences in bulimia. Although much is known regarding the various biological and endocrine parameters involved in eating disorders and the alterations in these following starvation and weight loss, little is known, as yet, about the underlying predisposing biological susceptibilities for eating disorders.

Anxiety disorders

There are numerous studies demonstrating the familial nature of anxiety disorders, with high rates of various anxiety disorders in parents of children with anxiety and also in children of adults with anxiety. Much of the quantitative genetic research has been conducted in adults, and there is evidence that panic disorder is a particularly heritable form of anxiety disorder. There is also evidence that earlier-onset cases may have a higher genetic loading. Other forms of childhood anxiety generally demonstrate heritability in the range of 40–50%, which is consistent with the adult literature. However, some of the findings are conflicting, which may be related to the differences in diagnosis of childhood anxiety disorders across studies and also differences in the gender distribution across them. There is significant evidence that anxiety disorders are more common in girls than in boys.

Adults and children with a variety of anxiety disorders exhibit startle reflex abnormalities. These may represent an underlying biological marker for anxiety, given that unaffected relatives of children with anxiety disorder also demonstrate abnormalities of startle reactions (Merikangas *et al*, 1999). A further underlying biological marker may be the increased sensitivity to a variety of respiratory stimulants such as CO_2 and sodium lactate among individuals with anxiety and panic disorder. Family studies of unaffected first-degree relatives have also demonstrated similar responses to respiratory stimuli, providing evidence that this may also be a biological trait marker for anxiety.

Conclusion

Biological factors are important in the aetiology and development of many, if not all, child psychiatric conditions. The field of child psychiatry, although initially reluctant to examine this important contribution, appears to be making up for lost time. Examination of recent child psychiatry literature demonstrates increasing application of a wide variety of biological approaches to the understanding of the aetiology of child psychiatric disorders. In addition, publication of the draft human genome sequence has accelerated this process further, allowing researchers to begin to unravel the biological underpinnings of human disease. Ultimately, this will lead to a greater understanding of the pathogenesis of psychiatric conditions and improved therapeutic interventions.

References

Anderson, G. M., Freedman, C. X., Cohen, D. J., *et al* (1987) Whole blood serotonin in autistic and normal subjects. *Journal of Child Psychology and Psychiatry*, **28**, 885–900.
Bailey, A., Le Couteur, A., Gottesman, I., *et al* (1995) Autism as a strongly genetic disorder: evidence from a British twin study. *Psychological Medicine*, **25**, 63–77.
Barton, M. & Volkmar, F. (1998) How commonly are known medical conditions associated with autism? *Journal of Autism and Developmental Disorders*, **28**, 273–278.
Botteron, K. N., Vannier, M. W., Geller, B., *et al* (1995) Preliminary study of magnetic resonance imaging characteristics in 8- to 16-year-olds with mania. *Journal of the American Academy of Child and Adolescent Psychiatry*, **34**, 742–749.

Chappell, P. B., Scahill, L. D. & Leckman, J. F. (1997) Future therapies of Tourette syndrome. *Neurologic Clinics*, **15**, 429–450.

Chugani, D. C., Muzik, O., Behen, M., *et al* (1999) Developmental changes in brain serotonin synthesis capacity in autistic and non-autistic children. *Annals of Neurology*, **45**, 287–295.

Cook, E. H., Lindgren, V., Leventhal, B. L., *et al* (1997) Autism or atypical autism in maternally but not paternally derived proximal 15q duplication. *American Journal of Human Genetics*, **60**, 928–934.

Eliez, S. & Reiss, A. L. (2000) MRI neuroimaging of childhood psychiatric disorders: a selective review. *Journal of Child Psychology and Psychiatry*, **41**, 679–694.

Faraone, S. V. & Biederman, J. (1998) Neurobiology of attention-deficit hyperactivity disorder. *Biological Psychiatry*, **44**, 951–958.

Ferrier, I. N., Stanton, B. R., Kelly, T. P., *et al* (1999) Neuropsychological function in euthymic patients with bipolar disorder. *British Journal of Psychiatry*, **175**, 246–251.

Filipeck, P. A. (1999) Neuroimaging in the developmental disorders: the state of the science. *Journal of Child Psychology and Psychiatry*, **40**, 113–128.

Folstein, S. & Rutter, M. (1977) Genetic influences and infantile autism. *Nature*, **265**, 726–728.

Friedman, L., Findling, R. L., Kenny, J. T., *et al* (1999) An MRI study of adolescent patients with either schizophrenia or bipolar disorder as compared to healthy control subjects. *Biological Psychiatry*, **46**, 78–88.

Goodyer, I. M., Herbert, J. & Altham, P. M. (1998) Adrenal steroid secretion and major depression in 8–16-year-olds. III. Influence of cortisol:DHEA ratio at presentation on subsequent rates of disappointing life events and persistent major depression. *Psychological Medicine*, **28**, 265–273.

Gordon, C. T., Frazier, J. A., McKenna, K., *et al* (1994) Childhood-onset schizophrenia: an NIMH study in progress. *Schizophrenia Bulletin*, **20**, 697–712.

Grigorenko, E. L. (2001) Developmental dyslexia: an update on genes, brains and environment. *Journal of Child Psychology and Psychiatry*, **42**, 91–126.

International Molecular Genetics Study of Autism Consortium (2001) A genomewide screen for autism: strong evidence for linkage to chromosomes 2q, 7q and 16p. *American Journal of Human Genetics*, **69**, 570–581.

Jones, I., Kent, L. & Craddock, N. (2002) The genetics of affective disorders. In *The Genetics of Psychiatric Disorders* (eds P. McGuffin, I. Gottesman & M. Owen), pp. 211–245. Oxford: Oxford University Press.

Jonkman, L. M. Kemner, C., Verbaten, M. N., *et al* (1997) Effects of methylphenidate on event-related potentials and performance of attention-deficit hyperactivity disorder children in auditory and visual selective attention tasks. *Biological Psychiatry*, **41**, 690–702.

Liu, J., Nyholt, D. R., Magnussen, P., *et al* (2001) A genome wide scan for autism susceptibility loci. *American Journal of Human Genetics*, **69**, 327–340.

McGuffin, P. & Gottesman, I. I. (1985) Genetic influences on normal and abnormal development. In *Child and Adolescent Psychiatry: Modern Approaches* (2nd edn) (eds M. Rutter & L. Hersov), pp. 17–33. Oxford: Blackwell Scientific.

Merikangas, K. R., Avenevoli, S., Dierker, L., *et al* (1999) Vulnerability factors among children at risk for anxiety. *Biological Psychiatry*, **46**, 1523–1535.

Mezzacappa, E., Tremblay, R. E., Kindlon, D., *et al* (1997) Anxiety, antisocial behavior and heart rate regulation in adolescent males. *Journal of Child Psychology and Psychiatry*, **38**, 457–470.

Milberger, S., Biederman, J., Faraone, S. V., *et al* (1997) ADHD is associated with early initiation of cigarette smoking in children and adolescents. *Journal of the American Academy of Child and Adolescent Psychiatry*, **36**, 37–44.

Pauls, D. L. & Leckman, J. F. (1986) The inheritance of Gilles de la Tourette syndrome and associated behaviors: evidence for autosomal dominant transmission. *New England Journal of Medicine*, **315**, 993–997.

Peterson, B. S., Skudlarski, P., Anderson, A. W., et al (1998) A functional magnetic resonance imaging study of tic suppression in Tourette syndrome. Archives of General Psychiatry, 55, 326–333.

Pine, D. S., Wasserman, G. A., Miller, L., et al (1998) Heart rate period variability in boys at risk for delinquency. Psychophysiology, 35, 521–529.

Rosenburg, D. R., Chgani, D. C., Musik, O., et al (1998) Altered serotonin synthesis in fronto-striatal circuitry in pediatric obsessive–compulsive disorder. Biological Psychiatry, 43, 24.

Rubia, K., Overmeyer, S., Taylor, E., et al (1999) Hypofrontality in attention deficit hyperactivity disorder during higher-order motor control: a study with functional MRI. American Journal of Psychiatry, 156, 891–896.

Salee, F. R., Hilal, R., Dougherty, D., et al (1998) Platelet serotonin transporter in depressed children and adolescents: H-paroxetine platelet binding before and after sertraline. Journal of the American Academy of Child and Adolescent Psychiatry, 37, 777–784.

Scourfield, J. & McGuffin, P. (2001) Genetic aspects. In Schizophrenia in Children and Adolescents (ed. H. Remschmidt), pp. 119–134. Cambridge: Cambridge University Press.

Simonic, I., Nyholt, D. R., Gericke, G. S., et al (2001) Further evidence of linkage of Gilles de la Tourette syndrome susceptibility loci on chromosomes 2p11, 8q22 and 11q23–24 in South African Afrikaners. American Journal of Medical Genetics, 105, 163–167.

Smalley, S. L., Asarnow, R. F. & Spence, M. A. (1988) Autism and genetics: a decade of research. Archives of General Psychiatry, 45, 953–961.

Swedo, S. E., Leonard, H. L., Garvey, M., et al (1998) Pediatric autoimmune neuropsychiatric disorders associated with streptococcal infections: clinical description of the first 50 cases. American Journal of Psychiatry, 155, 264–271.

Tannock, R. (1998) Attention deficit hyperactivity disorder: advances in cognitive, neurobiological, and genetic research. Journal of Child Psychology and Psychiatry, 39, 65–99.

Teicher, M. H., Anderson, C. M., Polcari, A., et al (2000) Functional deficits in basal ganglia of children with attention-deficit/hyperactivity disorder shown with functional magnetic resonance imaging relaxometry. Nature Medicine, 6, 470–473.

Thapar, A. & McGuffin, P. (1994) A twin study of depressive symptoms in childhood. British Journal of Psychiatry, 165, 259–265.

Thapar, A. & Scourfield, J. (2002) Childhood disorders. In Psychiatric Genetics and Genomics (eds P. McGuffin, M. J. Owen & I. I. Gottesman), pp. 147–180. Oxford: Oxford University Press.

Thomas, M. A., Ke, Y., Levitt, J., et al (1998) Frontal lobe proton MR spectroscopy of children with schizophrenia. Journal of Magnetic Resonance Imaging, 8, 841–846.

Tourette Syndrome International Consortium for Genetics (1999) A complete genome screen in sib-pairs affected with Gilles de la Tourette syndrome. American Journal of Human Genetics, 65, 1428–1436.

Videbech, P. (1997) MRI findings in patients with affective disorder: a meta-analysis. Acta Psychiatrica Scandinavica, 96, 157–168.

Wade, T., Martin, N. G. & Tiggemann, M. (1998) Genetic and environmental risk factors for the weight and shape concerns characteristic of bulimia nervosa. Psychological Medicine, 28, 761–771.

Watkins, J. M., Asarnow, R. F. & Tanguay, P. E. (1988) Symptom development in childhood onset schizophrenia. Journal of Child Psychology and Psychiatry, 29, 865–878.

Willcutt, E. G., Pennington, B. F. & DeFries, J. C. (2000) A twin study of comorbidity between attention-deficit hyperactivity disorder and reading disablity. American Journal of Human Genetics (Neuropsychiatric Genetics), 96, 293–301.

Wong, D. F., Singer, H. S., Brandt, J., et al (1997) D2-like dopamine receptor density in Tourette syndrome measured by PET. Journal of Nuclear Medicine, 38, 1243–1247.

237

CHAPTER 16

Psychosocial factors

Tim Morris

Many psychological and social factors are implicated as aetiological or risk factors in child mental health problems. Individuals are often exposed to multiple factors over a period of time. A developmental perspective (Cicchetti & Cohen, 1995) is needed as children develop over time and change as a result of their experiences. Development results in relatively ordered and lasting change occurring in physical structure, thought processes, behaviour and emotions (Jones, 2003). The processes of change in psychopathology have to be interpreted in the context of different expressions of problems and disorders at different developmental points. Some difficulties might continue in different forms through time, whereas others might represent a discontinuity in a previous developmental path. It is therefore difficult to evaluate the direct effects of single factors in isolation and for this reason it is useful to have a framework for considering each factor in relation to an individual child, at a particular point in time.

One framework is that of predisposing, precipitating and perpetuating factors: predisposing factors may make children more vulnerable to developing a disorder, precipitating factors may trigger the onset of a disorder and perpetuating factors may maintain a disorder. It is worth remembering that in some cases the same factor, e.g. parental marital conflict, can operate at each level. Not all exposed individuals will develop mental health problems. Protective factors and resilience in adversity may therefore also be important in a more complete under-standing of psychosocial aetiologies.

Even with the same factors it is still possible to see a diversity of outcome for a child. Different factors may in some cases lead to a similar end result or, conversely, a single factor may lead to multiple outcomes, as shown in Figure 16.1.

One major reason for this diversity in outcomes is the situations in which children find themselves. Psychosocial factors do not operate in isolation of other aetiological factors (Chapters 15 and 17), nor do children exist in isolation. The context (Carr, 1999) within which they

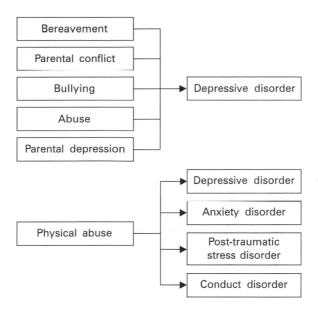

Fig. 16.1 Diversity of outcome.

live is likely to be at least as important as any particular psychosocial stressor. It is therefore helpful to consider psychosocial factors across a range of domains that children experience (Fig. 16.2). It is within this context that we will consider psychosocial risk factors. Box 16.1 shows the range of psychosocial influences on a child.

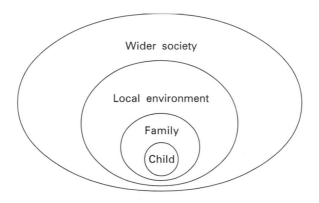

Fig. 16.2 The child in context.

Box 16.1   Psychosocial influences on mental health problems

Child factors
Age and gender
Ethnicity
Temperament
Individual strategies

Family factors
Family type
Family size and ordinal position
Parenting style
Family disruption
Reconstituted families
Residential and foster care
Parental mental illness
Parental criminality
Siblings
Extended family members

Local environmental factors
Peers
Schools
Life events
Poverty and social class
Neighbourhoods
Substance misuse

Wider societal factors
War and civil conflict
Immigration and asylum
Television and other media

Child factors

Age and gender

Chapter 5 reviewed the epidemiology of child psychiatric disorder and identified differences in prevalence rates at different ages and between the genders. The overall rates of emotional disorders are similar for boys and girls, although self-harm and anorexia nervosa are more common in adolescent girls. Autism, attention-deficit hyperactivity disorder (ADHD) and antisocial behaviour are more common in boys. Although biological and developmental factors are important in explaining these differences, psychosocial factors such as gender stereotyping and gender-role behaviour (Rippon, 1994) also play a part. In turn, individual differences will determine vulnerability and resilience to psychosocial risk factors. Age and gender differences in the first two decades of life provide a model to explore the complex interaction of psychosocial and neurobiological explanations of different disorders (Moffitt *et al*, 2001).

240

Ethnicity

Rates of mental disorder are different within particular ethnic groups in the UK. In children under 16 years old, 12% of Black children, 10% of White children and 8% of Asian children were found to have a disorder. The lowest prevalence was found within children from an Indian ethnic group, with an overall rate of 4%. These findings are difficult to interpret given the small size of the sample of minority group children (Ford *et al*, 2003), but ethnicity in relation to mental health is as important for children as it is in the debate within adult mental healthcare (Littlewood & Lipsedge, 1997). The psychosocial impact of being a member of a minority group alters across generations, presenting different issues in the first, second and subsequent generations (Lau, 2000). Professionals dealing with these children need to be able to identify pathological or maladaptive patterns of behaviours (Dwivedi, 2002) within a culturally sensitive perspective.

Temperament

Temperamental style refers to the way that an individual responds to a range of situations. Chess & Thomas (1995) in their 25-year longitudinal study grouped children into three temperamental types. Easy-temperament children were 40% of the sample. These children had regular patterns of feeding, sleeping and toileting. They approached new situations with a positive response and formed supportive networks. Their long-term prognosis was good and their temperament acted as a protective factor. Difficult-temperament children were 10% of the sample. They had irregular early childhood routines. They had negative responses to new situations and elicited negative responses from others. They were at greater risk of subsequent problems, and developed conduct and adjustment disorders. Fifteen per cent of the sample were classified as 'Slow to warm up'. They had temperamental characteristics in between the others and the prognosis was also halfway between the easy and difficult temperament groups. It was not possible to classify the remaining 35% of infants in this sample into these three categories.

These temperamental styles have been used to explain associations between an infant's behavioural responses and long-term adjustment in later life. The broad categories of temperament mean that the links between early childhood temperament and specific adult personality types are unclear, but there are links to more general measures of psychological function. More specific temperamental characteristics such as activity, sociability and emotionality may have a genetic basis (Plomin *et al*, 1988), but psychosocial experiences may then modify the expression of these characteristics over time.

Individual strategies

Children continue to develop their own styles of response to stimuli. Particular strategies and styles of responding interact with psychosocial factors in a dynamic way. A number of different models have been used to describe these functions. At a subconscious level, defence mechanisms may be seen as positive or negative depending on the circumstances and the developmental level of the child. Children's sense of self-efficacy is also important, with those with an internal locus of control and high self-efficacy being best able to cope with adversity. These positive traits are likely to develop when the child has positive and successful experiences. Children who experience difficulties or failure may attribute these difficulties to stable factors beyond their control, which reduces their sense of being able to change things. Unhelpful attributional styles and cognitive bias may lead to further difficulties. For example, children who have experienced parental aggression may expect aggressive behaviour from others. When faced with other people, they may interpret behaviour as hostile when it was not. They may then react to this perceived hostility with their own provocative and hostile behaviour. This may trigger an aggressive interaction, and also reinforces the initial cognitive interpretation. Similar cognitive biases have been found in other disorders such as depression, where distortions in cognitions are similar to those found in adults. A child's overall level of cognitive function as broadly measured by IQ mediates some of these responses, whereby children with lower levels of measured IQ have higher rates of mental health problems. Children with specific learning difficulties such as language delay and disorder have higher rates of conduct and disruptive behaviour disorders, and this may be as a result of early difficulties in social understanding and communication leading to hostile patterns of interaction.

Family factors

Children usually live within family units. Within these units, there are multiple relationships. Early parent–child attachment (Chapter 10), parental behaviour (Chapter 17) and the characteristics of the family are important and interrelated. Although a single factor can be associated with adverse mental health outcomes, frequently factors such as marital discord, divorce and inconsistent parental style cluster together, making the relative contribution of each difficult to assess.

Family type

Children may thrive in a range of different family types, e.g. married couples, same-sex couples, extended family networks, multifamily communes and reconstituted families. There is little evidence that family type in itself is associated with greater rates of child mental health problems, providing the quality of the relationships is good and there is no social adversity. The finding that the children of lone parents have double the rates of mental health problems of children in two parent families can be explained by the reasons for single-parent status, and the social and emotional hardship that may ensue. There is no clear difference in risk whether the single parent is male or female.

Family size and ordinal position

Children in larger families with five or more children have a significantly higher risk of mental health problems in terms of emotional and conduct disorders than those where there are one, two or three children. This may be the result of increased difficulty in monitoring and supporting each child, but may also be accounted for by increasing economic disadvantage.

The eldest child and only children tend to do better at school and at work. This may be explained by increased parental interaction and stimulation with this child. There is little evidence that 'middle children' are particularly disadvantaged by their ordinal position or that the sex order of the children has any particular implications for mental health.

Parenting style

A variety of different parental styles and characteristics may be considered within the normal range, and yet have an impact on child mental health. Different children may respond best to different parenting approaches. This 'goodness of fit' between the child and parents is likely to have a long-term effect, especially as patterns of interactions develop.

Parenting that is emotionally warm offers clear and consistent boundaries, and age-appropriate control is associated with the development of independent, confident individuals. Harsh, inconsistent parenting and the development of coercive interchanges are associated with the development of childhood conduct disorders (Patterson, 1982). For example, punitive methods of control such as smacking may be used to stop minor problems. The initial success of this approach may reinforce the parenting response. When faced with subsequent child behaviour, increasingly punitive methods may be used. A reinforcing sequence of events may then ensue (Forehand & McMahon, 1981). This may not only have a detrimental effect on parent–child relationships, but also affect the children's behaviour when they are with other people. Children who have experienced coercive parenting may have poorly developed social skills, be rejected by their peers and have low self-esteem in addition to conduct problems. Parents may also be perceived (Perris *et al*, 1994) as being overprotective, overinvolved and intrusive. These factors have been associated with depressive disorders, agoraphobia and with obsessive–compulsive disorders, although there are inconsistent results.

Family disruption

Disruption of the birth family most commonly occurs following parental separation or divorce. Approximately 40% of marriages end in divorce, and 1 in 4 children under 16 have this experience. Not only do children have to cope with the event at the time of separation and beyond, but they are likely to have experienced adverse circumstances in the family home leading up to an actual separation. Children are likely to be exposed to parental discord, which may range from verbal arguments to witnessing domestic violence. In the extreme cases, serious injury or death of a parent may occur (Harris-Hendriks *et al*, 2000). The direct and indirect effects of these family conflicts before separation (Cummings & Davies, 1994) have been increasingly recognised and correlated with subsequent adjustment problems in children.

The parental conflict does not necessarily end following the separation. Although the child will typically live for most of the time with one parent, it is usual for contact to be maintained with the other parent; the arrangements for such contact are often a source of ongoing parental conflict. Children may then become a focal point of this conflict and be placed in the invidious position of trying to support each parent against the other. If the child can maintain a good relationship with both parents, who work together to avoid conflict, this minimises the risk of an adverse psychosocial outcome (Hetherington & Stanley-Hagan, 1999). Thus, the consequences of divorce and separation for the child depend on the pre-separation environment and on what happens after the separation. Long-term adjustment for children reared in high-conflict families where parents separate is better than where parents remain together, indicating that divorce in certain circumstances may be a protective factor (Kelly, 2000).

Reconstituted families

Remarriage and other reconstituted family types are common. Many children live with a step-parent and need to form a relationship with this adult. Other children may also be involved, and an extended network of parents, step-parents, siblings, half-siblings and grandparents may develop. Younger children have greatest difficulty in the first year after remarriage, but behavioural problems decrease after 2 years. Adolescents have more difficulty coping with the changes associated with remarriage. A third of these reconstituted families also later separate. Children thus have to cope with multiple changes in family composition, which can amplify the psychosocial risk of family disruption.

Residential and foster care

A small proportion of children may need to live away from their family, and this represents an important high-risk group. Between 60% and

80% of these young people have mental health problems (McCann *et al*, 1996) that are considered to need treatment (Philips, 1997). Residential and foster care, however, comprise a heterogeneous group of psychosocial factors and the impact for an individual child depends upon the reason non-family care is needed, its duration and the type of facility used.

When young people are in local authority care or are being provided with accommodation by the local authority, then they are considered within the Children Act 1989 (Department of Health, 1991) to be 'looked after'. This usually happens when their family is considered unsuitable to care for them or can no longer do so. This may be as a result of a short-term problem such as parental illness or more chronic problems such as abuse, severe social difficulties, specific educational difficulties or uncontrollable behavioural problems.

The range of non-family provision includes family foster placement, residential schools, and individual and group care homes. Foster placements constitute the majority of placements for children looked after by local authorities. They are typically short-term and precipitated by times of crisis. This often works well when the child can return to a stable home environment. Some children remain in placements for a considerable time. When a child or adolescent is looked after for over 6 months the chances of return to the original family are much reduced (Coleman, 1999). Looked after children can also experience multiple and frequent changes of foster carer over a short period, often because their behaviour is difficult to manage within a family setting. Frequent moves may perpetuate the original problems and precipitate others.

Residential schools are used particularly when there are specific difficulties with mainstream schools providing education, such as when a child has moderate or severe learning difficulties or autism. Residential schools may also be helpful when there are severe emotional and behavioural disorders. In this context, the aim of the residential placement, in addition to education, is to improve or prevent further deterioration of a child's mental health difficulties.

A minority of children now live in residential care homes, and this sort of provision is mainly used when other options have not been successful. The overall provision of care homes for young people in the UK has reduced over the past 20 years. There has also been a gradual move from larger general units to more specialised smaller units (Berridge & Brodie, 1998). This has produced some benefits, but overall children in long-term residential care do less well across most areas of psychological function than children in non-residential care.

When the care provided is poor the developmental outcome is understandably poor. When the care is exceptionally deprived, as has been described in some Romanian orphanages (Rutter *et al*, 1999), then development may be significantly impaired, and some of these children have problems resembling autistic patterns of behaviour. This level of deprivation is exceptional, but it does emphasise the potential impact of psychosocial factors on long-term development. Residential care facilities have also provided the setting for children to experience other negative events, such as sexual, physical and emotional abuse. Where this abuse occurs in residential settings, the children who experience it are likely to develop mental health problems.

The impact of being in care continues into adulthood, with up to a third of the adult homeless and prison population having been in care in childhood. The social role changes in late adolescence involving leaving school, establishing adult relationships (Maughan, 2001) and independent living can precipitate mental health difficulties, especially for those in transition from care (McNeish *et al*, 2002), as after-care arrangements can be patchy. These adolescents may be particularly vulnerable, with increased risks of substance misuse, poverty and social disadvantage. This group of young people may also be vulnerable in their relationships with others, which sometimes results in a perpetuation of disadvantage across generations.

Parental mental illness

Parental mental illness operates through a number of mechanisms to increase the risk of mental health disorders in the offspring (Göpfert *et al*, 1996). There will be multiple influences from genetic, environmental, social and parenting domains. Factors having an impact on the child may exert their effects in the prenatal or postnatal period, or affect the individual's development during later childhood.

In the prenatal period, the clearest impact is through the direct effects on the foetus of parental substance misuse. Heroin is associated with intrauterine growth retardation and cocaine may directly affect neuronal development. Both cocaine and heroin are associated with neonatal addiction and withdrawal syndromes. The more commonly used substances, alcohol and tobacco, are also known to have a negative impact on foetal development: alcohol causing foetal alcohol syndrome and tobacco leading to small stature.

Prescribed drugs for parental mental illness such as mood stabilisers, antipsychotic drugs and antidepressants may also have a negative impact on a foetus. The most serious consequences for child development may occur even before a woman is aware she is pregnant, and therefore the possibility of pregnancy should be considered in all women of child-bearing age who are prescribed psychotropic medication, particularly mood stabilisers. Prenatal influences occur not only as a result of the substances ingested but also as a result of social disadvantage, poor nutrition and lack of obstetric care, which may occur with many mental illnesses. The babies of mothers with mental illness are more likely to be born prematurely or be ill at birth.

In the postnatal period, maternal depression is the most researched difficulty. Transient low mood sometimes called 'baby blues' is common, but does not have long-term consequences. A serious postnatal illness will affect the quality and nature of parenting that the child experiences (Stern, 1998). Depressed mothers may be insensitive to the needs of their infant, and may be critical and intolerant of infant behaviour. The infant may develop an attachment disorder or at a later stage a range of mental health problems may be evident. Postnatal depressive disorders are not confined to mothers, and 9% of fathers may fit the criteria for depression 6 weeks after the birth (Riley, 1995), making them less emotionally and practically involved with the newborn child.

Outside the perinatal period, a parental mental illness operates as a general risk factor for child mental health problems. Girls with a depressed parent are most likely to develop a depressive disorder, whereas boys may respond by developing oppositional and defiant behaviour. Parental personality disorders are likely to have a significant effect on children and are associated with increased levels of childhood conduct disorder. Mental illnesses are, however, often chronic or relapsing conditions with long-term psychosocial consequences. The risk may therefore be mediated through exposure to parental conflict, family disorganisation, emotional unavailability, and hostility towards the child rather than a specific illness-related response. Where one parent is ill, the child may be protected by a good relationship with the other parent. Should both parents be mentally ill, the effects on a child will be greater.

Parental criminality

Criminality in parents is associated with conduct disorders in children. The association is strongest if both parents have a criminal record. The association may be mediated through child-rearing practices such as inadequate supervision, negative attitude, hostility and cruelty towards the children. In cases where a parent is imprisoned there is frequently a loss of contact during the sentence and usually an increase in social deprivation. Recurrent imprisonment may significantly disrupt the parent–child relationship.

Siblings

The role of siblings has been less well explored than many other factors but relationships with siblings are often key within a family (Dunn, 1998). The arrival of a sibling may precipitate negative feelings such as jealousy and anger and when these are persistent a sibling rivalry disorder may develop. Poor relationships between siblings and overt sibling conflict may persist for many years and are associated with increased stress for a family. Aggression and/or violent acts directed by one sibling against another constitute the most common form of family violence (Browne & Herbert, 1997). Parents may be less concerned about violence and aggression between siblings than they would be about similar behaviour between unrelated peers.

Where one child in a family has a disability or other difficulties, then other children may receive less parental attention and support. When a mental health problem in one child is presented to services, then exploration of difficulties in siblings may be useful. The shared environment of the siblings may produce different problems in the siblings. Frequently children who are referred present with difficult to manage, oppositional and defiant disorders, whereas those with internalised disorders may be less noticed by parents and referring agencies. Differences in the way siblings are treated by parents in conflict situations may be one of the processes that compromise sibling relationships (Dunn & Davies, 2001). Sibling relationships can, however, be constructive and positive. These relationships may be particularly helpful when children are managing transitions in school and in coping with parental conflict, where the support available from a sibling can act as a protective factor (Cummings & Davies, 2002).

Extended family members

Extended family members, particularly grandparents, may have a key role in the lives of children. They can provide a supportive network for working families and can play a major part in childcare and parenting style decisions. These family members can be a resource for children and can provide supportive and a sustaining relationship when there is conflict within a parental or parent–child relationship. The wider family also provides a reference point when there is concern about a child, and this can be a key influence when accessing professional help. The extended family can also be a source of difficulty. Coercive patterns of parenting may be seen across several generations of families and relationship patterns may be seen to repeat (Hoffman, 1981). Members of the extended family may be in positions of trust with their relatives, but interfamilial and transgenerational abuse may occur.

Local environmental factors

Peers

The development of supportive peer relationships is a key development task across childhood and adolescence. Adolescents come to rely increasingly on their peers for support, and these relationships guide their actions. Children with mental health problems have fewer stable friendships and have difficulty joining peer groups. A lack of friendship is reported in 9% of 11- to 15-year-olds with any mental disorder, rising to 12% for those with ADHD. Children with autistic-spectrum disorders have particular difficulties developing and maintaining peer relationships and may have some insight into this difficulty. Children or adolescents who associate with a deviant peer group, for example individuals with conduct or behavioural disorders, are more likely to develop such problems. These peer relationships are also a powerful perpetuating factor when a child has a pre-existing mental health disorder.

Schools

Children spend many thousands of hours in school (Rutter *et al*, 1982). It is therefore unsurprising that school has a considerable influence on mental health. The overall composition of the student body, the quality of the school organisation and the efficiency of classroom management techniques influence student behaviour. School can be a positive experience and provide children with a supportive environment where they can develop independent life skills and enhanced self-esteem. A positive school experience may offset other negative factors elsewhere in a child's life.

Where students are unsupported or resources are poor, then this acts as a maintaining factor for children with mental health problems. Children with learning difficulties may not receive the help they need and develop further behavioural and emotional difficulties.

Bullying is a particular issue in the school environment and regularly affects approximately 10% of school children (Salmon *et al*, 1998). This can take a variety of forms, from physical threats and assaults to isolation and social exclusion. More recently, modern technologies have enabled newer ways of bullying and intimidation via text and e-mail messaging. Female bullies are more likely to use indirect methods such as social exclusion, but these can have as negative an outcome as the physical methods used by males. Victims of bullying are likely to be socially isolated and less aggressive than their peers (Thompson, 2000). Children with disabilities or with other overt differences may be particular targets of bullies.

Life events

Single traumatic adverse life events may precipitate not only post-traumatic stress disorders, but also adjustment disorders and depression. There is three times the risk of developing any disorder after a single event and this rises to 100 times the rate if the child experiences three recent adverse experiences. Common life events such as bereavement increase the risk of an individual developing a disorder both in childhood and in later adult life. The overall increase in risk is small, but the risk is greatest in those who are younger and/or female and in cases where the death was sudden. Good care after the bereavement reduces the subsequent risk.

Poverty and social class

There is a clear association between the levels of family income and mental disorder, with a low income being associated with increased rates of disorder. Children in families in social class V (unskilled work) have rates of mental disorder three times those of social class I (professionals). Where parents have never worked, the rates are over four times those of social class I. Poverty is, however, closely related to social class as measured by the occupation of the head of the household, and these two variables are unlikely to operate separately from each other. Where other more complex measures of social conditions are used, such as the ACORN classification (Meltzer *et al*, 2000), then the associations with mental health are similar.

Neighbourhoods

Living in an urban rather than a rural environment does not in itself change the rates or type of mental disorders seen in children; rather it is the quality of the environment. Where the local neighbourhood is run down, with community disorganisation, neglect, poor housing stock, a lack of safe play areas and overcrowding, then rates of mental disorder are increased. These conditions are much more common in deprived inner-city areas. These areas also suffer to a greater degree from significant criminal and antisocial activity and an increased availability of illicit drugs. Families who live in these deprived areas are often multiply disadvantaged and unable to move to less deprived areas.

Substance misuse

Alcohol, solvents and illegal drugs are the most common substances to have a negative effect on mental health. Parental substance misuse has effects on the child from conception. Developmental disorders may be a result of the toxic effects of these substances. Alcohol and substance misuse also has an effect on family functioning. Much of the later negative effects of parental substance mis use are likely to be mediated through inconsistent parenting and an adverse social environment.

Young people commonly also use alcohol and illicit drugs. Alcohol use is widespread (see Chapter 13). Solvent misuse has a high potential for immediate harm. Although regular use is uncommon, 10% of 14-year-old boys and girls have used solvents on at least one occasion (Beinart *et al*, 2002). Illegal drugs are used increasingly commonly, particularly in older adolescence. Cannabis use is now prevalent and it is estimated that the majority of young people have tried it on at least one occasion. Ecstasy, cocaine and heroin are less prevalent but are a significant cause of mental health disorders. The misuse of drugs is also a factor in the development of other problems such as criminal behaviour and prostitution.

Wider societal factors

Broader societal factors may also have an effect on mental health problems, although clear associations are difficult to demonstrate robustly. Societies' values are not fixed (Pollock, 1983); expectations of 'normal' behaviour and hence deviance move across generational and subcultural boundaries. In a multicultural society conflicts can arise out of different perceptions of behaviour. These factors may have an impact on the various domains that children find themselves in, and are difficult to ignore. Societal influences are no longer restricted to a local area or country. The impact of war and civil conflict on the mental health of children is well recognised (Yule, 2000), with a wide range of problems in addition to the expected post-traumatic reactions. Through immigration and asylum, people affected by such experiences may become part of communities across a dispersed geographic area. Indirect exposure to the impact of such experiences are also likely as information, experiences and views from around the world are now available directly and quickly via television and other media. The media also has influences across other domains relevant to mental health. A great deal of interest has been expressed in the role of these media (Kaliebe & Sondheimer, 2002) as an aetiological factor. Images of thinness in advertising and television have been implicated as having an impact on the prevalence of anorexia nervosa. Violent imagery has similarly been described in relation to particular violent incidents and an apparent rise in overall youth delinquency (Villani, 2001). The showing of particular events on television may have an impact: depicting suicidal acts has been associated with an increase in suicidal behaviour (Hawton & Williams, 2002), with young people being particularly susceptible to these media influences.

Conclusion

It is clear that various psychosocial aetiological factors operate in the development of and resilience to mental health disorders in childhood. The relationship between factors, which tend to accumulate over time, and different mental health problems is complex. A developmental perspective is needed, with different factors having differing effects at different developmental stages. A key task is not only to understand the relative contribution of these factors but also to explore the causal processes in the development of disorders over time.

References

Beinart, S., Anderson, B., Lee, S., et al (2002) *Youth at Risk? A National Survey of Risk Factors, Protective Factors and Problem Behaviour among Young People in England, Scotland and Wales*. London: Communities that Care.

Berridge, D. & Brodie, I. (1998) *Children's Homes Revisited*. London: Jessica Kingsley

Browne, K. & Herbert, M. (1997) *Preventing Family Violence*. London: Wiley.

Carr, A. (1999) *A Handbook of Child and Adolescent Clinical Psychology: A Contextual Approach*. London: Routledge.

Chess, S. & Thomas, A. (1995) *Temperament in Clinical Practice*. New York: Guilford.

Cicchetti, D. & Cohen, D. (eds) (1995) *Developmental Psychopathology: Theory and Methods*. New York: Wiley.

Coleman, J. (1999) *Key Data on Adolescence*. Brighton: TSA.

Cummings, E. M. & Davies, P. T. (1994) *Children and Marital Conflict*. New York: Guilford.

Cummings, E. M. & Davies, P. T. (2002) Effects of marital conflict on children: recent advances and emerging themes in process-oriented research. *Journal of Child Psychology and Psychiatry*, **43**, 31–63.

Department of Health (1991) *Working Together Under the Children Act 1989: A Guide to Arrangements for Inter-Agency Co-operation for the Protection of Children from Abuse*. London: HMSO.

Dunn, J. (1998) *The Beginnings of Social Understanding*. Oxford: Blackwell.

Dunn, J. & Davies, L. (2001) Sibling relationships and interparental conflict. In *Child Development and Interparental Conflict* (eds J. Grych & F. Fincham). New York: Cambridge University Press.

Dwivedi, K. N. (2002) *Meeting the Needs of Ethnic Minority Children* (2nd edn). London: Jessica Kingsley.

Ford, T., Goodman, R. & Meltzer, H. (2003) The British child and adolescent mental health survey 1999: the prevalence of DSM–IV disorders. *Journal of the American Academy of Child and Adolescent Psychiatry*, **42**, 1203–1211.

Forehand, R. L. & McMahon, R. J. (1981) *Helping the Noncompliant Child: A Clinicians Guide to Parent Training*. New York: Guilford.

Göpfert, M., Webster, J. & Seeman, M. V. (1996) *Parental Psychiatric Disorder: Distressed Parents and Their Families*. Cambridge: Cambridge University Press.

Harris-Hendriks, J., Black, D. & Kaplan, T. (2000) *When Father Kills Mother*. London: Routledge.

Hawton, K. & Williams, K. (2002) Influences of the media on suicide. *BMJ*, **325**, 1374–1375.

Hetherington, M. E. & Stanley-Hagan, M. (1999) The adjustment of children with divorced parents: a risk resilience perspective. *Journal of Child Psychology and Psychiatry*, **40**, 129–140.

Hoffman, L. (1981) *Foundations of Family Therapy: A Conceptual Framework for Systems Change*. New York: Basic Books.

Jones, D. P. H. (2003) *Communicating with Vulnerable Children. A Guide for Practitioners*. London: Gaskell.

Kaliebe, K. & Sondheimer, A. (2002) The media: relationships to psychiatry and children. *Academic Psychiatry*, **26**, 205–216.

Kelly, J. B. (2000) Children's adjustment in conflicted marriage and divorce: a decade review of research. *Journal of the American Academy of Child and Adolescent Psychiatry*, **39**, 963–973.

Lau, A. (2000) *South Asian Children and Adolescents in Britain*. London: Whurr.

Littlewood, R. & Lipsedge, M. (1997) *Aliens and Alienists: Ethnic Minorities and Psychiatry*. London: Routledge.

Maughan, B. (2001) Prospect and retrospect: lessons from longitudinal research. In *Research and Innovation on the Road to Modern Child Psychiatry*, vol. 1 (eds J. Green & W. Yule). London: Gaskell.

McCann, J. B., James, A., Wilson, S., *et al* (1996) Prevalence of psychiatric disorders in young people in the care system. *BMJ*, **313**, 1529–1530.

McNeish, D., Newman, T. & Roberts, H. (2002) *What Works for Children? Effective Services for Children and Families*. Buckingham: Open University Press.

Meltzer, H., Gatward, R., Goodman, R., *et al* (2000) *Mental Health of Children and Adolescents in Great Britain*. London: HMSO.

Moffitt, T. E., Caspi, A., Rutter, M., *et al* (2001) *Sex Differences in Antisocial Behaviour: Conduct Disorder, Delinquency and Violence in the Dunedin Longitudinal Study*. Cambridge: Cambridge University Press.

Patterson, G. R. (1982) *Coercive Family Process*. Eugene, OR: Castalia Press.

Perris, C., Arrindell, W. A. & Eisemann, M. (1994) *Parenting and Psychopathology*. Chichester: John Wiley.

Philips, J. (1997) Meeting the psychiatric needs of children in foster care: social workers' views. *Psychiatric Bulletin*, **21**, 609–611.

Plomin, R., De Fries, J. C. & Fulker, D. W. (1988) *Nature and Nurture During Infancy and Early Childhood*. Cambridge: Cambridge University Press.

Pollock, L. (1983) *Forgotten Children*. Cambridge: Cambridge University Press.

Riley, D. (1995) *Perinatal Mental Health: A Source Book for Health Professionals*. New York: Radcliffe Medical Press.

Rippon, E. (1994) Sex and gender differences: issues for psychopathology. In *Seminars in Psychology and Social Sciences* (eds D. Tantam & M. Birchwood) pp. 203–223. London: Gaskell.

Rutter, M., Maughan, B., Mortimore, P., *et al* (1982) *Fifteen Thousand Hours: Secondary Schools and Their Effects on Children*. Boston: Harvard University Press.

Rutter, M., Andersen-Wood, L., Beckett, C., *et al* (1999) Quasi-autistic patterns following severe early global privation. *Journal of Child Psychology and Psychiatry and Allied Disciplines*, **40**, 537–549.

Salmon, G., James, A. & Smith, D. M. (1998) Bullying in schools: self-reported anxiety, depression, and self esteem in secondary school children. *BMJ*, **317**, 924–925.

Stern, D. N. (1998) *The Motherhood Constellation: A Unified View of Parent–Infant Psychotherapy*. London: Karnac.

Thompson, D. A. (2000) Bullying and harassment in and out of school. In *Young People and Mental Health* (eds P. Aggleton, J. Hurry & I. Warwick). Chichester: Wiley.

Villani, S. (2001) Impact of media on children and adolescents: a 10 year review of the research. *Journal of the American Academy of Child and Adolescent Psychiatry*, **40**, 392–401.

Yule, W. (2000) From pogroms to 'ethnic cleansing': meeting the needs of war affected children. *Journal of Child Psychology and Psychiatry and Allied Disciplines*, **41**, 695–702.

CHAPTER 17

Disorders of parenting and child abuse

Stephen Earnshaw

The history of child advocacy is a relatively recent one. The National Society for the Prevention of Cruelty to Children (NSPCC) was founded in Britain in 1884. This was against a background of social reform and the increasing recognition of the importance of childhood and the need to protect children's rights. However, public awareness still tended to be confined to the most extreme forms of physical abuse and neglect. The next major shift in public awareness did not take place until the 1960s. Kempe *et al* (1962) described the 'battered child' syndrome, and this led to increasing recognition of the problem on both sides of the Atlantic.

The recognition of child sexual abuse is the most recent of all. It was not until the 1970s that there was a sudden increase in the rate of reporting in the USA, followed shortly afterwards by a similar trend in Britain.

Definitions

There is no universally accepted definition of abuse and consequently there are many around. Definitions have been derived for different purposes (e.g. legal, clinical or research), but most share the following key elements:

1. evidence of commission of an act (or in the case of neglect, omission of action) that is likely to result in damage to the child;
2. evidence of harm (or likely harm) to the child resulting from this;
3. evidence of a power imbalance in the relationship (e.g. adult/child or older child/younger child).

Definitions imply a clear distinction between abusive and non-abusive experiences, which is not borne out in clinical practice. It is helpful to think in terms of a spectrum of experience with a threshold line. Either side of this line are grey areas representing clinical uncertainty, where mistakes can be made. Importantly, the threshold line is not fixed, and will vary with changes in the legal framework and social policy.

Disorders of parenting fall in the grey areas and represent situations that give rise to concern. They are not disorders in the traditional sense, as the 'disorder' rests in the patterns of interaction. In this way, they are conceptually similar to attachment disorders.

In clinical practice one encounters many families whose styles of relating to one another give rise to concern. It is vital that the areas of concern can be clearly defined and quantified. Parenting assessments and the role of the child and adolescent psychiatrist are discussed in the latter part of the chapter.

Categories of abuse

1. Physical abuse.
2. Sexual abuse.
3. Neglect.
4. Emotional abuse.

Epidemiology

The epidemiology of abuse is particularly problematic given the issues of definition, levels of reporting and varying rates of registration. Officially quoted figures in the UK suggest that approximately 32 000 children are on the Child Protection Register at any one time (Department of Health, 1999). This is likely to underrepresent the true prevalence of abuse.

According to figures based on registration (Department of Health, 2000a), the most common form of abuse is neglect, with an incidence of 1.2/1000. This is followed by physical abuse (0.8/1000), sexual abuse (0.6/1000) and emotional abuse (0.5/1000).

The frequency in the population is not known with any certainty. In a review of 16 North American studies (Gorey & Leslie, 1997) the estimated prevalence in the adult population of sexual abuse occurring in childhood was 12–17% for females and 5–8% for males. The authors go on to suggest that there are insufficient figures to make a similar estimate for physical abuse and no studies on which to base figures for emotional abuse and neglect.

In clinical practice it is not uncommon for children to be the victim of several different types of abuse, but they will only be registered for the predominant one.

Physical abuse (non-accidental injury)

Non-accidental injury (NAI) involves actual physical harm to a child. This may include hitting, shaking, burning or scalding, throwing, suffocating or drowning, and poisoning. In the UK (except for Scotland) there is no law preventing the physical punishment of children by their parents; consequently, judgements will need to be made about what constitutes reasonable physical force.

Presentation

The way in which the parents respond to an injury may arouse suspicion and suggest the need for further clarification or investigation. Any of the following factors should alert clinicians to possible abuse:

1. an unexplained delay in seeking treatment;
2. parents who struggle to give a reasonable explanation or give one that is incompatible with the pattern of injury;
3. conflicting accounts about how the injury was sustained;
4. parents who show an inappropriate level of concern in relation to the injury or are defensive when questioned;
5. refusal to consent to further medical investigation;
6. a pattern of previous presentation to services with physical injuries;
7. concerns about the nature of parent/child interactions;
8. children who look frightened, withdrawn, sad or show 'frozen watchfulness'.

Physical examination or investigation may reveal characteristic injuries, which are well described in standard paediatric textbooks. This is a clear indication for a detailed physical examination with accurate recording of the findings. Locally agreed protocols should be in place for ensuring that this is done satisfactorily.

Family characteristics

Certain family and social characteristics are often noted:

1. parents may be young and lacking in social support;
2. one partner may not be the birth parent of all the children;
3. parents may have come from violent family backgrounds or have been physically abused themselves;
4. parents may lack an understanding of a child's developmental needs and have unrealistic expectations;
5. the child may have been unwanted or born prematurely;
6. the child may be regarded as temperamentally difficult;
7. the family may live in adverse social circumstances.

It is important to appreciate that the presence of any of these risk factors is not indicative of abuse and that they must be viewed in the context of the overall clinical picture.

Case example 1

Accident and emergency staff were suspicious about an 18-month-old child's scalds. Jodie's parents were both in their late teens and it was difficult to get a clear account of what had happened. The father said that Jodie must have poured the hot drink on herself, while the mother said that she was unclear what had happened. The casualty records showed that the child had been brought to the department several times in the last month, by her mother, with minor physical injuries.

Jodie was examined by a consultant paediatrician, who felt the pattern of the splashes were consistent with hot liquid being thrown on her. There were also a number of cigarette burns on her body of varying ages. The father refused to allow Jodie to be admitted to the paediatric ward and the couple tried to take their daughter home. The local social services department were contacted and an emergency protection order was secured. Jodie was kept on the paediatric ward overnight while a short-term foster placement was found.

At the child protection case conference, the father continued to maintain that the injuries were accidental and both parents refused to cooperate with the social services assessment. A care order was subsequently granted and Jodie was placed with a foster family.

Jodie's mother subsequently told social workers that her partner had caused the injuries and that she was prepared to work with the department to get Jodie back. She left her partner and with a lot of support from the family's social worker Jodie was able to return home.

Sexual abuse

Child sexual abuse continues to have all the problems relating to definition that have been outlined already. It involves forcing or encouraging a child (irrespective of their level of development or understanding of the act) to take part in sexual activity. This includes penetrative acts (e.g. vaginal, anal, digital and oral penetration) and non-penetrative acts (e.g. masturbation, fondling, observing sexual behaviour or pornography and encouraging them to behave in a sexually inappropriate way).

The abusive act is founded on the basis that a minor cannot have consensual sex with an adult (Faulk, 1994). The issue of valid consent is complex in adolescents (see Chapter 6) and where there is a small age difference between the young people involved (Jones, 2000).

Children from all social backgrounds can be affected, and there is no skew towards lower socio-economic status, as is seen in cases of physical abuse and neglect.

Girls are about 2.5 to 3 times more likely to be abused than boys (Putnam, 2003). The perpetrators are usually male adults who are known to the victim (e.g. fathers, stepfathers, other relatives, neighbours and family friends). In one study, 85% of victims knew their abuser, but only 31% was intrafamilial abuse, and 5% was by strangers. Abuse by women is much less common and it may be that they are more likely to be co-abusers. Women are more likely to abuse boys than girls.

Sexual abuse can come to light in a number of different ways. The most common way is for the child to make a disclosure of abuse to another child or a trusted adult (e.g. relative or teacher). There will often be tremendous pressure on the child not to disclose, and disclosures may be partial or misleading. Pressure can come in the form of coercion or threats from the abuser or family and disclosures may subsequently be retracted.

Alternatively, an adult may make an allegation or it may come to light in association with other forms of abuse. Distressed or developmentally inappropriate sexualised behaviour can arouse suspicions.

There is often no physical sign of sexual abuse, although certain physical findings may raise concern. Any suspicious findings should be viewed in context (Bamford & Roberts, 1993).

Case example 2

A 14-year-old girl first presented to child mental health services with an overdose following an episode of binge drinking. Katy had evidence of a depressive disorder and started cognitive–behavioural therapy with a female worker. As the therapy progressed, she was able to disclose sexual abuse by a family friend over a period of approximately a year.

These concerns were discussed with her parents prior to alerting social services. The parents initially struggled to accept what Katy had said and felt that she was 'attention-seeking'. This coincided with her taking another overdose. However, with the help of the professionals involved, their position changed and they became more supportive of their daughter.

Police and social services jointly interviewed Katy and the videotaped evidence was passed to the Crown Prosecution Service. Katy's younger sister was also interviewed, and it emerged that the man had started to make advances towards this child too.

As Katy's mood improved she was able to undertake specific post-abuse work, while the parents had parallel sessions with another worker. She made good progress and was discharged after 18 months.

Neglect

Neglect is the persistent failure to meet a child's basic needs. These may be physical, social or psychological (either alone or in combination). It involves acts of omission rather than commission and is therefore distinguished from other forms of abuse. Neglect can involve failure to provide adequate food, clothing and shelter; failure to protect the child from danger and physical harm; and not allowing a child to have access to proper medical or mental healthcare and schooling.

Neglect can include failure to provide adequate cognitive stimulation, i.e. lack of communication and joint activities with the child. Failure to provide an emotionally warm environment (i.e. ensuring that a child has a secure, stable and nurturing relationship with a significant adult) starts to blur at the boundary with the next category of emotional abuse.

Case example 3

Nursery school staff were concerned about a 4-year-old boy's unkempt state, and alerted social services. During a home visit, serious concerns emerged about the level of supervision provided by his mother. He could leave the house when he chose, even though they lived near a main road. The child was frequently left unsupervised in the house while his mother was at her boyfriend's home. There was no food in the house, and his clothes smelt strongly of urine.

The social worker agreed to visit the house regularly to provide support. On one occasion, she found Jack alone in his room covered in his own excrement. There was a urine-soaked mattress in the corner but no other furniture. His mother was found unconscious following an opiate overdose. Jack was placed in emergency foster care.

His mother agreed to cooperate with a drug treatment programme and the family were rehoused in another part of the town. Jack was able to return home gradually and his mother remained drug free, with support.

Emotional abuse

Emotional or psychological abuse involves repeatedly conveying to a child that they are worthless, unlovable, unwanted, defective or in danger. Parents can be hostile, critical, rejecting or indifferent to the child. Parents may make threats to abandon the child, e.g. by putting them into care or taking an overdose unless the child changes his or her behaviour. Equally, parents can be emotionally abusive by being overprotective and emotionally smothering, which can prevent normal social contact with peers. Perhaps most damaging of all, parents can be unpredictable and emotionally inconsistent, for example oscillating between showing affection and rejection.

In some families, the child can be singled out for blame and siblings encouraged to 'scapegoat' their brother or sister. Children can be made to shoulder the burden of household tasks, which may be developmentally inappropriate.

Children can get caught up in disputes between their parents. They can come under considerable pressure to side with one parent against the other and may be blamed for domestic difficulties.

It can be more difficult to establish that emotional abuse has taken place, but it is no less pernicious than other forms of abuse.

Case example 4

A 10-year-old boy was referred to the child mental health service because of behavioural difficulties and faecal soiling. John had moderate learning difficulties, and both parents were in their mid-fifties. The pregnancy was unplanned and John had been born after a prolonged labour. His father had a history of recurrent depression and his mother had limited mobility because of arthritis. Both parents were socially isolated and had no surviving family.

John was currently struggling in a mainstream school as his parents were opposed to him transferring to a special school. They explained to the child mental health worker that they thought their son's difficulties were due to him being 'lazy and useless'. They were critical of his current school for not being strict enough with him.

John had a poor self-image and referred to himself as stupid. When he couldn't do work at school, he would punch himself in the head and call himself useless.

If he couldn't do his homework, he would be locked in his bedroom all evening without food or water. It was on these occasions that he would soil. Following a discussion with the parents, a social services assessment was requested.

As part of the assessment there was a series of joint home visits by the social worker and the child mental health worker. With time they were able to establish a good rapport with the parents, who came to accept their son's learning difficulties and agreed to him transferring to a special school. This helped the parents, as they were able to meet other people who had children with learning difficulties.

Both parents agreed to undertake work with the child mental health team looking at their parenting. They were able to develop a better understanding of John's developmental needs and started to make links between their own experiences of being parented and the way they related to their son. They also explored their anxieties about their son's long-term future.

Another worker worked with John on an individual basis and he was able to make good progress with self-esteem work. This was reinforced by his class teacher. After 12 months of intensive input, there had been marked changes within the family and social services were able to close their involvement.

Long-term effects of child abuse

There can obviously be both physical and psychological sequelae of child abuse and neglect. In this chapter I focus on the psychological outcomes, which are often the most enduring.

When considering the consequences of abuse, it needs to be understood that there is a wide range of possible outcomes. This is a result of the number of potential variables that might affect the developmental course. These include child factors such as developmental stage, type of abuse, characteristics of the abuse, duration of the abuse and the context in which the abuse has taken place. Any potential consequences of the abuse will need to be disentangled from other environmental influences and any fallout once the abuse came to light, e.g. family break-up or financial difficulties. These factors must all be borne in mind when attempting to make sense of any outcome studies.

Cicchetti & Toth (1995) looked at the long-term outcomes of children who had been the victims of physical abuse and neglect. These authors found a wide range of effects: aggressive and disruptive behaviour; insecure and atypical attachments; affect dysregulation; peer relationship problems, such as aggression and social withdrawal; and academic underachievement. They also highlighted a number of adverse clinical outcomes: these include oppositional defiant and conduct disorders, attention-deficit hyperactivity disorder, depression and post-traumatic stress disorder.

The effects of emotional abuse and neglect are likely to be varied and dependent on the nature of the abuse and the developmental stage of the child. As with other forms of abuse involving caretakers, effects are mediated through the attachment relationship (see Chapter 10). The child needs to make sense of the dissonance that exists when the attachment figure is the abuser and often internalises a sense that they are to blame and of being worthless and unlovable.

There are likely to be long-term consequences for the child's psychosocial development, and emotional abuse and neglect are likely to have a worse long-term prognosis than physical abuse. They have persisting problems with peer group relationships, affect regulation, attentional problems and impulse control. They are at risk of developing significant emotional and behavioural difficulties. They also show delays in language development (Coster et al, 1989)

In extreme cases, children may show rocking or other self-stimulatory behaviours. There may also be repetitive self-injurious behaviour such as scratching, biting, hitting or self-laceration. The child may also show its level of distress through soiling or enuresis.

Putnam (2003) describes three basic groups of outcome for child sexual abuse: psychiatric disorders, dysfunctional behaviours and neurobiological dysregulation.

The psychiatric disorders are major depression and dysthymia (the strongest association), borderline personality disorder, somatisation disorder, substance misuse disorders, post-traumatic stress disorder, dissociative identity disorder and bulimia nervosa.

Age-inappropriate sexualised behaviour is the most closely linked behavioural manifestation. There is also a link with increased arrest rates for sex crimes and prostitution. Finally, there are reports of neuroendocrine abnormalities such as increased levels of cortisol in sexually abused girls.

Powers & Eckenrode (1990) surveyed runaway and homeless youths in New York State, the majority of whom were 15- to 16-year-old girls: 60% reported they had been physically abused by their families; 42% had experienced emotional abuse, 48% neglect and 21% sexual abuse.

It is vital to appreciate that child abuse is cyclical and that victims of childhood abuse are at increased risk of ending up in abusive relationships or becoming abusers themselves (Glasser et al, 2001).

261

Psychosocial short stature

This represents a group of children with significant impairment of linear growth secondary to prolonged abuse or neglect. These children's height will characteristically be below the third centile and the mechanism is thought to be impaired control of linear growth by the hypothalamo–pituitary axis. Growth hormone levels are often low, but this is not always the case.

The clinical picture typically includes:

1. impairment of biological rhythms, such as sleep and appetite: these children will often have hyperphagia, with hoarding of food, pica and associated polydipsia;
2. disorders of self-regulation, e.g. encopresis, enuresis and inattention;
3. disorders of affect regulation, e.g. low self-esteem, poor self-image and depression;
4. cognitive impairment, e.g. language delay, low IQ score and poor academic attainment;
5. disorders of social relationships: these children have major difficulties with reciprocal social relationships and will often have significant behavioural difficulties.

These children typically show a dramatic 'catch-up' of growth when they have been removed from the abusive experience for a significant period. The condition is often confused with non-organic failure to thrive (NOFTT), not least because both groups have impaired growth in early childhood. Growth is less impaired in NOFTT and is due to inadequate nutrition rather than significant abuse. It is usually the result of disordered feeding patterns, and there are none of the associated behavioural characteristics. Growth is typically delayed in the first couple of years, with less capacity for 'catch-up' subsequently.

Factitious disorder by proxy (Munchhausen syndrome by proxy)

This is a condition that has had many different names, from the eponymous Meadow's syndrome (Meadow, 1977) through to the current title of 'factitious disorder by proxy', as proposed by the American Psychiatric Association. The name 'Munchhausen syndrome by proxy' was coined by analogy with Munchhausen syndrome in adults. The current UK Department of Health guidance refers to 'fabrication or induction of illness by a carer', which is an adequate description of the condition.

Factitious illness involves a three-way relationship between a health professional, parent (almost always a mother) and child. It presents in three main ways:

1. false reporting, exaggeration or fabrication of a child's signs and symptoms (this might include the false reporting of symptoms that are difficult to verify, such as headache or urinary frequency);
2. fabrication of signs and symptoms, and falsification of medical charts, records and specimens of bodily fluids;
3. direct induction of illness by a variety of means.

Factitious disorder by proxy illustrates well the lack of a clear boundary between abusive and non-abusive parenting; it exists at one end of a continuum of health-seeking behaviour. The term is probably best reserved for clearly abusive experiences that can result in physical harm or death. The mother in such cases will often have a personality disorder.

Case example 5

Luke was a 3-year-old boy who was admitted to the paediatric ward for further investigation. He had been a regular attender at his local general practice since his birth, usually with minor complaints. It often proved difficult to reassure Luke's mother that all was well.

Recently he had suffered from recurrent eye infections, which had failed to respond to antibiotics. While on the ward his mother stayed with him night and day. On one occasion she was observed by the night staff to be rubbing contaminated ointment into Luke's eyes. The ward sister confronted the mother with this, who responded by trying to remove Luke from the ward. The mother was persuaded to let him stay and was interviewed the following day by the paediatrician and social worker. Luke was placed with a foster carer and a child protection case conference was held.

Luke's mother was able to acknowledge her role in the eye infections, and agreed to cooperate with a psychological assessment. She had become depressed since the death of her own mother, who she had always felt was critical of her parenting of Luke.

With the support of the mother's therapist and social worker, Luke was able to return home without further concerns being raised.

Child protection

The need to protect the child overrides all other considerations (including confidentiality) and there is a professional duty in the UK to pass on these concerns to the statutory authorities (social services, NSPCC or the police). Readers should familiarise themselves with their local procedures. It is recommended that concerns are discussed with a senior colleague, provided that the delay does not put the child at further risk. Every National Health Service trust will have a doctor and a nurse with special responsibility for child protection.

Social services have a statutory duty to ensure further enquiries take place to determine if there is a need to act to safeguard the child or to promote the child's welfare. They will undertake an initial assessment, followed, if indicated, by an extended assessment. This will usually involve checking the child protection register, consulting with other agencies and assessing the child's and family's needs. This is likely to include an interview with the child, the carers and relevant others. There is a standardised format for conducting joint videotaped interviews involving police and social services.

The framework for assessment of children in need and their families (Department of Health, 2000b) makes the important distinction between children in need of services and a subgroup of children in need because of concerns about 'significant harm'.

Significant harm is a concept introduced in the Children Act 1989 as the threshold criterion justifying compulsory intervention in family life in the best interests of the child. The Act defines 'harm' as meaning 'ill-treatment or the impairment of health or development'.

For the reasons already discussed, it will be appreciated that clinical judgement must be exercised in determining whether significant harm has occurred or not.

There may be a need for immediate intervention to protect the child. In such cases an application can be made to the courts for an emergency protection order. This is a short-term order, granted if the courts are satisfied that children are likely to suffer significant harm unless they remain where they are (e.g. a paediatric ward), or are removed to a place specified by the applicant.

If child protection concerns remain after the assessment phase, then a child protection case conference will be convened. This brings together the family and professionals with the aim of collating information, determining whether significant harm has taken place and agreeing on a child protection plan. A decision will also be made about whether to place the child's name on the child protection register.

The local authority has the option of initiating care proceedings if it is thought the child needs the protection of a care order.

Assessment of parenting

Parenting involves allowing a child to move from a position of dependency to one of relative independence. A parent's role is to steer a child towards the most appropriate developmental pathway and to act as a buffer against adverse experiences. They endeavour to maximise the child's developmental potential by providing 'good enough' experiences along the way.

An overarching definition or theory of parenting has remained elusive and there is a shift towards focusing on specific aspects of parenting and associated child outcomes (O'Connor, 2002). This is entirely consistent with clinical practice, where sweeping judgements about good and bad parents should be avoided. Consultations focus on particular facets of parenting such as parental roles, ability to set consistent limits, and sensitivity to the child's developmental needs.

Child mental health professionals will often be asked to comment on parenting issues, either through their clinical work with families or as part of a specially commissioned report. Reports will usually be requested in order to help social services departments or courts make decisions about a child's care.

Assessing parenting capacity is a complex process. As a psychiatrist, you might be asked to comment on the likely impact of a variety of conditions on parenting capacity. These conditions can include psychiatric disorders, personality disorders, drug and alcohol misuse, learning difficulties and domestic violence.

It is vital to have a framework for undertaking formal assessments, as you will be asked to comment on key issues in a child's life such as where they live and the nature of the contact they have with their parents. It is important that the information is presented in a clear and systematic way, and that conclusions are clearly supported by evidence.

The Framework for Assessment (Department of Health, 2000b) is used by social workers to undertake assessments of children in need and includes a section on parenting capacity. Reder & Lucey (1998) describe a more clinically oriented approach, which is qualitatively more sophis-ticated. Their assessment focuses on the following headings:

1. **The parent's relationship to the role of parenting**. This includes the parent's ability to provide age-appropriate physical and emotional care, the parent's attitudes to discipline and limit-setting, and the parent's ability to acknowledge any parenting problems and take responsibility for them.
2. **The parent's relationship to the child**. This includes the range of feelings a parent has towards a child, and the parent's ability to empathise with the child and to put the child's needs first.
3. **Family influences**. The family's ability to deal with stress, whether the child is drawn into discordant relationships, the psychological 'meaning of the child' to the parents and the interaction between parent and child temperamental characteristics.
4. **Interaction with the external world**. The nature of support networks and the parent's relationship with professionals.
5. **The potential for change**. The family's likelihood of making use of therapeutic support and the response to previous interventions.

The role of the child and adolescent psychiatrist

The training of child psychiatrists places them in an ideal position to offer an informed opinion in cases of child abuse or parenting disorders.

Child psychiatrists have a broad understanding of child development and developmental psychopathology, adult psychopathology, family functioning and paediatrics. They are able to weigh up risk and resilience factors, and present a balanced view of the likely impact on the child and the types of interventions required.

Good inter-agency communication is vital, and each agency needs to be clear about its respective role in the care plan. Social services will usually take the lead role.

There may be a number of phases, each of which will require a different intervention.

1.   **The initial phase**. This begins when the abuse first comes to light and there is a statutory investigation. Police and social services will undertake this investigation, but a child psychiatrist might be involved in more complex cases where a mental health assessment is indicated. The psychiatrist may also be involved in planning the joint interview and initial care plan.

2.   **Separation from family**. This is work undertaken if the child requires a temporary placement away from the family. A child psychiatrist may have a role in supporting and advising on the placement.

3.   **Rehabilitation**. In this phase the child is reintegrated into the family. There may be a key role for a child psychiatrist undertaking individual and family work (see below).

4.   **Alternative placement**. This is where work is directed towards finding a new place for the child to live if rehabilitation is not possible. Again, there may be a role for a child psychiatrist in supporting and advising social services on placement issues.

The reader is referred to Stevenson (1999) for a detailed discussion of the complex area of treatment. Putnam (2003), meanwhile, makes an important distinction between the therapeutic needs of symptomatic and asymptomatic children. A psychoeducational approach is probably the treatment of choice for the latter, coupled with close monitoring. Symptomatic children require focused interventions, generally of the cognitive–behavioural type.

The psychological needs of non-abusing parents in the aftermath of an enquiry need addressing (Forbes *et al*, 2003), and this is an important prognostic indicator for the child.

The field of child protection is one of the most emotionally demanding areas in which psychiatrists have to work. It is vital that they have the support of a team and a forum for discussing cases if they are to remain objective. Without this backup, there is a real risk that clinical judgements can be distorted by the powerful emotions these cases generate.

References

Bamford, F. & Roberts, R. (1993) Sexual abuse II. In *ABC of Child Abuse* (ed. R. Meadow). London: BMJ Publishing Group.

Cicchetti, D. & Toth, S. L. (1995) A developmental psychopathology perspective on child abuse and neglect. *Journal of the American Academy of Child and Adolescent Psychiatry*, **34**, 541–565.

Coster, W. J., Gersten, M. S., Beeghly, M., *et al* (1989) Communicative functioning in maltreated toddlers. *Developmental Psychology*, **25**, 1020–1029.

Department of Health (1999) *Children and Young People on Child Protection Registers, Year Ending 31 March 1999*. London: Government Statistical Service.

Department of Health (2000a) *Health and Personal Services Statistics for England (1999)*. London: Stationery Office.

Department of Health (2000b) *Framework for Assessment of Children in Need and Their Families*. London: Stationery Office.

Faulk, M. (1994) Offences against the person and forensic psychiatry. In *Basic Forensic Psychiatry* (2nd edn) (eds M. Faulk, M. Roberts, J. O'Grady, *et al*). Oxford: Blackwell.

Forbes, F., Duffy, J. C., Mok, J., *et al* (2003) Early intervention service for non-abusing parents of victims of child sexual abuse. Pilot study. *British Journal of Psychiatry*, **183**, 66–72.

Glasser, M., Kolvin, I., Campbell, D., *et al* (2001) Cycle of child sexual abuse: links between being a victim and becoming a perpetrator. *British Journal of Psychiatry*, **179**, 482–494.

Gorey, K. M. & Leslie, D. R. (1997) The prevalence of child sexual abuse: an integrative review. Adjustment for potential response and measurement bias. *Child Abuse and Neglect*, **21**, 391–398.

Jones, D. P. H (2000) Child abuse and neglect. In *New Oxford Textbook of Psychiatry* (eds M. G. Gelder, J. J. Lopez-Ibor & N. C. Andreasen). Oxford: Oxford University Press.

Kempe, C. H., Silverman, F. N., Steele, B. F., *et al* (1962) The battered child syndrome. *Journal of the American Medical Association*, **181**, 17–24.

Meadow, R. (1977) Munchhausen syndrome by proxy: the hinterland of child abuse. *Lancet*, ii, 343–345.

O'Connor, T. G. (2002) Annotation: the 'effects' of parenting reconsidered: findings, challenges and applications. *Journal of Child Psychology and Psychiatry*, **43**, 555–572.

Powers, J. L. & Eckenrode, J. (1990) Maltreatment among runaway and homeless youths. *Child Abuse and Neglect*, **14**, 87–98.

Putnam, F. W. (2003) Ten year research update review: child sexual abuse. *Journal of the American Academy of Child and Adolescent Psychiatry*, **42**, 269–278.

Reder, P. & Lucey, C. (1998) Significant issues in the assessment of parenting. In *Assessment of Parenting: Psychiatric and Psychological Contributions* (eds P. Reder & C. Lucey). London: Routledge.

Stevenson, J. (1999) The treatment of the long-term sequelae of child abuse. *Journal of Child Psychology and Psychiatry*, **40**, 89–111.

Further reading

Bernet, W. (1997) Practice parameters for the forensic evaluation of children and adolescents who may have been physically or sexually abused. American Academy of Child and Adolescent Psychiatry. *Journal of the American Academy of Child and Adolescent Psychiatry*, **36** (suppl. 10), 37S-56S.

Eminson, M. & Postlethwaite, R. (2000) *Munchhausen by Proxy Abuse.* Oxford: Butterworth-Heinemann.

Jones, D. P. H. & Ramchandani, P. (1999) *Child Sexual Abuse: Informing Practice from Research.* Abingdon: Radcliffe Medical Press.

Jones, D. P. H (2003) *Communicating With Vulnerable Children: A Guide for Practitioners.* London: Gaskell.

Reder, P. & Lucey, C. (1998) *Assessment of Parenting: Psychiatric and Psychological Contributions.* London: Routledge.

CHAPTER 18

Principles of treatment, service delivery and psychopharmacology

Bobby Smyth and Simon G. Gowers

Children attending child psychiatric services rarely present with a single discrete disorder. In the real world of clinical child and adolescent psychiatry, it is usual for a child and family to present with an array of difficulties. Consequently, although diagnosis is a useful starting point, treatment plans are usually based on a diagnostic formulation. The formulation will encompass the child's presenting difficulties, the child's and family's strengths and weaknesses, and the strengths and weaknesses in the wider system (i.e. school, neighbourhood, etc.), and will generate hypotheses about the factors that have acted as predisposers, precipitators and perpetuators of the current problems. Ideally, the treatment offered will match the issues identified in the formulation, taking into account the current evidence base for the effectiveness of interventions for the primary diagnosis.

Tiered service delivery

It is estimated that only about one in ten children with a psychiatric disorder will be seen by community child and adolescent mental health services (CAMHS) in the UK. However, the majority of such children do attend their general practitioner, although they will often present with physical complaints (Kramer & Garralda, 2000). General practitioners have been encouraged to maintain a high level of suspicion regarding the existence of psychiatric disorder in their young patients. There is preliminary evidence that brief, effective interventions can be delivered to children with mental health problems in the primary care or Tier 1 setting (Coverly et al, 1995; Kramer & Garralda, 2000).

Tier 2 is the least well-defined tier of child mental health services (Health Advisory Service, 1995). Ideally, Tier 2 treatments will be provided to children whose needs have not been met by Tier 1. It is envisaged that those working at Tier 2 have a role in training and consulting to colleagues in primary care (Appleton, 2000). In addition, they provide time-limited treatment to children and families whose needs do not require input from a multidisciplinary team.

Tier 3 comprises the specialist multidisciplinary CAMHS. Tier 4 consists of very specialised and intensive treatments, including in-patient and day facilities (see Chapter 20).

Multidisciplinary teams

Child and adolescent psychiatry teams are normally multidisciplinary, and they therefore include individuals from diverse professional backgrounds. There will often be a child and adolescent psychiatrist, a child psychologist, child mental health nurses, social workers and child mental healthcare workers. In addition to diversity of professional background, team members will often bring expertise in specialist treatments such as systemic family therapy, various individual therapies, parent training, psychopharmacology, group therapy, community outreach and consultation. Consequently, child and adolescent psychiatry teams are almost as heterogeneous as the families who attend for treatment. The treatment offered to a particular family will vary to some extent from one service to another, depending on the skills and professional backgrounds of the team members (Audit Commission, 1999).

Inter-agency working

In view of the complex difficulties with which children may present and the fact that they often receive input from many services, collaborative inter-agency working is to be encouraged. The input provided by the CAMHS may take the form of direct work with the child or family, or consultation to one or more of the other agencies involved. Partners in this joint working may include community paediatrics, educational psychology, adult mental health, social services, voluntary sector agencies, school nurses, youth offending teams, learning disability services and health visitors.

Increasingly, many aspects of this inter-agency working have been formalised into UK government policy, such as the National Service Framework. For example, CAMHS are one of many services that are expected to provide specific input into meeting the needs of targeted vulnerable groups, such as looked after children, young offenders and young drug users.

Commissioning CAMHS

It is clear that CAMHS can theoretically deliver a very wide range of services. However, delivery of the full range of services mentioned above has significant resource implications, both financially and professionally. Davey & Littlewood (1996) have outlined a 'menu' of services from which mental health commissioners can choose. The options vary from a cheap, minimalist 'one-star' service to an expensive but comprehensive 'five-star' service. If funding is provided for a one-star service, there can be no expectation that this service will be in a position to provide the wide array of treatments, court assessments, community outreach, consultation, preventive work and inter-agency work mentioned above.

Treatment context

The treatment offered and the setting in which it is delivered should be appropriate to a child's developmental stage. Therapeutic work with younger children should be conducted in a child-friendly environment and will usually involve play (Joseph, 1998). On the other hand, adolescents may feel patronised if seen in a room full of children's toys and decorated in a 'childish' fashion (Wilson, 1991).

The service should strive to work with families with a collaborative and positive approach. In other words, the service's response to the initial referral and to the first and subsequent appointments should occur in a manner that is child-centred and family-centred rather than service-centred.

The service will need to be sensitive to the barriers to treatment attendance and engagement that can occur owing to racial, cultural, socio-economic and gender differences. The potential difficulties that such differences can generate will be reduced by their acknowledgement both within the staff group and also in work directly with families. Consequently, both engagement and the therapeutic alliance can be enhanced (Reder & Fredman, 1996; Flaskas, 1997).

Parental rights and responsibilities and consent to treatment

Treatment cannot be provided to a child or family without obtaining the appropriate consent. Whether or not a child is competent to give consent, it is good practice to provide a developmentally appropriate explanation of the treatment to the child (Department of Health, 2001). Where a child is not competent, consent can be provided by the person and/or the agency holding parental responsibility. Where a child is competent, he or she can consent to a treatment, irrespective of the wishes of those with parental responsibility. Once again, it is best practice to attempt to obtain agreement from those in parental responsibility even if the child is competent.

A paradox currently exists on this matter. Although competent children can consent on their own, they cannot refuse a treatment in circumstances where those with parental responsibility have provided consent. The legal arguments on the issue of consent are based upon the Children Act 1989, the Mental Health Act 1983 and case law. It seems likely that the recently enacted human rights legislation will lead to challenges to the current status quo. A more detailed discussion is included in Chapter 6.

Confidentiality

Children and families have a right to expect confidentiality. Nevertheless, it is usual for information to be shared with other professionals, e.g. the referrer. Where information is being communicated to others, this fact should be made clear to families at the outset (Royal College of Psychiatrists, 2000). The Department of Health is increasingly advocating a policy of greater transparency by all medical services, including the routine copying of letters about patients to the patients themselves. Although it is certainly not yet standard practice in CAMHS to copy letters to families, some services have been successfully working in this way for many years (Gauthier, 1999).

Where children attend for individual therapy, it is also necessary to discuss issues of confidentiality. At the outset of therapy, it should be made clear to the child and parents the type and detail of information that will be fed back to parents. It will be necessary for the therapist to breach confidentiality if they acquire information that indicates the child, or somebody else, is at significant risk and they believe that sharing the information might reduce the risk. In cases of doubt, advice should be obtained from a colleague. Specific details may need to be shared with parents and/or external agencies such as social services. The breaching of confidentiality may also be necessary during family therapy or in individual work with parents for similar reasons.

The provision of therapy to children who have been abused, whether physically or sexually, is fraught with difficulty in circumstances where charges are being brought against an alleged perpetrator. The therapeutic process is often affected by the criminal, legal and child protection process. Confidentiality may be lost to the extent that therapists may be required to copy all therapy notes to the Crown Prosecution Service; however, the therapist must at all times endeavour to act in the best interests of the child. During therapy, clinicians are advised to avoid discussing the detail of the incidents of abuse, in case such discussion might 'contaminate' the evidence that the child may be asked to provide in court. The dangers of CAMHS engaging in 'anti-therapeutic therapy' in such circumstances have been eloquently discussed by Fulniss (1991).

Ending treatment

Treatment can end for a variety of reasons. Ideally, it will end in a planned manner, as a result of a mutual agreement between therapist, child and family. Frequently, children and families simply drop out of treatment. They may do so because problems or symptoms have abated, or they might perceive the treatment as being unhelpful.

There are circumstances in which the therapist should make a unilateral decision to end treatment, even if the family are willing to continue attending. In circumstances where the family seem unable or unwilling to participate usefully in treatment, ending should be strongly considered. Occasionally, the child or family may consciously or unconsciously seek to create the illusion of doing something, while actually changing nothing and maintaining the (pathological) status quo. This might arise, for example, where a family have been directed to attend therapy by a court in the process of child care proceedings, but can also occur where the families have actively sought help. By persisting with treatment in such circumstances, the therapist may simply be perpetuating the difficulties (Fulniss, 1991).

Unsuccessful treatment

Irrespective of their medical specialty, doctors will inevitably encounter patients who have very poor outcomes and some who die. Psychiatry in general, and child psychiatry in particular, appears to have greater difficulty than most specialties in accepting bad outcomes (Lask, 1986). For example, there is a tendency by society, families and the profession to view the death of an adolescent with anorexia nervosa or the suicide of an emotionally disturbed young person as a professional failure and always preventable. In contrast, the same burden of expectation is neither placed upon nor accepted by physicians and surgeons. They will usually view bad outcomes as a consequence of an illness process rather than a reflection of their inadequacies. Although complacency should not be tolerated, the myth that every psychological problem has a solution, if only the therapist were good enough, requires challenging (Lask, 1986; Graham, 2000).

Effective treatments and evidence-based medicine

Doctors should provide treatments for which there is evidence. The best evidence traditionally is provided by a systematic review or a meta-analysis of several randomised controlled trials (RCTs). The number of good-quality RCTs is steadily growing (Fonagy et al, 2002); however, there are a number of difficulties in conducting and interpreting randomised controlled trials in child psychiatry:

- Children are often excluded from trials if they have a comorbid disorder, although comorbidity is the norm in clinical practice (Audit Commission, 1999).
- Patients enter into an RCT on the basis of having a specific disorder. However, the context in which this disorder occurred is ignored. (It may be appropriate for an orthopaedic surgeon to largely ignore the precipitant of a fractured tibia when deciding upon a treatment. However, the precipitating and perpetuating factors associated with an anxiety disorder in a child may have a greater bearing on the treatment approach used by a child psychiatrist than the diagnosis itself.)
- Usually the efficacy of treatment is examined rather than its effectiveness in 'real world' clinical settings (Hotopf et al, 1999).
- Randomised controlled trials are impractical for rare disorders.
- In trials examining treatments other than medication, it is usually not possible to mask patients and researchers to the treatment being received.
- There are difficulties in ensuring the integrity and consistency of psychological treatments in RCTs.
- Randomised controlled trials are usually short in duration, and consequently fail to provide guidance on the long-term effectiveness and safety of treatments.

Owing to these limitations of traditional RCTs in child psychiatry, it has been argued that greater importance should be attached to qualitative research (Graham, 2000) and, despite their limitations (Muir Gray, 1997), descriptive studies. Others have defended the merits of the randomised controlled trial, but suggest that it may on occasions need to be adapted to make it more pragmatic and consequently more relevant (Hotopf et al, 1999; Harrington et al, 2002).

Increasingly, following appraisal of existing research evidence, consensus statements on treatment of specific disorders are being established by expert groups such as FOCUS (Fox & Joughin, 2002), the National Institute for Clinical Excellence (2001), the American Academy of Child and Adolescent Psychiatry (McClennan & Werry, 1997) and others (Hughes et al, 1999). Fonagy et al (2002) have provided an excellent summary of the current state of the evidence base.

Prevention

The overlapping concepts of health promotion and health education are generally included alongside disease prevention in thinking of ways of reducing morbidity from child mental health problems.

Health promotion is defined by the World Health Organization as the process of enabling people to increase control over, and to improve, their health. The key goal of health promotion is to enhance positive health (well-being and fitness), while preventing ill-health. Health promotion also acknowledges that physical, social and mental components are inter-linked. The UK Department of Health now recommends that this should be one of the major activities of child mental health services (Department of Health, 1995). Health education is concerned with the fostering of motivation and skills that promote health, alongside the actual giving of information. Health education has to influence not just the general public, but also those organisations and bodies in a position to formulate health protection policies and regulations.

Disease prevention involves decreasing (or eliminating) risk, or aetiological factors, that contribute to or cause disease. Preventive strategies have traditionally been thought of as occurring prior to (prevention), during (treatment) and after (maintenance) index episodes of illness (Harrington & Clark, 1998).

Primary prevention

Primary prevention involves activities that reduce the incidence of disorder in those who have not yet developed it. An example of this in paediatrics would be immunisation to prevent measles. In child and adolescent psychiatric practice, primary prevention is necessarily targeted on risk factors and risk mechanisms. Taking depression as an example, the key risk factors can be summarised as personal characteristics, social characteristics and current adversities.

Secondary prevention

Secondary prevention involves the early detection of illness and its standard treatment. Again borrowing examples from physical medicine, the Papanicolaou smear test for pre-cancerous change in the cervix and post-operative antibiotic treatment both represent secondary prevention. Psychiatric disorders are rarely amenable to early detection at a point when no symptoms are present, because their diagnosis largely depends upon the report of symptoms (Greenfield & Shore, 1995). Thus, the focus must be on detection at an early stage when only a few symptoms are present, or when they have existed for only a short time.

Secondary prevention thus relies on screening tests for treatable disorders being implemented in appropriate populations. For screening to be economic, the following criteria must be applied:

- the disorder screened for must have a treatment intervention;
- early detection and treatment must reduce morbidity (and/or mortality);

- the screening test must be of high sensitivity (to avoid false negatives);
- the screening test must have high specificity (to avoid false positives);
- the prevalence of the disorder in the target population must be high.

Tertiary prevention

Tertiary prevention involves maintenance, treatment or rehabilitation to reduce the debilitating impact, discomfort or severity of a disorder once it has developed. It might also involve the reduction of the complications of the disorder. An example from physical medicine would be the provision of a regimen of regular exercises following a shoulder or back injury. In psychiatric practice, examples include maintenance treatment with lithium to prevent relapse in adolescent bipolar illness, educational or vocational rehabilitation of adolescents with chronic psychotic disorders to reduce social impairment, and on occasions the use of psychotropic medications and psychotherapy.

Types of preventive activity

Preventive activities may be universal or selective. Universal preventive strategies are applied to everyone, without any attempt to target groups at risk of a disorder. Childhood measles, mumps and rubella (MMR) immunisation is a good example of this approach. Universal prevention has the following advantages:

- it is less stigmatising;
- it can dramatically reduce incidence (as in the complete eradication of smallpox);
- where the burden of care affects whole families (as in depression or schizophrenia), or where morbidity is associated with symptoms rather than a full-blown disorder (as in depression), everyone benefits a little.

Selective prevention aims to target high-risk groups. These may be vulnerability- or event-focused (Newton, 1988), or indicated (Mrazek & Haggerty, 1994). Vulnerability-focused interventions seek to improve the resilience of adolescents at risk of mental illness, perhaps by working with the individual or their family. Event-centred interventions aim to have an impact on happenings that may be linked to mental illness. Thus, the effects of bereavement, sexual abuse and other traumas can be ameliorated using debriefing and other techniques aimed at externalising the traumatic experience. Finally, indicated interventions are those targeted towards high-risk individuals who have minimal but discernible symptoms known to be consistent with the later onset of a mental disorder. Interventions in the prodrome of early-onset schizophrenia would fall into this category.

Selective interventions have the following advantages:

- they are more cost-effective;
- they minimise the risk of harm to non-affected individuals;
- the interventions can be tailored to particular circumstances.

Psychopharmacology

Evidence is growing that pharmacological agents are of use in the treatment of a wide variety of child and adolescent psychiatric disorders. The number of psychopharmacological agents has also grown rapidly since the 1990s. Research suggests that children who suffer from hyperkinetic disorder, depressive disorder, obsessive–compulsive disorder, anxiety disorder, Tourette syndrome or a psychotic disorders may benefit from medications.

The prescribing of psychopharmacological medication to children increased dramatically during the last 30 years of the 20th century. There have been concerns that the prescribing of these agents in ordinary clinical practice is outpacing our scientific knowledge regarding their effectiveness and safety (Jenson et al, 1999; Riddle et al, 2001a). Increased prescribing has been most obvious in the USA. Safer & Krager (1988) have estimated that the number of prescriptions for stimulants to treat hyperactivity has doubled every 4 to 7 years from 1971. Also in the USA, Olfson et al (2002) found significant increases in the number of children and adolescents receiving psychotropic medication in 1996 compared with 1987. Stimulant use increased fourfold, with over 5% of 6- to 18-year-olds receiving such medication. Antidepressant use increased threefold, with 1% of 6- to 14-year-olds and 2% of 15- to 18-year-olds being prescribed an antidepressant in 1996.

British child psychiatrists have traditionally been more cautious prescribers of medication. In one British survey, a third of the child psychiatrists reported that they very rarely prescribed medication to children (McNicholas, 2001).

Deciding on the effectiveness and safety of medications

Clinicians who treat childhood psychiatric disorders are faced with the challenge of finding a sensible middle ground on the issue of prescribing medications. On the one hand, an excessively conservative approach to prescribing could deny children access to effective treatment of their disorder, and thereby prevent a return to normal psychological, social and emotional development. Alternatively, a more liberal approach to prescribing might unnecessarily expose children to the adverse con-sequences of ineffective medications, perhaps adding to both short-term and long-term disability, while also delaying access to effective non-pharmacological treatments.

Finding a middle ground is a challenge that all doctors face when presented with prescribing decisions. However, in child psychiatry this challenge is complicated by a number of factors:

1. Research trials on new medications usually excluded children prior to 2000, for a number of reasons. First, there are understandable concerns about exposing children to possible risk and difficulties in obtaining informed consent. Unfortunately, their exclusion from these clinical trials has resulted in an absence of data on the efficacy and safety of medications in children. Efficacy in childhood disorders cannot be assumed on the basis of demonstrated efficacy in adult populations. The failure of tricyclic antidepressants to treat depression in childhood highlights this point (Hazell *et al*, 1995). There are also inherent dangers in assuming safety of medications in child populations on the basis of the results of studies among adults (e.g. aspirin, chloramphenicol). The USA made changes to its legislation at the end of the 1990s to address this issue. Pharmaceutical companies are now required to conduct trials on children where a medication is likely to be prescribed to children. It is likely that the rest of the world will benefit from the improved and increased research that this legislation will generate.

2. The lack of research conducted by pharmaceutical companies prior to the release of a medication has been compounded by a relative lack of subsequent research on children. There are only a small number of randomised controlled trials (RCTs) examining pharmacological treatments of child psychiatric disorders. Those RCTs that have been conducted often exclude subgroups of children on the basis of gender, age or comorbidity. This limits the generalisability of the findings. The strengths and weaknesses of the RCT as a means of assessment of child psychiatric treatments (Harrington *et al*, 2002) have been discussed earlier in this chapter.

3. Much of the research on pharmacological treatments of child psychiatric disorders has been conducted in the USA. Diagnostic criteria in the USA are frequently different from those used in Europe. This is most obvious in the case of hyperactivity: the ICD–10 diagnosis of hyperkinetic disorder requires that hyperactivity be pervasive (World Health Organization, 1992), which is not the case in the DSM–IV diagnosis of attention-deficit hyperactivity disorder (American Psychiatric Association, 1994). Similarly, many children diagnosed with bipolar affective disorder in the USA might not receive such a diagnosis in Britain (Carlson, 1990). This difference in use of diagnostic terms, in addition to social and cultural differences, hampers interpretation of American research.

4. There is a relative lack of long-term research studies. The few 'long-term' studies that have been conducted usually involve follow-up periods of only 6–18 months. As many child psychiatric disorders require treatment over many years, psychiatrists currently have a very limited evidence base on which to make decisions regarding effectiveness and safety in such circumstances.

5. The brain continues to develop during childhood and adolescence. It is possible that the developing brain may be more susceptible to the beneficial effects or the adverse consequences of medications that influence neurotransmitter systems (Huttenlocher, 1990; Vitiello, 1998). Consequently, Riddle et al (2001a) have argued that studies examining treatment effectiveness and safety should look separately at groups of children in early, middle and late childhood.

The history of adult psychopharmacology indicates that medications that have passed through the rigorous licensing process are often subsequently withdrawn owing to the late emergence of serious adverse effects (Lasser et al, 2002). Such rare adverse events may take decades to materialise. Thioridazine provides a recent example (Reilly et al, 2002). Despite increased prescribing to children, paediatric patients receive most psychotropic medications much less frequently than adults, owing to the reduced prevalence of serious psychiatric disorder and caution in prescribing to this age group. Consequently, rare adverse events that are childhood-specific may take longer to emerge. Clinicians noting adverse events should report these to central agencies to ensure their earliest possible detection (Committee on Safety of Medicines in the UK and MedWatch in the USA).

The failure to include children in the early trials of medication resulted in pharmaceutical companies being unable to obtain a licence to market these medications as treatments of disorders in children. Nevertheless, clinicians can and do prescribe medications 'off licence'. In the USA, it has been estimated that more than 80% of the medications prescribed to children and adolescents were unlicensed for use in that age group (Riddle et al, 2001a). Around half of all prescriptions issued by British child psychiatrists are done so outside of the manufacturers' licence (Johnson & Clark, 2001). Because of this widespread and necessary practice, the Royal College of Paediatrics and Child Health (1999) has produced a formulary as guidance for clinicians. This provides a pragmatic guide and ensures a degree of internal consistency in prescribing practices.

Given the limited quality of the evidence base for the pharmacological treatment of childhood psychiatric disorders, there is a trend towards the establishment of consensus-based treatment algorithms (McClennan & Werry, 1997; Hughes et al, 1999). These can be a useful resource in guiding the lone clinician.

Deciding whether or not to prescribe a medication

Following the diagnosis of a disorder for which there exists a pharmacological treatment, the clinician should not automatically proceed to recommending medication as part of the treatment plan. It must be borne in mind that Western society is ambivalent about the prescribing of psychotropic medication to children. Individual families differ greatly in their views on such prescribing. The building of a therapeutic alliance between clinician and child and family will require that respect for these views be demonstrated. The attitudes and expectations of family members regarding medication should be explored and discussed. For example, prescribing of medication may fuel a family's view that the 'problem' lies entirely within the child and that the solution lies entirely with the drug. In child psychiatry this is rarely the case, and prescribing could be counterproductive while such views predominate. Medication will often only form part of a wider treatment package, which may involve psychoeducation, and individual and family therapy.

Characteristics of the individual child will need to be considered prior to prescribing. The presence or absence of confounding, atypical or comorbid symptoms or disorders may influence prescribing options. Coexisting medical conditions may alter pharmacokinetics or act as a contraindication to medication.

Prior to commencing pharmacotherapy, consideration needs to be given to the environment in which the child lives. With very disorganised families, there may be increased concern that medications will not be reliably administered; this would have implications for medications with characteristics such as a narrow therapeutic index (e.g. lithium) or significant complications following sudden discontinuation of treatment (e.g. clonidine). It might be inappropriate to consider prescribing medication that might be misused (e.g. methylphenidate) to a child who lives with a relative known to misuse substances. Medication requiring a midday dose usually involves substantial cooperation from the child's school, which may not always be forthcoming. Consequently, one needs to consider wider contextual issues in addition to the diagnosis.

Drug formulation issues may also influence prescribing options. Preparation in a liquid format will allow greater flexibility in the prescribed dosage and may simplify administration of a medication. Many psychotropic medications are teratogenic (for example lithium and carbamazepine); girls who are sexually active should be warned of this risk and advised to use appropriate contraception.

Deciding what dosage to prescribe – pharmacokinetics

Physiologically, children should not be viewed as 'small adults'. Children metabolise drugs at rates different from those in adults. Children generally have a higher glomerular filtration rate than do adults. Consequently, medications that are cleared by the kidney, such as lithium, will tend to have a shorter half-life. The lithium dose to bodyweight ratio tends to be higher for children than for adults, for example (Viesselman *et al*, 1993). Similarly, metabolism of drugs by the liver cytochrome P450 isoenzymes also appears more efficient in children. Consequently, the dose to weight ratio of drugs such as the selective serotonin reuptake inhibitors (SSRIs) may be higher in children, although the preliminary data suggest substantial individual variability (Emslie *et al*, 1999).

A further implication of the shorter half-life of many medications in children is that steady-state levels will be reached more quickly. There is an absence of childhood-specific data on drug–drug interactions, even though polypharmacy is a frequent occurrence (McNicholas, 2001; Olfson *et al*, 2002).

Issues to consider following the decision to prescribe

Following the agreement between clinician and family to prescribe a psychotropic medication to a child, the clinician faces a series of additional decisions. These subsequent decisions are predictable at the outset, and should be given consideration when prescribing is initiated.

- The side-effects to be monitored should be determined and thought given to the likely course of action should they occur. Many clinicians choose to monitor side-effects through parent- and/or child-completed questionnaires. If doing so, it is wise to complete the first or baseline questionnaire prior to commencement of medication and then repeat regularly during treatment.
- It can be helpful to identify target symptoms at the outset of treatment so that the presence or absence of a clinical response can be clearly determined.
- The duration of time to wait for a clinical response to the medication should be decided upon.
- Consideration should be given to the options available if there is no response after an adequate trial of medication.
- Following a treatment response, thought should be given to the length of time the child should remain on the medication to avoid relapse. This time will be influenced by:
  - the severity of the index episode of illness;
  - the past history of recurrence;
  - a family history of recurrent similar illness;
  - current contextual factors for the child or family, e.g. forthcoming events such as examinations, which may increase the likelihood and adverse consequences of a relapse.

Classes of medication

Stimulants

The two principal stimulant medications used to treat hyperkinetic disorder and attention-deficit hyperactivity disorder (ADHD) are methylphenidate and amphetamine. A third stimulant, pemoline, has fallen out of favour owing to its hepatotoxicity. Multiple studies have demonstrated the short-term efficacy of stimulant medications in treating the core symptoms of hyperkinetic disorder. These studies also indicate the safety of methylphenidate and amphetamine (Greenhill *et al*, 1999). However, studies have generally failed to demonstrate any significant associated gains in academic or social functioning (Riddle *et al*, 2001*a*).

Two of the most comprehensive RCTs in child psychopharmacology have examined the use of stimulant medication in the treatment of ADHD. Gillberg's study showed that amphetamine was significantly better than placebo over a 15-month period (Gillberg *et al*, 1997). The US Multimodal Treatment of ADHD (MTA) study compared medication, behavioural management, a combination of both, and 'normal' community treatment. Children were followed up for 24 months (MTA Cooperative Group, 1999; Jenson *et al*, 2001). The medication treatment arm was protocol-driven. In terms of core ADHD symptoms, medication proved superior to either community treatment or behavioural treatment alone. The addition of behavioural treatment to medication provided an improvement in some outcomes. The majority of those receiving normal community treatment also received stimulant medication. The key elements of the MTA medication protocol appear to be the use of slightly higher dosages on average, the use of three daily doses rather than two, and regular communication with teachers during assessment of the medication response. Preliminary analysis of the MTA study data indicates that its results are also generally applicable to the ICD–10 diagnosis of hyperkinetic disorder. Weaknesses of the two studies include the fact that they excluded pre-school children, adolescents and females. However, there are smaller studies that suggest the efficacy and safety of stimulant medications in these groups (Riddle *et al*, 2001*a*).

Side-effects of stimulants include appetite suppression, sleep disturbance, stomach aches and headaches. Initially, children may experience increased tearfulness. Early concerns that long-term pre-scribing might lead to growth retardation have proved generally unfounded (Kramer *et al*, 2000). Nevertheless, it is advised to monitor weight and height during treatment and to review if either begins to drop across the centiles. The value of taking a drug 'holiday' is now controversial. Blood pressure should be monitored during treatment in view of the risk of hypertension. Although there has been concern that stimulants might precipitate or aggravate pre-existing tics, more recent research has failed to support this view (Riddle *et al*, 2001*a*).

In Britain, paediatricians frequently diagnose and manage children with hyperkinetic disorder. During the mid-1990s, a majority of child psychiatrists expressed concern about this situation. However, half reported that they did not prescribe stimulant medications to their patients. The majority believed that stimulant medications were under-utilised in Britain at that time (Bramble, 1997).

In standard form, both methylphenidate and amphetamine have a short half-life of 2–4 hours. Consequently, these medications must be administered two or three times per day. Sustained-release preparations have been developed and were extensively used in the USA during the 1990s. Theoretically, once-daily administration could improve compliance. Criticisms include the slower onset of action, the lower peak plasma level possibly diminishing efficacy, and the longer duration of action increasing side-effects (Ford et al, 2000). The most recent sustained-release preparations of methylphenidate have quite sophisticated drug delivery systems, providing serum levels during the day that mimic those seen with the multiple doses of standard methylphenidate. Despite this progress, standard preparations should still be used as first-line treatment.

Selective serotonin reuptake inhibitors

The five SSRIs are fluoxetine, paroxetine, fluvoxamine, citalopram and sertraline. In the late 1990s, there appeared to be a growing evidence base that suggested that SSRIs have an important role in the treatment of a variety of childhood psychiatric disorders (Emslie et al, 1999). Emslie et al (2002) demonstrated the superiority of fluoxetine over placebo in the treatment of depression in children and adolescents. Researchers demonstrated the short-term efficacy of fluvoxamine and sertraline in the treatment of obsessive–compulsive disorder (OCD) in children and adolescents in separate RCTs (March et al, 1998; Riddle et al, 2001b). In both studies, recovery following treatment with the SSRI was more often partial than complete. A multicentre RCT has demonstrated the efficacy of fluvoxamine in the treatment of anxiety disorders in childhood (RUPP Anxiety Study Group, 2001). Preliminary data suggest that SSRIs may have a role in the treatment of selective mutism (Black & Uhde, 1994) and tic disorders, including Tourette syndrome (Kurlan et al, 1993).

The major difference between the selective serotonin inhibitors is the variation in half-life. Riddle et al (2001a) concluded that there was no evidence of meaningful or significant differences in terms of treatment efficacy between the SSRIs.

Many of the studies mentioned above provided data that highlighted the apparent short-term and medium-term safety of the SSRIs. However, in 2003, meta-analysis of efficacy and unwanted effects raised doubts about the balance of benefit to risk of these drugs. Common side-effects of SSRIs include nausea, sleep disturbance, agitation, sexual dysfunction and weight gain. The former two side-effects are usually self-limiting. Discontinuation of SSRIs with a short half-life, e.g. paroxetine, commonly results in a withdrawal syndrome. Unlike the tricyclic antidepressants, SSRIs are relatively safe in overdose. Nevertheless, owing to concerns about the potential for increasing suicidality, paroxetine was withdrawn for children and adolescents by the Committee on the Safety of Medicines in 2003. Later in the same year, concerns about the limited evidence base for the effectiveness of SSRIs in child and adolescent depression led to withdrawal of all drugs in this class for use in those under 18 years old, other than fluoxetine. The debate about the risks and benefits of these drugs is likely to be ongoing.

Tricyclic antidepressants

Tricyclic antidepressants(TCAs) are not a first-line treatment for any childhood psychiatric disorder (Geller et al, 1999). Clomipramine has demonstrated short-term efficacy in the treatment of paediatric OCD (de Veaugh-Geiss et al, 1992). Nevertheless, its side-effect profile has caused most clinicians to opt for SSRIs in the first instance. Imipramine can be effective in the short-term treatment of nocturnal enuresis, but relapse is the norm following discontinuation of treatment (Geller et al, 1999). A meta-analysis of studies examining the use of TCAs in the treatment of childhood depression confirmed their lack of efficacy in this age-group (Hazell et al, 1995). There is evidence to support the use of TCAs in the treatment of ADHD and they are consequently recommended as second- or third-line treatment options.

Common side-effects include drowsiness, dry mouth, blurred vision, constipation and sleep disturbance. Electrocardiographic (ECG) changes may occur and there have been a small number of sudden deaths of children taking TCAs, although causality is disputed. Cardiotoxicity is a major problem in overdose.

Mood stabilisers

Lithium has traditionally been the agent of first choice in the treatment of bipolar affective disorder. It is the only mood stabiliser with RCT data to support its use in the treatment of this disorder in adolescents (Geller et al, 1999). Lithium has been evaluated for treatment of aggression in childhood, with mixed results. Populations have been heterogeneous, and diagnostic criteria unclear (Ryan et al, 1999).

Therapeutic serum levels recommended in the treatment of bipolar affective disorder are similar to those in adults, at 0.6–1.0 mmol/l for prophylaxis and rising to 1.2 mmol/l in the acute phase of illness (McClennan & Werry, 1997). Owing to the faster renal clearance seen in children, they tend to require a higher lithium dose per kilogram than adults, and will also reach steady-state serum levels more quickly.

Unplanned discontinuation of lithium therapy has been shown to substantially increase the risk of relapse of bipolar affective disorder in a study of adolescents followed for 18 months (Strober *et al*, 1990).

Thanks to the use of valproate and carbamazepine as anticonvulsants, there is substantial experience with the long-term prescribing of both of these drugs to children and adolescents. There is, however, an absence of data on the therapeutic serum level for these medications in the treatment of bipolar affective disorder (Clark, 2001*b*). The levels used in treatment of epilepsy are sometimes quoted and adopted.

The side-effects of valproate include nausea, tremor, weight gain, hair loss and ataxia. Hepatotoxicity is rarely seen. Long-term treatment with valproate commenced in childhood and adolescence has been associated with polycystic ovaries (Isojarvi *et al*, 1993). Care is advised in sexually active girls, because valproate is associated with neural tube defects if prescribed in the first trimester of pregnancy.

Carbamazepine has side-effects which include rashes, drowsiness, ataxia, nausea and blurred vision. These side-effects may be related to peak serum level and can therefore be reduced by prescribing slow-release preparations. Very rare but serious side-effects include agranulo-cytosis, aplastic anaemia and hepatotoxicity. Consequently, it is advised that a full blood count and liver function tests be performed prior to commencement of therapy and intermittently thereafter (McClennan & Werry, 1997; James & Javaloyes, 2001). Carbamazepine is a potent inducer of the cytochrome P450 isoenzymes. Like the other mood stabilisers, carbamazepine can be teratogenic.

If there is a failure to respond to a first-line mood stabiliser after a trial period of 4–5 weeks, a combination of medication, such as lithium and valproate, can be used (Clark, 2001*b*; James & Javaloyes, 2001).

Atypical antipsychotics

As psychosis and schizophrenia are rare in children and adolescents, it is difficult to recruit adequate numbers of patients into research studies. Consequently, the efficacy and safety data on atypical antipsychotics are sparse in this age group. Nevertheless, these drugs are increasingly used as first-line treatments of psychotic disorders in childhood. Clozapine is one of the very few medications for which there is evidence. It has demonstrated superior short-term outcome to haloperidol in treatment-resistant schizophrenia in adolescents (Kumra *et al*, 1996). Atypical antipsychotic agents are advised in the treatment of psychotic symptoms associated with severe affective disorders (Clark, 2001*b*; James & Javaloyes, 2001).

Risperidone is recommended in the treatment of tic disorders and there is some evidence to support such use (Robertson & Stern, 1998). There is evidence for the efficacy of risperidone in the reduction of stereotypies, aggression and impulsivity in childhood autism, although there is no enhancement of pro-social behaviour or communication skills (McDougle *et al*, 1997). Further evaluation on the use of risperidone in autism is ongoing by the Research Units of Paediatric Psychopharmacology, a subsection of the National Institute of Mental Health in the USA.

Side-effects of atypical antipsychotics vary between medications. Sedation, weight gain and sleep disturbance are common within this group of medications. The weight gain associated with atypicals appears to be greater than that seen with other psychotropic medication (Riddle *et al*, 2001*a*). Galactorrhoea may occur. Risperidone produces troublesome extrapyramidal side-effects at higher dosages (Campbell *et al*, 1999). Clozapine should be avoided if there is a history of seizures. The most serious side-effect of clozapine is agranulocytosis and this occurs with sufficient frequency to require intensive monitoring. Other side-effects of clozapine include hypersalivation and dizziness.

Other antipsychotics

There is evidence, albeit limited, to support the use of haloperidol in the treatment of childhood schizophrenia (Spencer & Campbell, 1994). The side-effect profile of medications such as haloperidol have caused them to be superseded by atypical antipsychotics as first-line treatments (Clark, 2001*a*). Haloperidol has been shown to be superior to placebo in reducing stereotypies, tantrums and hyperactivity in children with autism (Campbell *et al*, 1999). Pimozide, sulpiride and haloperidol have evidence to support their efficacy in the treatment of Tourette syndrome (Robertson & Stern, 1998). In the past, these medications have been evaluated for the treatment of aggression and conduct disorder in children, with variable results. The risk–benefit profile suggests that such prescribing is rarely justifiable (Campbell *et al*, 1999).

Common side-effects include sedation and parkinsonism. Acute dystonic reactions are more common in adolescents than in adults. Although many medications in this class can produce galactorrhoea, it is most commonly associated with sulpiride. Pimozide prolongs the QT interval in ECG studies and consequently it is recommended to conduct baseline followed by monthly ECGs during dose titration (Green, 1995). Tardive dyskinesia is a potential long-term serious side-effect of this class of medication.

Alpha-2 adrenergic agonists

A meta-analysis has demonstrated that clonidine has a moderate effect size (0.6) in the treatment of ADHD, and consequently it is identified as a second- or third-line treatment for this disorder (Connor *et al*, 1999). Controlled studies have failed to demonstrate its efficacy in the treatment of tic disorders. Uncontrolled studies have provided some preliminary evidence that another drug in this class, guanfacine, may be effective in the treatment of ADHD and tic disorders. However, it would be premature to recommend routine use of this medication.

The most common side-effect of clonidine is sedation, although this tends to diminish over a few weeks. Hypotension may occur. Clonidine should not be discontinued abruptly as there is a risk of a rebound hypertensive episode. Discontinuation over a period of 3–4 days is recommended. There is an unresolved controversy over a small number of sudden deaths occurring during the co-administration of methylphenidate and clonidine (Riddle et al, 2001a).

Anxiolytics

Benzodiazepines have very little part in the treatment of child psychiatric disorders (Riddle et al, 1999). It is probably unjustified to prescribe benzodiazepines for anxiety disorders or symptoms in childhood. These drugs do have a role in short-term sedation prior to and during distressing medical procedures. Short-acting benzodiazepines, such as lorazepam, are recommended for acute tranquillisation of adolescents with major psychiatric disorders such as schizophrenia, mania or psychosis, where severe agitation is a prominent element of the clinical presentation (Clark, 2001a; James & Javaloyes, 2001).

Dose-related sedation is the most common side-effect of the benzodiazepines. Tolerance and dependence develop, and these drugs can be misused. Withdrawal symptoms develop if they are administered over several weeks. Behavioural disinhibition, manifested by irritability and aggression, can occur when taking benzodiazepines (Riddle et al, 1999).

Buspirone is used to treat anxiety disorders in adults. Unlike benzodiazepines, it does not provoke tolerance or dependence. Despite the absence of controlled studies, it has been used in the treatment of childhood anxiety disorders (Riddle et al, 1999). Side-effects are generally mild and include nausea, sedation and dizziness.

Naltrexone

Small controlled studies indicate that naltrexone may have a role in reducing overactivity in autism (Riddle et al, 1999). However, these studies did not demonstrate a reduction in self-injurious behaviour or enhancement of social skills, both of which had been suggested by earlier open studies.

Melatonin

Small clinical trials indicate the efficacy of melatonin in the treatment of sleep disorder in children with neurological disability (Jan et al, 1999). It is also frequently prescribed to children without neurological disorder, despite limited evidence. Melatonin is not licensed in any age group in Britain. The relative lack of side-effects has contributed to the willingness of child psychiatrists to prescribe melatonin. Its half-life is 35–50 minutes and children are usually commenced on a regimen of 2–5 mg, taken 30 minutes before bedtime.

Novel therapies

It is anticipated that future decades will witness a greater understanding of the aetiology and pathophysiology of child psychiatric disorders. This is likely to be followed by development of more focused, and perhaps very novel, treatments. For example, it has been proposed that a subtype of post-infection obsessive–compulsive disorder might respond to treatment with plasma exchange (Perlmutter *et al*, 1999).

Alternative therapies

There is evidence of a growing schism in Western societies on the issue of drug treatments. On one hand, many parents avidly seek information regarding treatment options and keenly monitor scientific advances. Unfortunately, some of the information obtained may be less than reliable. They have high expectations that doctors offer the most up-to-date medical treatments. On the other, there are many parents who are fundamentally suspicious of traditional 'science'. They prefer alternative therapies such as homoeopathy and reflexology. There is preliminary evidence that some 'natural' remedies such as St John's wort may indeed be effective in the treatment of mild depression in adults (Woelk, 2000).

Other physical treatments

Electroconvulsive therapy

Child psychiatrists are more reluctant than adult psychiatrists to recommend electroconvulsive therapy (ECT), and it is generally considered to be a treatment of last resort. However, it is recommended as a treatment to consider in very severe affective disorder (Clark, 2001b; James & Javaloyes, 2001). Prior to proceeding with ECT, it is suggested that an independent second opinion be sought.

Resources

Medicines Control Agency Committee on Safety of Medicines (UK): http://www.mca.gov.uk/
Royal College of Psychiatrists FOCUS Project: http://www.rcpsych.ac.uk/cru/focus/
Medwatch (USA): http://www.fda.gov/medwatch/
National Institute of Mental Health and Research Units of Pediatric Psychopharmacology (USA): http://www.nimh.nih.gov/home.cfm
American Academy of Child and Adolescent Psychiatry: http://www.aacap.org/about/index.htm

References

American Psychiatric Association (1994) *Diagnostic and Statistical Manual of Mental Disorders* (4th edn) (DSM–IV). Washington, DC: American Psychiatric Association.

Appleton, P. (2000) Tier 2 CAMHS and its interface with primary care. *Advances in Psychiatric Treatment*, **6**, 388–396.

Audit Commission (1999) *Children in Mind: Child and Adolescent Mental Health Services*. London: Audit Commission.

Black, B. & Uhde, T. W. (1994) Treatment of elective mutism with fluoxetine: a double-blind placebo-controlled study. *Journal of the American Academy of Child and Adolescent Psychiatry*, **33**, 377–382.

Bramble, D. (1997) Psychostimulants and British child psychiatrists. *Child Psychology and Psychiatry Review*, **2**, 159–162.

Campbell, M., Rapoport, J. L., Simpson, G. M. (1999) Antipsychotics in children and adolescents. *Journal of the American Academy of Child and Adolescent Psychiatry*, **38**, 537–545.

Carlson, G. A. (1990) Child and adolescent mania: diagnostic considerations. *Journal of Child Psychology and Psychiatry*, **31**, 331–342.

Clark, A. (2001a) Proposed treatment for adolescent psychosis: schizophrenia and schizophrenia-like psychosis. *Advances in Psychiatric Treatment*, **7**, 16–23.

Clark, A. (2001b) Proposed treatment for adolescent psychosis: bipolar illness. *Advances in Psychiatric Treatment*, **7**, 143 149.

Connor, D. F., Fletcher, K. E. & Swanson, J. M. (1999) A meta-analysis of clonidine for the treatment of attention-deficit hyperactivity disorder. *Journal of the American Academy of Child and Adolescent Psychiatry*, **38**, 1551–1559.

Coverly, C., Garralda, M. E. & Bowman, F. (1995) Psychiatric interventions in primary care for mothers whose school-children have psychiatric disorder. *British Journal of General Practice*, **45**, 235–237.

Davey, R. & Littlewood, S. (1996) You pays your money and you takes your choice: helping purchasers to commission an appropriate child and adolescent mental health service. *Psychiatric Bulletin*, **20**, 272–274.

Department of Health (1995) *A Handbook on Child and Adolescent Mental Health*. London: HMSO.

Department of Health (2001) *Seeking Consent: Working with Children*. London: Department of Health.

De Vaugh-Geiss, J., Moroz, G., Biederman, J., *et al* (1992) Clomipramine hydrochloride in childhood and adolescent obsessive–compulsive disorder: a multicentre trial. *Journal of the American Academy of Child and Adolescent Psychiatry*, **31**, 45–49.

Emslie, G. J., Walker, J. T., Pliszka, S. R., *et al* (1999) Nontricyclic antidepressants in children and adolescents. *Journal of the American Academy of Child and Adolescent Psychiatry*, **38**, 517–528.

Emslie, G. J., Heiligenstein, J. H., Wagner, K. D., *et al* (2002) Fluoxetine for acute treatment of depression in children and adolescents: a placebo-controlled, randomized clinical trial. *Journal of the American Academy of Child and Adolescent Psychiatry*, **41**, 1205–1215.

Flaskas, C. (1997) Engagement and the therapeutic relationship in systemic therapy. *Journal of Family Therapy*, **19**, 263–282.

Fonagy, P., Target, M., Cottrell, D., *et al* (2002) *What Works for Whom; A Critical Review of Treatments for Children and Adolescents*. New York: Guilford.

Ford, T., Taylor, E. & Warner-Rogers, J. (2000) Sustained release methylphenidate. *Child Psychology and Psychiatry Review*, **5**, 108–113.

Fox, C. & Joughin, C. (2002) *Childhood-Onset Eating Problems: Findings from Research*. London: Gaskell.

289

Fulniss, T. (1991) *The Multi-professional Handbook of Child Sexual Abuse: Integrated Management, Therapy and Legal Interventions*. London: Routledge.

Gauthier, J. (1999) Writing to families. *Psychiatric Bulletin*, **23**, 387–389.

Geller, B., Reisling, D., Leonard, H. L., *et al* (1999). Critical review of tricyclic antidepressant use in children and adolescents. *Journal of the American Academy of Child and Adolescent Psychiatry*, **38**. 513–516.

Gillberg, C., Melander, H., von Knorring, A. L., *et al* (1997) Long-term stimulant treatment of children with ADHD symptoms. A randomised double-blind placebo controlled trial. *Archives of General Psychiatry*, **54**, 857–864.

Graham, P. (2000) Treatment interventions and findings from research: bridging the chasm in child psychiatry. *British Journal of Psychiatry*, **176**, 414–419.

Green, W. H. (1995) Antipsychotic drugs. In *Child and Adolescent Clinical Psychopharmacology* (2nd edn) (ed. W. H. Green). London: Lippincott, Williams & Wilkins.

Greenfield, S. F. & Shore, M. F. (1995) Prevention of psychiatric disorders. *Harvard Review of Psychiatry*, **3**, 115–129.

Greenhill, L. J., Halperin, J. M. & Abikoff, H. (1999) Stimulant medications. *Journal of the American Academy of Child and Adolescent Psychiatry*, **38**, 503–512.

Harrington, R. & Clark, A. (1998) Prevention and early intervention for depression in adolescence and early adult life. *European Archives of Psychiatry and Clinical Neuroscience*, **248**, 32–45.

Harrington, R. C., Cartwright-Hatton, S. & Stein, A. (2002) Randomised trials. *Journal of Child Psychology and Psychiatry*, **43**, 695–704.

Hazell, P., O'Donnell, D., Heathcote, D., *et al* (1995) Efficacy of tricyclic drugs in treating child and adolescent depression: a meta-analysis. *BMJ*, **310**, 897–901.

Health Advisory Service (1995) *Child and Adolescent Mental Health Services: Together We Stand. The Commissioning Role and Management of Child and Adolescent Mental Health Services*. London: HMSO.

Hotopf, M., Churchill, R. & Lewis, G. (1999) Pragmatic randomised controlled trials in psychiatry. *British Journal of Psychiatry*, **175**, 217–223.

Hughes, C. W., Emslie, G. J., Crimson, M. L., *et al* (1999) The Texas children's medication algorithm project: report of the Texas consensus conference panel on medication treatment of childhood major depressive disorder. *Journal of the American Academy of Child and Adolescent Psychiatry*, **38**, 1142–1154.

Huttenlocher, P. R. (1990) Morphometric study of human cerebral development. *Neuropsychologia*, **28**, 517–527.

Isojarvi, J. I., Laatkainen, T. J., Pakarinen, A. J., *et al* (1993) Polycystic ovaries and hyperandrogenism in women taking valproate for epilepsy. *New England Journal of Medicine*, **329**, 1383–1388.

James, A. C. D. & Javaloyes, A. M. (2001) Practitioner review: the treatment of bipolar disorder in children and adolescents. *Journal of Child Psychology and Psychiatry*, **42**, 439–449.

Jan, J. E., Freeman, R. D. & Fast, D. K. (1999) Melatonin treatment of sleep–wake disorders in children and adolescents. *Developmental Medicine and Child Neurology*, **41**, 491–500.

Jenson, P. S., Bhatura, V. S., Vitiello, B., *et al* (1999) Psychoactive medication prescribing practices for US children: gaps between research and clinical practice. *Journal of the American Academy of Child and Adolescent Psychiatry*, **38**, 557–565.

Jenson, P. S., Hinshaw, S. P., Swanson, J. M., *et al* (2001) Findings from the NIMH Multimodal Treatment study of ADHD (MTA): implications and applications for primary care providers. *Journal of Developmental Behaviour and Paediatrics*, **22**, 60–73.

Johnson, J. & Clark, A. F. (2001) Prescribing of unlicensed medicines or licensed medicines for unlicensed applications in child and adolescent psychiatry. *Psychiatric Bulletin*, **25**, 465–466.

Joseph, B. (1998) Thinking about a playroom. *Journal of Child Psychotherapy*, **24**, 359–366.

Kramer, T. & Garralda, M. E. (2000) Child and adolescent mental health problems in primary care. *Advances in Psychiatric Treatment*, **6**, 287–294.

Kramer, J. R., Loney, J., Ponto, L. B., *et al* (2000) Predictors of adult height and weight in boys treated with methylphenidate for childhood behavior problems. *Journal of the American Academy of Child and Adolescent Psychiatry*, **39**, 517–524.

Kumra, S., Frazier, J. A., Jacobson, L. K., *et al* (1996) Childhood-onset schizophrenia: a double-blind clozapine-haloperidol comparison. *Archives of General Psychiatry*, **53**, 1090–1097.

Kurlan, R., Como, P. G., Deeley, C., *et al* (1993) A pilot controlled study of fluoxetine for obsessive compulsive symptoms in children with Tourette's syndrome. *Clinical Neuropharmacology*, **16**, 167–172.

Lask, B. (1986) Whose responsibility? *Journal of Family Therapy*, **8**, 205–206.

Lasser, K. E., Allen, P. D., Woolhandler, S. J., *et al* (2002) Timing of new black box warnings and withdrawals for prescription medications. *JAMA*, **287**, 2215–2220.

March, J. S., Biederman, J., Wolkow, R., *et al* (1998) Sertraline in children and adolescents with obsessive compulsive disorder: a multicentre randomised controlled trial. *JAMA*, **280**, 1752–1756.

McClennan, J. & Werry, J. S. (1997) Practice parameters for the assessment and treatment of children and adolescents with bipolar disorder. *Journal of the American Academy of Child and Adolescent Psychiatry*, **36**, 157S–176S.

McDougle, C. J., Holmes, J. P., Bronson, M. R., *et al* (1997) Rispiridone treatment of children and adolescents with pervasive developmental disorders: a prospective open label study. *Journal of the American Academy of Child and Adolescent Psychiatry*, **36**, 685–693.

McNicholas, F. (2001) Prescribing practices of child psychiatrists in the UK. *Child Psychology and Psychiatry Review*, **6**, 166–171.

Mrazek, P. J. & Haggerty, R. J. (eds) (1994) *Reducing Risks for Mental Disorders: Frontiers for Preventive Intervention Research*. Washington, DC: National Academy Press.

MTA Cooperative Group (1999) A 14 month randomised clinical trial of treatment strategies for attention deficit/hyperactivity disorder. *Archives of General Psychiatry*, **56**, 1073–1086.

Muir Gray, J. A. (1997) *Evidence-Based Health Care*. Edinburgh: Churchill Livingstone.

National Institute for Clinical Excellence (2001) *The Guideline Development Process – Information for the Public and the NHS*. London: NICE.

Newton J. (1988) *Preventing Mental Illness*. London: Routledge.

Olfson, M., Marcus, S. C., Weissman, M. M., *et al* (2002) National trends in the use of psychotropic medications by children. *Journal of the American Academy of Child and Adolescent Psychiatry*, **41**, 514–521.

Perlmutter, S. J., Leitman, S. F., Garvey, M. A., *et al* (1999) Therapeutic plasma exchange and intravenous immunoglobulin for obsessive-compulsive disorder and tic disorders in childhood. *Lancet*, **354**, 1153–1158.

Reder, P. & Fredman, G. (1996) The relationship to help: interacting beliefs about the treatment process. *Clinical Child Psychology and Psychiatry*, **1**, 457–467.

Reilly, J. G., Ayis, S. A., Ferrier, I. N., *et al* (2002) Thioridazine and sudden unexplained death in psychiatric in-patients. *British Journal of Psychiatry*, **180**, 515–522.

Riddle, M. A., Bernstein, G. A., Cook, E. H., *et al* (1999) Anxiolytics, adrenergic agents and naltrexone. *Journal of the American Academy of Child and Adolescent Psychiatry*, **38**, 546–556.

Riddle, M. A., Kastelic, E. A. & Frosch, E. (2001*a*) Pediatric psychopharmacology. *Journal of Child Psychology and Psychiatry*, **42**, 73–99.

Riddle, M. A., Reeve, E. A., Yaryura-Tobias, J. A., *et al* (2001*b*) Fluvoxamine for children and adolescents with obsessive compulsive disorder: a randomised controlled multicentre trial. *Journal of the American Academy of Child and Adolescent Psychiatry*, **40**, 222–229.

Robertson, M. M. & Stern, J. S. (1998) Tic disorders: new developments in Tourette syndrome and related disorders. *Current Opinion in Neurology*, **11**, 373–380.

Royal College of Paediatrics and Child Health (1999) *Medicines for Children*. London: Royal College of Paediatrics and Child Health.

Royal College of Psychiatrists (2000) *Good Practice Guidelines: Confidentiality*. London: Royal College of Psychiatrists.

RUPP Anxiety Study Group (2001) Fluvoxamine for the treatment of anxiety disorders in children and adolescents. *New England Journal of Medicine*, **344**, 1279–1285.

Ryan, N. D., Bhatara, V. S. & Perel, J. M. (1999) Mood stabilisers in children and adolescents. *Journal of the American Academy of Child and Adolescent Psychiatry*, **38**, 529–536.

Safer, D. J. & Krager, J. M. (1988) A survey of medication treatment for hyperactive/inattentive students. *JAMA*, **260**, 2256–2258.

Spencer, E. K. & Campbell, M. (1994) Children with schizophrenia: diagnosis, phenomenology, and pharmacotherapy. *Schizophrenia Bulletin*, **20**, 713–725.

Strober, M., Morrell, W., Lampert, C., *et al* (1990) Relapse following discontinuation of lithium maintenance therapy in adolescents with bipolar illness: a five year naturalistic, prospective follow up. *American Journal of Psychiatry*, **147**, 457–471.

Viesselman, J. O., Yaylayan, S., Weller, E. B., *et al* (1993) Antidysthymic drugs (antidepressants and antimanics). In *Practitioner's Guide to Psychoactive Drugs for Children and Adolescents* (eds J. S. Werry & M. G. Aman), pp. 239–268. New York: Plenum.

Vitiello, B. (1998) Pediatric psychopharmacology and the interaction between drugs and the developing brain. *Canadian Journal of Psychiatry*, **43**, 582–584.

Wilson, P. (1991) Psychotherapy with adolescents. In *Textbook of Psychotherapy in Psychiatric Practice* (ed. J. Holmes). New York: Churchhill Livingstone.

Woelk, H. (2000) Comparison of St John's wort and imipramine for treating depression: randomised controlled trial. *BMJ*, **321**, 536–539.

World Health Organization (1992) *International Statistical Classification of Diseases and Related Health Problems (ICD–10)*. Geneva: WHO.

CHAPTER 19

Psychosocial approaches and psychotherapies

Alison Wood and Steve Hughes

This chapter aims to give an overview of psychological treatment approaches used in child and adolescent mental health practice. We have included social and educational approaches, as well as the more 'traditional' therapies, and acknowledge that these interventions will be used by various professionals working within all levels of child and adolescent mental health services (CAMHS). We give a brief summary of the theoretical basis for each intervention, indications and contra-indications for its use, and a review of the evidence base pertaining to that treatment approach.

Treatment planning

Assessment in child and adolescent psychiatry has been covered in Chapter 7. A detailed initial assessment, involving individual interview with the young person referred, a parental/carer interview, liaison with other professionals involved (including education and social services) and a psychiatric formulation, is essential to treatment planning. Treatment plans should be individual and problem-oriented. A proportion of young people referred to child and adolescent psychiatrists will have multiple and complex problems, requiring multimodal treatment programmes. There may be involvement from several members of the multidisciplinary team. The aim of treatment planning is to set goals of treatment and plan how these will be met and by whom. Symptom reduction is the prime goal of treatment. A second essential goal of treatment is the promotion of normal development. This may be obvious for young people presenting with developmental disorders such as autistic-spectrum disorders; however, it is helpful to consider the emotional and social development of any child with a psychiatric disorder in terms of fostering normal development and facilitating normal growth. Continuing in this theme, fostering autonomy and self-reliance is a goal that focuses on the importance of empowering and educating young people and their families to deal with future problems. Finally, there is increasing acceptance of the importance of generalisation of treatment gains and of maintaining improvements. Psychiatric services frequently are able to provide only short-term interventions, meaning that continuing progress will be the responsibility of community services and individuals. Finally, environments and contexts are important. Rather than change the child, changing the environment might be the intervention that is most helpful.

All therapeutic interventions should be applied by practitioners who have had appropriate training and are receiving ongoing supervision. Treatments should be contingent on progress and based on sound empirical evidence.

Case example

A 13-year-old girl was referred for a psychiatric assessment with multiple symptoms of depression following the death of her grandmother. Following the assessment, it emerged that her two siblings were also experiencing difficulties in adjustment and the loss of the grandmother had resulted in the girl's mother being admitted to a psychiatric hospital with a hypomanic episode. Treatment planning must take into consideration contexts and systems. The girl's treatment programme involved individual pharmacotherapy for depression and cognitive–behavioural therapy. Liaison with social services and adult psychiatric services preceded the mother's discharge from hospital and it was then possible to engage the family in psychoeducational sessions and family therapy. The role of the psychiatrist was to prescribe and monitor medication and facilitate the psychoeducational sessions. A community psychiatric nurse (CPN) worked individually with the girl using a cognitive approach, and family sessions were conducted jointly by the psychiatrist and the CPN with the support of the family therapy team. Initially there were concerns about the risk of self-harm and regular risk assessments were conducted. It was possible to treat the family on an out-patient basis. Social services were involved in seeking alternative placements within the extended family for the children.

The above case example illustrates the importance of combining multiple treatment approaches. Psychotherapy is often defined as treatment by psychological means. These interventions rely primarily upon a direct and personal relationship between the patient and therapist. For each intervention there are specific techniques or strategies used within a particular style of therapeutic relationship. We have chosen interventions that are well established and/or have an evidence base. The following interventions are described in this chapter:

- social and educational management
- behavioural treatments
- cognitive–behavioural therapy
- interpersonal therapy
- psychodynamic approaches

- creative therapies
- family therapy
- group therapy.

Social and educational management

This section refers to psychological therapies or interventions that take place in non-medical settings. Child and adolescent mental health services should be community-oriented in their approach to management of common child and adolescent mental health problems. A successful example of work in non-medical settings is multisystemic therapy (Henggeler *et al*, 1998). This intensive treatment approach relies on an extremely thorough initial psychiatric assessment and detailed formulation of the young person's current difficulties. Interventions are then offered across a number of environments. Treatments are conducted within the family home, in school and in the local community at various levels. The therapeutic programme is coordinated by a specialist therapist working intensively with the family, being enabled to do so by carrying a very small case-load and receiving multidisciplinary supervision. The behaviour that is tackled by this approach includes severe emotional and behavioural disturbances imposing risk to individuals. Treatment involves regular risk assessments and a close collaborative relationship with professionals from social and educational services and with other clinicians. The programme was developed in the 1970s for working with chronic delinquency, but has subsequently been modified to provide an alternative to in-patient treatment for children and adolescents presenting with a range of severe and worrying problems (Rowland *et al*, 2000).

Social management

Relatively frequently, the psychiatric assessment of a child presenting with a mental health disorder raises concerns about the child's environment, be it with their biological family, reconstituted family or in a residential setting. The formulation of that young person's difficulties includes a need to explore alternative environments or placements for that child, and treatment will involve joint work between child and adolescent mental health services and social services towards assessing risk and resolving these difficulties. Children may therefore be placed in foster care, accommodated by social services in residential settings or may be homeless. The therapeutic potential of foster care is recognised widely and in the UK all children who cannot be placed within their families are fostered wherever possible. Foster care includes shared care in which foster carers share the care of children with their birth families. This is particularly useful with disabled children and for emergency or short-term placement. There are now specialist foster care programmes for children with particularly severe emotional and behavioural problems.

Over the years there have been long-standing and continuing concerns regarding social services' residential establishments for children and adolescents. They do not offer satisfactory long-term alternatives to family life and there has been a major movement towards fostering of children in public care. The provision of children's home accommodation has shrunk and now stands at around 10 500 places in England. Around 400 of these offer secure provision (Nichol, 2002). Surveys of the mental health of young people in children's homes and foster care show consistently that nearly all of these children manifest some form of psychopathology (McCann *et al*, 1996). There is therefore a major role for child and adolescent mental health services in working closely with social services to assess and treat where appropriate these vulnerable young people. Assessment and consultation work for local social services departments forms an important part of routine child and adolescent mental health practice. This includes the assessment of individual children and adolescents with a view to writing court reports or making recommendations regarding placements or treatment, and consultation work with individual residential children's homes or institutions, offering advice in the overall management of young people with emotional and behavioural problems.

Educational management

Young people who present with mental health disorders usually have difficulties in both school and family settings. It is therefore important in both assessment and treatment for child psychiatrists to collaborate closely with professionals from education. Child and adolescent mental health practitioners will need to liaise with mainstream schools and special schools (e.g. for young people with emotional and behavioural problems; for young people with autistic-spectrum disorders; for young people with specialist speech and language disorders, and for children with severe and moderate learning disability). Interventions in col-laboration with school can take place at different levels. Initially, the child and adolescent mental health practitioner will need to seek information regarding the functioning of patients in school. Information is sought regarding their academic abilities, their peer relationships and their relationships with adults as observed in a school setting by trained teachers. In addition, it will be important that the school has knowledge of a young person's difficulties and an understanding of the formulation of these so that they can be involved where appropriate in treatment interventions, or at least be supportive of treatments. In some instances, children, adolescents and their parents are unwilling for schools to be involved and clearly their consent is essential. For children presenting with complex psychiatric difficulties, it is good practice to conduct an observation of the child within a school setting and to collaborate closely with educational staff. Children presenting with autistic-spectrum disorders, for example, can present very differently within clinic and school settings.

One example of an aetiological factor in children's emotional and behavioural problems is bullying. There has been much work over recent decades documenting the extent and destructiveness of bullying and also on attempts to characterise bullies and victims and understand how to manage these situations. Much of this work has been conducted by Dan Olweus in Norway (Olweus, 1993). Group dynamics within the school are of great importance in understanding bullying, as most occurs in unstructured times and is related to supervision at breaks and lunchtimes. Interventions need to be delivered at the whole school level, at the classroom level and to the individual child. Children can be seriously affected by bullying and this can be a focus of psychotherapeutic work, either individually or in groups.

Many of the psychological interventions described in this chapter are applicable for use in schools. Group interventions and individual treatments can be administered by CAMHS professionals within schools. Over the past few years, there have been schemes where CAMHS workers are involved in training and collaborating with school nurses, educational welfare officers and special needs teachers so that increasing understanding and management of common children's emotional and behavioural problems can take place at the community level. This philosophy is growing, and is having a positive influence on teachers and their abilities to manage quite severe behavioural problems within the classroom.

Behavioural treatments

Behaviour therapies are derived from empirically developed learning theories, which hold that human behaviour, whether normal or abnormal, is acquired and maintained by the same processes. Theoretical models include classical conditioning, operant conditioning (Gross, 1996) and social learning theory (Bandura, 1977). Behavioural therapies can be applied to modify or extinguish problem behaviours and to increase desired behaviours.

Assessment and formulation

A thorough assessment of the factors mediating behaviour begins by obtaining a detailed history of the child and his or her environment. Baseline information is gathered about antecedents, behaviours and consequences (ABC) and the settings in which they occur:

- **Antecedents** Antecedents are events or circumstances (stimuli) that occur immediately prior to the behaviour and have a role in its precipitation.
- **Behaviours** These include nature, frequency, severity, duration, pervasiveness, persons involved, times, places and situations.
- **Consequences** What happens after the behaviour? How it is managed? This reveals information about positive and negative reinforcement. Consequences in turn become antecedents to further behaviour.
- **Settings** These include individual factors (age, gender, developmental level, temperament, thoughts, feelings) and wider contextual variables such as family, school and social circumstances, attachments, reinforcement history, attitudes and life events (distal antecedents). An assessment of strengths and interests is important in order to tailor rewards.

Objective information is gathered using observations in clinic, home and school. The use of 'ABC' diaries allow parents (and the therapist) to increase their objective awareness of the factors mediating behaviour. Standardised measures provide an objective means of quantifying behaviour. A further vital component of assessment is 'functional analysis' or 'applied behaviour analysis', which is based on the premise that all behaviour serves a function (Herbert, 2002). It is therefore necessary to determine how the behaviour helps the child. For example, if a child often has tantrums in crowded places, resulting in removal to a quieter place, it may be that the child is fearful of such situations and the function of the behaviour is to ensure removal and consequent anxiety reduction.

A comprehensive formulation incorporates the above information, generating hypotheses to explain the function of the behaviour and how it is maintained. It is vital that the specific ABC information is interpreted with regard to setting variables.

Treatment planning and implementation

The treatment plan aims to change the target behaviour by altering the environmental variables, and is devised by the therapist in collaboration with the parents (and child), using the hypotheses generated by the formulation, and drawing on individual and family strengths. Strategies endeavour to initiate and increase desired behaviours and to reduce undesired behaviours.

To reduce undesired behaviours, it is essential to develop and differentially reinforce alternative desired behaviours to replace them. These new behaviours must serve an identical function and be more effective in their aim for treatment to succeed. Clear, realistic step-wise goals of treatment should be agreed, and parents and teachers must be actively involved in the treatment process. It is necessary to prioritise problem behaviours if there are many of them, and the plan must be appropriate to the child's developmental level. Progress should be regularly monitored and evaluated.

Behavioural techniques to increase desired behaviour

Positive reinforcement

Operant approaches are central to behavioural interventions. Positive reinforcers or rewards include praise, star/reward charts, adult attention, privileges, activities and material rewards, which are often used in combination. Material rewards need not be large or expensive. Parents often neglect praise for everyday behaviour, but it provides very powerful reinforcement to children. Ideal rewards are immediate, practical, tangible, consistent, resistant to satiation, in proportion to achievement and administered in small amounts, for the achievement of small step-wise goals (Gelfand & Hartmann, 1984).

Rewards differ from (and are far more effective than) 'bribes', in that they are awarded following the completion of desired behaviour, rather than offered as an inducement in advance. The reward threshold must be readily achievable, so that the child perceives early success. Gradually increasing intervals between rewards and increasing the requirements to achieve them modifies behaviour until the final desired behaviour is achieved (shaping) (Gross, 1996).

Behavioural techniques to decrease undesired behaviour

Environmental manipulation

Antecedent stimuli, which directly precipitate an undesired behaviour response, are removed or altered in order to prevent the adverse response (stimulus change).

Punishment and sanctions

Unpleasant consequences of behaviour such as withholding of rewards or loss of privileges can be useful, but only if used in conjunction with positive reinforcement of desired behaviour. Sanctions must be immediate, time-limited, proportionate, reasonable and perceived as negative by the child. However, punitive measures must be used carefully. Their efficacy is short-lived as the child quickly habituates and it is easy to generate a cycle where the child actually receives much attention (positive reinforcement) for undesired behaviour.

Extinction and time out from positive reinforcement

If there is no reward for a behaviour, it will decrease (extinction). Ignoring undesired behaviour is therefore very effective if its function is to gain social attention. Parents must be warned that the intensity of the undesired behaviour often increases initially as the child attempts to elicit the expected response. Repeated removal of the child from this situation to a quiet, unrewarding setting (time out from positive reinforcement) may be effective, but must be used in conjunction with positive techniques to increase desired behaviour.

Graded exposure and systematic desensitisation

The child is gradually exposed to a planned hierarchy of feared stimuli, with simultaneous strategies to manage anxiety and increase the sense of control, such as positive reinforcement, muscle relaxation, breathing exercises and guided pleasant imagery. The child gradually habituates to the stimulus and anxiety is extinguished. Facing the fear in this supported way eliminates the negative reinforcement caused by escape or avoidance. Cognitive techniques are also used and heroic characters may be deployed to assist children in defeating their fears. Flooding involves placing the child in the most feared situation until anxiety has fully dissipated. The degree of anxiety generated, and the difficulties in safely managing this, mean graded exposure is usually the preferred approach.

Exposure and response prevention

This is a variation of systematic desensitisation and has been successfully used for compulsions in obsessive–compulsive disorder (Bolton *et al*, 1983). The child is gradually exposed to a hierarchy of situations in imagination or directly, that provoke compulsions, which are then resisted by the child with parental/therapist support. This might include, for example, touching an object perceived as contaminated, then not washing hands for a specified period. When anxiety has reduced, the stimulus intensity and ensuing compulsion-free periods are gradually increased.

Clinical applications and effectiveness

Cognitive theories have demonstrated the need to examine not only behaviour, but also associated thoughts and feelings. Many treatments now incorporate a cognitive aspect, although the behavioural elements remain highly important and many have been empirically well validated. Behavioural treatments are indicated in the management of most disorders presenting to CAMHS. Two clinical examples below illustrate that a behavioural component of treatment will often take place alongside other approaches.

Enuresis

Episodes of wetting are managed with the minimum of fuss to avoid any positive reinforcement. Fluid restriction and a planned urination in the night may be useful. Dry periods are rewarded with praise and star charts, etc. An enuresis alarm can be placed under the bed sheet, which sounds and wakes the child and parents if urination occurs. The child is then taken to the toilet and returned to bed. This technique involving both classical conditioning and operant learning is effective in over 80% of cases (Doleys, 1977), but may need periodic booster sessions.

Encopresis

Behavioural interventions are essential, in conjunction with medication and diet for underlying constipation (Herbert, 1996). Psychoeducation, scheduled toilet visits and addressing of fears (e.g. pain, toilet phobia) are accompanied by positive reinforcement of use of toilet and appropriate bowel opening with rewards and star charts. Inadvertent reinforcement of soiling is removed by managing accidents with the minimum of fuss.

Cognitive–behavioural therapy

Cognitive–behavioural therapy (CBT) is an active, problem-oriented treatment that can be conducted with individuals or groups and has a coherent theoretical foundation. Cognitive and behavioural approaches or procedures have the common distinguishing feature of simultaneous endorsement of the importance of the role of both cognitive and behavioural processes in shaping and maintaining psychological disorders. Cognitive–behavioural treatments have now been developed for most disorders encountered in psychiatric practice with adults (Hawton *et al*, 1992). More recent publications have described equivalent developments with children and adolescents (Reinecke *et al*, 1996; Graham, 1998).

Cognitive therapy is founded upon the assumption that behaviour is adaptive and that there is an interaction between the individual's thoughts, feelings and behaviours. A large theoretical body of knowledge is growing up around the use of CBT in the treatment of depressive disorders. Beck's cognitive theory of depression (Beck, 1967; Beck *et al*, 1979) outlines three concepts: negative automatic thoughts, cognitive distortions and dysfunctional beliefs. Although these relate specifically to the understanding of depressive disorders, the concepts are valuable when considering the wider use of CBT for child and adolescent psychiatric disorders. Negative automatic thoughts are superficial 'here and now' thoughts, which can negatively influence mood states. Individuals with depressive disorders describe thoughts of personal failure and self-criticism, thoughts that their future is hopeless and not amenable to change, and misinterpretations of the world around them. Cognitive distortions are habitual errors in the logic of thinking that alter reality and lead to the types of automatic thoughts described above. The most common are 'all or nothing' thinking, selective abstraction, personalisation and fortune-telling. Cognitive errors are thought to

301

arise out of dysfunctional core beliefs or schemas. These are the deepest level of cognition. Core beliefs are absolute statements about ourselves, others and the world. They are relatively stable patterns of thinking that govern the ways in which external situations are interpreted.

In addition to cognitive theory, behavioural theory and social learning theory are encompassed within the theoretical rationale underlying CBT.

Fundamental to CBT is the nature of the therapeutic relationship. 'Collaborative empiricism' refers to the therapist's stance as educator and facilitator, stimulating and inspiring patients to solve problems and recover from their particular predicaments. This approach transposes well to adolescents, who often have a short attention span, dislike authority and need to be in control.

A typical cognitive–behavioural treatment programme is a short-term, time-limited therapeutic programme which is individual and problem-oriented and is planned to take place over an 8–12 week period. Initially, an in-depth assessment is completed of the adolescent's presenting problems within the context of the individual's life situation. The treatment programme usually begins with the identification of the treatment goals or objectives, together with a further exploration and assessment of cognitive and behavioural phenomena. The central part of the programme comprises cognitive, behavioural and interpersonal techniques, and the final part aims to summarise progress and identify the needs of other therapeutic work. It is important to involve parents and carers in this process. Each individual session should be of 30–50 minutes' duration, and starts with setting an agenda and reviewing 'homework' tasks. At the end, each session is summarised and followed by setting a further homework task.

Young people with severe difficulties, e.g. acute depression or bulimia nervosa, may require twice-weekly therapy sessions. However, it is usual to plan 4–8 weekly sessions in the first instance, followed by a review of progress. Throughout the planning and execution of the treatment programme, therapist and patients collaborate to use empirical methods to identify and resolve specific problems. Cognitive–behavioural therapy may be administered by any professional with therapeutic experience of working with adolescents who has had appropriate training; ongoing therapeutic supervision is essential.

Assessing suitability for CBT

A cognitive approach is applicable to most disorders in adolescent psychiatry. Cognitive–behavioural therapy can be used in children as young as 7–8 years old. Assessing suitability and planning CBT involves identifying aspects of presenting problems, individual factors and situational issues that best fit with this method of psychotherapeutic working. A cognitive–behavioural approach is suitable for young people presenting with conditions such as clinical depression, eating disorders, obsessive–compulsive disorder or any problem in which cognitive distortions such as a negative self-appraisal are key components. Cognitive–behavioural therapy is also indicated for the treatment of anxiety and panic, attention-deficit hyperactivity disorder, conduct disorders, post-traumatic stress disorder, and the treatment of chronic pain and somatisation (Graham, 1998). Cognitive–behavioural therapy may also have a place in the treatment of young people with psychotic disorders. The young person must be able to identify a suitable focus for work and agree to 'give the treatment a try'. It is necessary that the young person has the ability of meta-cognition and is able to take responsibility for change. The approach is mainly verbal and a degree of insight and emotional literacy are necessary. The practicalities of treatment involve the ability to read and write, attending regularly for appointments, and a willingness to carry out homework tasks. Cognitive–behavioural therapy is contraindicated for adolescents with severe learning disabilities, those who externalise their difficulties and those whose verbal skills and cognition are immature. This last group of young people may benefit from CBT in combination with other therapies. Young people also require support from parents or carers in CBT. Practical assistance is required in facilitating the young person's attendance at appointments, and parental interest and support are necessary even if parents are not directly involved in therapy. It is necessary that the environment is safe and reasonably stable. Many young people presenting with psychiatric disorders have unstable and damaging home circumstances; these patients may identify cognitions that are profoundly negative but founded in reality. In such cases CBT may still be a helpful approach; however, a thorough risk assessment regarding all of these factors should be part of the initial assessment.

Components of a CBT programme

The initial phase of CBT includes assessment and socialising the young person into a cognitive method of working. A comprehensive assessment will involve interviewing the young person alone and with the family, and will result in a detailed analysis of the presenting problems, family situations, social relationships, and intellectual and school functioning. It is helpful to develop a cognitive–behavioural formulation to include a description of the main areas of difficulty, and an explanation of how the problem developed, including predisposing factors and strengths as well as immediate precipitants and a summary of maintaining factors. The CBT programme will be based on this formulation. The initial phase of CBT is in many ways a continuation of assessment. The rationale of CBT is presented to the young person, and the young person and therapist identify goals of therapy. Cognitive–behavioural therapy lays particular emphasis on agendas, goals and priorities. Goals should be owned by the young person and an initial rating of severity is useful. Self-monitoring is introduced whereby the young person has to note that an event (emotion, thought or behaviour) has occurred. This leads to the conclusion of diary tasks where baseline recordings of the presenting problems and identified goals can be made.

During the middle phase of CBT, a combination of cognitive techniques, behavioural techniques and social problem-solving approaches are used to engage a young person in active work on change. Cognitive techniques include emotional recognition, eliciting and recording automatic thoughts, thought stopping and distraction techniques. It also involves identification of dysfunctional beliefs, identification of thinking errors, cognitive restructuring and cognitive reformulation. Behavioural techniques include activity scheduling, self-reinforcement, behavioural analysis, relaxation training, conducting behavioural experiments and desensitisation, and response prevention. Social problem-solving techniques include communication and interpersonal skills and social problem-solving. The middle phase of CBT should take up approximately 8 sessions and involve a process of evaluation with the therapist so that any deterioration or difficulties can be responded to.

The final phase of CBT will span two to four sessions, but may include maintenance sessions spaced out to occur less frequently and facilitate a healthy separation from the therapist. The final sessions offer an opportunity for the adolescent to summarise what he or she has gained from the therapy, to re-rate individual goals and to identify continuing problems. The focus of this closure phase is to help the young person predict future problems and how to deal with them in the light of their therapeutic gains.

Clinical effectiveness

There is considerable evidence in support of the use of CBT for depressive and anxiety disorders. A systematic review of CBT for depressive disorders (Harrington *et al*, 1998) showed significant benefit of CBT over alternative inactive interventions. There is also evidence of the benefit of CBT for obsessive–compulsive disorder (OCD). March (1995) conducted a review of 32 articles describing treatment of OCD, and concluded that CBT, alone or in combination with pharmacotherapy, is an effective treatment for OCD in children and adolescents. Cognitive–behavioural therapy for bulimia nervosa has been the subject of much research in adults (Fairburn *et al*, 1986). This has been shown to be highly effective. In contrast, there is little good evidence to support the use of CBT for conduct disorders and attention-deficit hyperactivity disorder (ADHD).

In summary, there is a wide diversity of techniques encompassed within CBT. Core procedures aim to alter distorted thought processes.

Cognitive models exist for many adolescent psychiatric disorders, the most coherent of which are those for depressive and anxiety disorders, bulimia nervosa, post-traumatic stress disorder and obsessive–compulsive disorder. Cognitive–behavioural therapy is probably not applicable to children who are under the age of 7–8 years. The cognitive–behavioural assessment and formulation are a crucial part of the treatment process, and a key task in introducing CBT to a young person is engaging them in collaborative working.

Interpersonal therapy

Interpersonal therapy was developed for adult use by Klerman *et al* (1984) and has been adapted for use in adolescence by Mufson and colleagues (Mufson *et al*, 1993; Mufson & Fairbanks, 1996). This form of individual therapy was formulated for the treatment of depression. It is probably not suitable for young people under the age of 11 years. The therapy is designed as a once-weekly treatment that takes place over 12 weeks. Three phases of treatment are described. During sessions 1–4, the aim is to assess symptoms, family relationships and social context. In the second phase, the therapist works with the young person and where necessary conjointly with other family members to address difficulties. The final phase of therapy addresses endings and closure. The style of therapy is that of a collaborative approach to problem-solving. There are links to brief focused psychodynamic therapy and cognitive–behavioural therapy. The underlying rationale of treatment is that depression in adolescence is related to problems in social relating. Specific issues relating to sexual relationships, peer relationships and adolescent identity are explored in therapy. Examples of themes used in sessions include grief, role disputes or transitions, interpersonal conflicts and particular difficulties related to family situations.

Interpersonal therapy is mainly described for use in depression; however, in adults it has also been used for patients presenting with bulimia nervosa. There is evidence accumulating for the efficacy of interpersonal therapy. In a randomised controlled trial (Mufson *et al*, 1999) depressed adolescents were offered interpersonal therapy or clinical monitoring. They were given a brief treatment manual. The group receiving interpersonal therapy had significantly fewer symptoms on the Hamilton Rating Scale for Depression at the end of therapy, and showed better problem-solving skills. This was a preliminary study and as yet no follow-up data have been reported.

In summary, interpersonal therapy is a relatively new but promising individualised therapeutic approach that is applicable to adolescent disorders. Therapy is mainly individual but does include parents peripherally in case management and supporting the therapy.

Psychodynamic approaches

In contrast to the behavioural therapies, psychodynamic approaches focus on the child's inner experience and, to a varying degree, elements of which the child is unaware. Psychodynamic approaches are non-directive. When treating young children, play is used both literally and metaphorically. Psychodynamic approaches can use different media for communication of emotionally laden material. Media used are directed at the developmental stage of the child and are those that are most easily accessed by the child. Therapy may involve use of art materials, drama and music, play and talking (the last particularly with adolescents). Psychodynamic psychotherapy seeks to help children process the cognitive and affective components of memories that may be distortions of actual events. Children are helped to obtain some sense of mastery and understanding of their lives and learn to manage themselves without having to resort to troublesome defensive (self-protective) strategies. The aim is to restore normal psychological development when possible and to strengthen internal psychological resources. Psychodynamic approaches all accept the idea of unconscious parts of the mind where normal everyday logic does not apply, and where links are made between thoughts, feelings and memories in idiosyncratic ways.

Psychoanalytic theory has been developed in work with adult patients looking back towards childhood. The theoretical underpinnings of child psychoanalysis have undergone change over many years from Freudian and Kleinian psychoanalysis, object relation theory and later the inclusion of attachment theory. This is a large field, which is outside the scope of this chapter.

Important concepts in working in this way with children are transference and countertransference. It is assumed that the patient lacks insight into his or her feelings and the therapist endeavours to offer interpretations. These are spoken hypotheses about possible conflicts or defences. Transference explains how the patient re-experiences aspects of his or her difficulties in the therapy relationship, and countertransference refers to feelings aroused in the therapist by the therapeutic relationship. These reactions can be powerful when working with children and adolescents. They can lead to very strong feelings of wishing to protect the child inappropriately, or less commonly of distaste towards the child.

As with other psychological approaches, supervision is crucial. The therapist needs time to reflect on therapeutic sessions and to discuss these in therapy supervision. Therapists are required to have undergone psychoanalysis prior to working in this way and must be able to be in contact with powerful emotions in both themselves and their patients. There are various types of psychodynamic approaches that are suitable for use with children.

Psychodynamic psychotherapy with children (psychoanalysis)

The setting of the therapy is viewed as crucial. Children are seen three to five times a week. It is thought important to see the child at the same time, in the same place and if relevant with the same materials. By establishing such boundaries, the therapist can develop a therapeutic space for anxieties to be explored. The therapy is non-directive. There are different schools of therapy, based initially on the work of Melanie Klein (Klein, 1932) and Anna Freud (first published in 1927; see Freud, 1946). Play therapy refers to the use of play as a medium for therapy and is the equivalent of an adult's attempts to free associate while lying on the psychoanalytic couch. Historically this was the only treatment available to child psychiatrists, and it was used for all conditions presenting to child and adolescent psychiatrists. For such therapy to be possible the young person must have considerable practical support and it is now available only in very specialist centres or in private practice.

Brief psychotherapy

Brief, less intensive forms of psychotherapy are now available, which use psychodynamic theory in a more flexible way. Patients are seen individually over 10–20 sessions (De Shazer, 1988). This is mainly applicable to adolescents. The approach aims to help the young person by using a solution-focused interview and aims to increase understanding by the young person of specific difficulties or problems. As opposed to psychodynamic psychotherapy, parents are involved and transference and countertransference interpretations are used less frequently. Clinically, brief psychotherapy has been found useful in overcoming specific crises, for example following self-harm, grief and family crises.

Clinical applications

Child psychotherapy in the UK has had to adapt to the National Health Service framework, with children rarely being seen more frequently than weekly. Child psychotherapists carry out significant consultation work with other professionals in social services, education and therapeutic communities. They have also found a place in specialist paediatric departments and provide direct assessment and ongoing work with patients as well as support for the staff, who are often working with children who have emotionally distressing conditions. Overall there is little research evidence that psychodynamic approaches to treatment are effective; however, it is recognised that research in this field is enormously complicated. For instance, patients taken on for such therapies are an extremely heterogeneous group; therapists are also heterogeneous in their backgrounds and training, and descriptions of treatment are difficult to come by. A review of the literature and meta-analysis (Roth & Fonagy, 1996) has shown that there are large and consistent differences between treatments in terms of effect size and that these differences are confounded by the use of measures to assess outcome that favour behavioural treatments.

In summary, psychodynamic theory is an integral part of child and adolescent psychiatric training. It informs much of our understanding of relationships, both therapeutic and institutional, and has a part to play in both individual therapeutic work with children and adolescents and group work. Psychoanalysis is no longer considered mainstream and is not practised in routine child and adolescent mental health settings. One difficulty with the psychodynamic approach is that it focuses therapy entirely on the child or adolescent and may have the effect of alienating parents, carers and other services involved with the child. Psychoanalytical theory is a rich source of understanding of relationships and therefore of relevance to many psychological treatments.

Creative therapies

Creative interventions use play, art, music or drama as a medium for therapeutic work. These approaches are 'non-verbal' and therefore particularly suitable for younger children and for young people whose verbal abilities are compromised by learning difficulties or other developmental disorders, such as the autistic-spectrum disorders. These therapies are generally regarded as very specialised and would be routinely available in in-patient settings, although they are not routinely on offer in district child and adolescent mental health services.

Art therapy can be given individually or to groups. Using the medium of art, young people are helped to deal with inner conflicts, gain insight and achieve harmony between inner and outer worlds (Simon, 1992). It is applicable to any young person with a mental health problem who can use art as a means of expression. It is useful in the assessment of child or adolescent functioning as well as an ongoing therapeutic model. Art therapy sessions usually take place weekly over a medium- to long-term period, with each session lasting about 45 minutes. Therapists may bring their own materials or conduct sessions in a designated art therapy room. Art therapy is particularly helpful for young people who find verbal therapies difficult or too threatening. There is little evidence available to support its use, other than anecdotal account.

Family therapy

Family therapy is based on the premise that problems presenting in a child are an expression of dysfunction in the family system, such as disordered communication, relationships or structures, and treatment should be directed at the family as a whole. We first describe the current practice of family therapy within child and adolescent mental health settings, followed by indications and contraindications for its use, and then describe briefly the influential schools of family therapy under-pinning modern family therapeutic practice.

Current practice

Family therapy practice varies widely. An eclectic, pragmatic approach that utilises the most appropriate theoretical elements according to the context of the problem and the needs and attitudes of the family is probably the most useful. Assessments should involve as many family members as possible, and should cover:

- the presenting difficulties as seen by each member of the family;
- family interactional patterns, including the family's structures, roles, communication, beliefs and problem-solving strategies;
- life cycle and transition issues;
- the family's social and cultural context.

Constructing a family tree (genogram) involves the whole family and invariably reveals rich information. In a family therapy clinic, the therapist and family are usually observed by other team members, either behind a one-way screen, or with a 'reflecting team' (Andersen, 1987) in the room to maximise the feedback given.

Indications and contraindications for family therapy

Family therapy is indicated in the treatment of most disorders presenting to CAMHS. The main advantage of family therapy is the recognition of interpersonal influences in the family system. However, sole use of family therapy by professionals who may lack knowledge of child psychiatric diagnoses may result in failure to recognise more con-stitutional disorders, e.g. autistic-spectrum disorders, ADHD, learning disability or psychosis. If children are only seen with other family members, information may not be disclosed, for example about abuse. In addition, it may be difficult for some families, who seek help with what they perceive to be the child's problem, to accept that change in the whole family system is required. Thus, many services perform a full psychiatric assessment prior to or in addition to the involvement of the family therapy team. Family therapy is expensive of both therapist and patient time.

The following schools of family therapy influence current practice:

- **Structural family therapy** This therapy model is based on the assumption that a well-functioning or 'healthy' family has a clear intergenerational hierarchy, with well-demarcated but permeable boundaries in roles and relationships (Minuchin, 1974). Enmeshment, where boundaries are unclear or highly permeable, prevents the autonomous functioning of individuals. Conversely, disengagement results from rigid, impermeable boundaries, and prevents communication or interaction between family members. Symptoms in the identified patient are viewed as the product of disorder in these structures and hierarchies, and the interactional behaviour patterns that result. Therapy aims to restore appropriate family organisation so that the problem resolves. The therapist is directive and observes family interactions, sometimes asking families to re-enact problems, to gain an awareness of the family structure and power distribution. Symptoms are reframed as reflecting the distorted structures and boundaries and are then challenged by the therapist. This may involve actively directing the family to set rules or re-enact the problem in an alternative way in the session.

- **Strategic family therapy** In this model, the presenting problem is not conceptualised as a reflection of dysfunctional structures, but as part of a sequence of repetitive and dysfunctional patterns of family communication. Symptoms are viewed as strategies used by the individual to control relationships when more adaptive methods fail (Haley, 1976). As with the structural model, the therapist is directive and only concerned with the present. The dysfunctional repeating sequence of behaviour is the focus of the therapy and is broken down into separate elements. The therapist devises practical strategies for each problem to provide alternative, functional interactional patterns.

- **Milan systemic family therapy** This approach began the 'second wave' of family therapy. It asserts that covert beliefs within families strongly influence behaviour and are responsible for dysfunctional interactions. Such beliefs are revealed using circular questioning techniques, based on an evolving hypothesis, which describes the function of the symptom in the family (Selvini Palazzoli *et al*, 1980). Circular questioning aims to explore how beliefs influence behaviours in the family. For example, the therapist may ask A about how they feel B's behaviour/symptom affects C. The different perceptions, beliefs and attitudes of each family member, which may often be only implicit in everyday life, are thus made explicit to all family members. These beliefs are then challenged, provoking reflection among family members.

- **Brief solution-focused therapy** For this approach, occasions and situations when the problem is *not* occurring or is less severe are examined in detail. By identifying these successful 'exceptions' and exploring the associated interactional sequences, the therapist helps the family recognise what is different about these occasions and demonstrates that they already possess the solutions. Change requires increasing the frequency of these successful sequences (De Shazer & Berg, 1992). Therapy is confined to five to ten sessions and uses precise, limited and readily achievable goals.

- **Social constructionist family therapy and the narrative approach**
  The 'third wave' of family therapy in the 1980s extended some of the concepts of the Milan school, emphasising the idea that reality is inherently subjective and multiple versions of the 'truth' can be equally possible. Social constructionists asserted that problems were personal stories that people used to explain what was happening and thus would differ in each family member. This approach also led to a shift away from the therapist being viewed as the 'expert' (Anderson & Goolishan, 1992).

More recently, the narrative approach has focused on the premise that people make sense of their experiences by constructing stories of their lives. Depending on gender, culture, social and family norms, some stories may achieve strong prominence over others. An individual's or family's behaviour and capacity to deal with problems or changes are therefore restricted, because alternatives that do not fit with these prevailing stories are discarded. The therapist aims to help the family rewrite their stories of distressing experiences, emphasising successes, such as how they fought their traumatic experiences. This serves to change the meaning of these experiences and reduces the constraining effects of the previous narrative (White & Epston, 1990).

Externalising strategies have been used, in which the problem is ascribed a 'will of its own'. In this way, the blame, conflict and pessimism associated with symptoms is reduced if the whole family can be united in a fight against that symptom.

Outcome studies

Family therapy has developed with a relative lack of empirical research. However, randomised controlled trials have shown effectiveness for anorexia nervosa in adolescents (Russell *et al*, 1987), conduct disorder (Shadish *et al*, 1993) and drug misuse (Carr, 2000). There are also some encouraging studies of the use of family therapy for emotional disorders, bereavement and psychosomatic problems, and evidence that family therapy improves family communication (Carr, 2000).

Group therapies

Group treatments have been widely used in adult psychiatry, but less commonly in child and adolescent psychiatry. This is changing. Treating young people in groups has many advantages. A significant advantage can be the economic use of therapeutic time through several patients being seen at once. In addition, contact with other children of similar ages allows feedback from peers, which is often respected more than that from therapists, particularly in adolescence. Group therapy can be short-term focused interventions or longer-term treatments. It usually focuses on a specific disorder or group of clients. Group approaches can be applied to parents as well as to children and adolescents. Group treatments can be delivered within the CAMHS, in both in-patient or residential units and out-patient settings, and are also used in schools and community centres. Groups are frequently used in the voluntary sector as a means of informal support.

Attempts have been made to classify the factors that may be operating in group approaches. Yalom (1985) delineated 11 primary curative factors: instillation of hope; universality; imparting of information; altruism; the corrective recapitulation of the primary family group; development of socialisation techniques; imitative behaviour; interpersonal learning; group cohesiveness; catharsis; and existential factors. In all descriptions of group psychotherapy as applied to children and adolescents, content and process are adapted to the appropriate developmental stage of the young people concerned. Groups therefore have a restricted age range. The ideal group size is between six and eight members. As with all therapeutic interventions, therapists require training and ongoing supervision. In general, it is useful to involve two therapists. There should be a period of planning before the group session timetabled, followed by the group session and then a session for reflection and feedback. Overall, there is a lack of empirical evidence in favour of group therapy interventions. We describe below some commonly used applications of group therapy within child and adolescent mental health services, including evidence of efficacy where this is available.

Psychodynamic groups

Group interventions can broadly be divided into interventions that are non-directive, where group process is the focus of therapeutic change, and focused groups, where the content is the primary therapeutic element. In practice most group treatments use both content and process elements in achieving benefit. Evans (1998) described active analytic group therapy for adolescents. This fairly long-term group treatment is applicable to most difficulties with an onset in adolescence, and was initially described as taking place within a residential setting. The group uses the adolescent peer group to improve coping mechanisms and toleration of anxiety, and to promote normal development. Other examples of group interventions where the process is regarded as key are psychodrama (a therapeutic approach using dramatic techniques for working through conflicts) and art therapy. There is little evidence base in support of these interventions.

Social skills groups

These group approaches focus on the content/material used, with less attention given to process. Social skills training for children and adolescents was developed during the early 1970s with attempts to teach the skills of social interactions, for example eye contact, smiling and body language (Spence & Marzillier, 1979). These approaches have developed to include cognitive and behavioural techniques. There are many social skills programmes, which are manualised and have been applied to different age groups of young people.

Oppositional defiant disorder and conduct disorder

The Dinosaur School curriculum (Webster-Stratton & Hammond, 1997) is a multimodal social skills programme for children 6–13 years of age. Treatment includes relaxation techniques, recognition of emotions and empathy training, social problem-solving skills training, anger management, friendship skills, communication skills and management in the classroom setting. There has been one randomised controlled study (Webster-Stratton & Hammond, 1997) which showed a reduction in aggressive behaviour at home and an improvement in peer social skills. These changes persisted until one-year follow-up. Other group interventions focused on anger management, interpersonal skills and aggression are available.

In general, group approaches involving children presenting with oppositional defiant and conduct disorder have been disappointing in their outcome.

Parent training groups

Parent training programmes teach behavioural principles of child management to parents and carers by following a specific curriculum over several weeks. This is the single most effective intervention for the treatment of conduct problems in children and is solidly based on extensively researched models of parent–child interaction. The content of programmes now goes beyond behaviour to address beliefs, emotions and the wider social context of children's behavioural difficulties. Group programmes address issues that can impair parents' effectiveness, such as poor self-confidence, depression, marital dysfunction and social isolation. Most programmes take place over 8 to 12 sessions lasting 1.5–2 hours each (Forehand & McMahon, 1981; Webster-Stratton & Herbert, 1994; Barkley, 1997). Many of these programmes use video material, role-play and a general sharing of experiences. A meta-analysis by Serkitch & Dumas (1996) calculated a mean effect size of 0.86 for child behaviour change. Other parent training programmes have been described focusing on maternal depression, marital difficulties, adult social skills and social isolation (Scott, 2002).

Groups for young people who have experienced sexual abuse

Group approaches can be structured or unstructured. Group sessions provide a safe forum for discussing experiences of sexual abuse and their sequelae. McGain & McKinzey (1995) found that group therapy was better than no treatment for young people who had suffered sexual abuse. Advantages of a group therapeutic approach over an individual approach were re-experiencing of the trauma, feeling accepted and working on self-esteem and confidence, and working on issues of self-protection and prevention.

Groups for offenders

Groups have been used for adolescents who commit major offences such as sexual abuse. Key issues underlying the use of such an intervention are that the adolescent is accountable for the offence and the approach is specific to that particular offence. Work is carried out on stages of offending, such as contemplation, committing the offence and sub-sequent feelings of guilt. There is an educational element to programmes in raising awareness of victims' responses and including strategies to help prevent re-offending (Bentovim *et al*, 1991).

Group interventions for depression and anxiety

Cognitive–behavioural group interventions have been used for teenagers with social phobias and have also been applied to the treatment of depression. Lewinsohn *et al* (1997) describe the 'coping with depression in adolescence' course. This is based on a social learning model of depression and focuses on training young people in social skills, cognitive restructuring and problem-solving. It is a school-based programme lasting for 10 sessions and has been widely used in North America. Randomised controlled trials have shown benefit of this approach.

Problems with group approaches

Group interventions are in general not suitable for young people with active psychotic symptoms who may not be able to develop a cohesive bond with the group; nor are they suitable for young people who are violent, aggressive or impulsive (in which case they should only be accepted on the condition that they will be able to comply with the group rules). Engagement in a group is crucial and young people should not be made to attend against their wishes. The exception to this may be groups for offenders where treatment is seen as part of probation/rehabilitation.

In summary, since the 1990s substantial developments have taken place in the delineation and manualisation of group interventions. These have been part of a process of seeking evidence for effectiveness and standardising approaches. Evidence is accumulating in favour of the efficacy of group interventions for many disorders presenting to child and adolescent psychiatrists. Groups make good use of limited resources, and in general are underused in child and adolescent mental health settings.

References

Andersen, T. (1987) The reflecting team. *Family Process*, **26**, 415–428.

Anderson, H. & Goolishan, H. H. (1992) *The Client is the Expert: A Not Knowing Approach to Therapy as a Social Construction*. Newbury Park, CA: Sage.

Bandura, A. (1977) Self-efficacy: toward a unifying theory of behavioural change. *Psychological Review*, **84**, 191–215.

Barkley, R. (1997) *Defiant Children: A Clinician's Manual for Assessment and Parent Training* (2nd edn). New York: Guilford.

Beck, A. T. (1967) *Depression: Clinical, Experimental and Theoretical Aspects*. New York: Hoeber Medical.

Beck, A. T., Rush, A. J., Shaw, B. F., *et al* (1979) *Cognitive Therapy of Depression*. New York: Guilford.

Bentovim, A., Vizard, E. & Hollows, A. (1991) *Children and Young People as Abusers: An Agenda for Action*. London: National Children's Bureau.

Bolton, D., Collins, S. & Steinberg, D. (1983) The treatment of obsessive-compulsive disorder in adolescence. A report of fifteen cases. *British Journal of Psychiatry*, **142**, 456–464.

Carr, A. (2000) Evidence-based practice in family therapy and systemic consultation. *Journal of Family Therapy*, **22**, 29–60.

De Shazer, S. (1988) *Clues: Investigating Solutions in Brief Therapy*. New York: Norton.

De Shazer, S. & Berg, I. K. (1992) Doing therapy: a post-structural revision. *Journal of Marital and Family Therapy*, **20**, 413–422.

Doleys, D. M. (1977) Behavioral treatments for nocturnal enuresis in children: a review of the recent literature. *Psychological Bulletin*, **84**, 30–54.

Evans, J. (1998) *Active Analytic Group Therapy for Adolescents*. London: Jessica Kingsley.

Fairburn, C. G., Kirk, J., O'Connor, M., *et al* (1986) A comparison of two psychological treatments for bulimia nervosa. *Behaviour Research and Therapy*, **24**, 629–643.

Forehand, R. L. & McMahon, R. J. (1981) *Helping the Noncompliant Child: a Clinician's Guide to Parent Training*. London: Guilford.

Freud, A. (1946) *The Psychoanalytic Treatment of Children*. London: Imago.

Gelfand, D. M. & Hartmann, D. P. (1984) *Child Behavior Analysis and Therapy*, 2. New York: Pergamon Press.

Graham, P. (ed.) (1998) *Cognitive–Behaviour Therapy for Children and Families*. Cambridge: Cambridge University Press.

Gross, R. (1996) *Psychology: The Science of Mind and Behaviour*. London: Routledge.

Haley, J. (1976) *Problem Solving Therapy*. San Francisco, CA: Jossey-Bass.

Harrington, R. C., Whittaker, J., Shoebridge, P., *et al* (1998) Systematic review of efficacy of cognitive behaviour therapies in childhood and adolescent depressive disorder. *BMJ*, **316**, 1559–1563.

Hawton, K., Salkovskis, P. M., Kirk, J., *et al* (eds) (1992) *Cognitive Behaviour Therapy for Psychiatric Problems: A Practical Guide*. Oxford: Oxford University Press.

Henggeler, S. W., Schoenwalk, S. K., Borduin, C. M., *et al* (1998) *Multisystemic Treatment of Antisocial Behavior in Children and Adolescents*. New York: Guilford.

Herbert, M. (1996) *Toilet Training, Bedwetting and Soiling*. Leicester: BPS Books.

Herbert, M. (2002) Behavioural therapies. In *Child and Adolescent Psychiatry* (4th edn) (eds M. Rutter & E. Taylor), pp. 900–920. Oxford: Blackwell Science.

Klein, M. (1932) *The Psychoanalysis of Children*. London: Hogarth Press.

Klerman, G., Weissman, M. Rounsoville, B., *et al* (1984) *Interpersonal Psychotherapy of Depression*. New York: Basic Books.

Lewinsohn, P., Clarke, G. N., Rohde, P., *et al* (1997) A course in coping: a cognitive–behavioural approach to treatment of adolescent depression. In *Psychosocial Treatments for Child and Adolescent Disorders* (eds E. D. Hibbs & P. S. Jensen), pp. 109–135. Washington, DC: American Psychiatric Association.

March, J. S. (1995) Cognitive behavioural therapy in children and adolescents with OCD: a review and recommendations for treatment. *Journal of the American Academy of Child and Adolescent Psychiatry*, **34**, 7–18.

McCann, J., James, A., Wilson, S., *et al* (1996) Prevalence of psychiatric disorder in young people in the care system. *BMJ*, **313**, 1529–1530.

McGain, B. & McKinzey, R. (1995) The efficacy of group treatment in sexually abused girls. *Child Abuse and Neglect*, **19**, 1157–1169.

Minuchin, S. (1974) *Families and Family Therapy*. Cambridge, MA: Harvard University Press.

Mufson, L. & Fairbanks, J. (1996) Interpersonal psychotherapy for depressed adolescents: a one-year naturalistic follow up study. *Journal of the American Academy of Child and Adolescent Psychiatry*, **35**, 1145–1155.

Mufson, L., Moreau, D. & Weissman, M. (1993) *Interpersonal Psychotherapy for Depressed Adolescents*. New York: Guilford.

Mufson, L., Moreau, D., Weissman, M., *et al* (1999) Efficacy of interpersonal psychotherapy for depressed adolescents. *Archives of General Psychiatry*, **56**, 573–579.

Nichol, R. (2002) Practice in non-medical settings. In *Child and Adolescent Psychiatry* (4th edn) (eds M. Rutter & E. Taylor), pp. 1077–1089. Oxford: Blackwell.

Olweus, D. (1993) *Bullying at School: What We Know and What We Can Do*. Oxford: Blackwell.

Reinecke, M. A., Dattilio, F. M. & Freeman, A. (eds) (1996) *Cognitive Therapy with Children and Adolescents: A Casebook for Clinical Practice*. New York: Guilford.

Roth, A. & Fonagy, P. (1996) *What Works for Whom? A Critical Review of Psychotherapy Research*. New York: Guildford Press.

Rowland, M., Henggeler, S., Gordon, A., *et al* (2000) Adapting multi-systemic therapy to serve youth presenting psychiatric emergencies: two case studies. *Child Psychology and Psychiatry Review*, **5**, 30–43.

Russell, G., Szmuckler, G., Dare, C., *et al* (1987) An evaluation of family therapy in anorexia and bulimia nervosa. *Archives of General Psychiatry*, **44**, 1047–1056.

Scott, S. (2002) Parent training programmes. In *Child and Adolescent Psychiatry* (4th edn) (eds M. Rutter & E. Taylor), pp. 949–967. Oxford: Blackwell.

Selvini Palazzoli, M., Boscolo, L., Cecchin, G., *et al* (1980) Hypothesising-circularity-neutrality: three guidelines for the conductor of the session. *Family Process*, **19**, 3–12.

Serkitch, W. & Dumas, J. (1996) The effectiveness of behavioural parent training to modify antisocial behaviour in children: a meta analysis. *Journal of Behaviour Therapy*, **27**, 171–186.

Shadish, W. R., Montgomery, L. M., Wilson, M. R., *et al* (1993) Effects of family and marital psychotherapies: a meta-analysis. *Journal of Consulting and Clinical Psychology*, **61**, 992–1002.

Simon, M. R. (1992) *The Symbolism of Style: Art as Therapy*. London: Tavistock.

Spence, S. & Marzillier, J. S. (1979) Social skills training with adolescent male offenders. I: Short-term effects. *Behaviour Research and Therapy*, **17**, 7–16.

Webster-Stratton, C. & Hammond, M. (1997) Treating children with early onset conduct problems: a comparison of child and parent training interventions. *Journal of Consulting and Clinical Psychology*, **65**, 93–109.

Webster-Stratton, C. & Herbert, M. (1994) Working with parents who have children with conduct disorders: a collaborative process. In *Troubled Families, Problem Children* (ed. C. Webster-Stratton), pp. 105–167. Chichester: John Wiley.

White, M. & Epston, D. (1990) *Narrative Means to Therapeutic Ends*. London: Norton.

Yalom, I. D. (1985) *The Theory and Practice of Group Psychotherapy*. New York: Basic Books.

CHAPTER 20

Liaison approaches

Andrew Weaver

This chapter describes how child and adolescent mental health services (CAMHS) can operate in ways other than directly assessing or treating young people. It encompasses accounts of both liaison and consultation, terms that are often used interchangeably by professionals and that can be defined in different ways (often depending on personal preference). The term 'liaison' derives from military usage, whereby a member of one force would act as an intermediary with another. A (now obsolete) use of the word actually referred to the way in which a sauce can be thickened by adding eggs. Taylor (1986) points out that, as in cooking, good liaison provides something more than just the sum of its constituent parts.

Consultation, on the other hand, links back to the word 'counsel', meaning advice. The professional relationship between the person seeking advice (the consultee) and the provider of that advice (the consultant) is not necessarily a hierarchical one (as opposed to clinical supervision). Both parties may have their own areas of expertise and training, although the consultant will have greater knowledge about facts or processes that the consultee is seeking advice on. A district social worker or teacher, for example, may ask for advice about the management of a child in their care. The consultant would not be treating the child directly or taking clinical responsibility, but helping the other professional utilise his or her own skills in improving the situation.

The process of consulting and liaising

Nicol (1994), in his chapter on practice in non-medical settings, views mental health consultation as one of the three core skills necessary in such practice, the others being direct work with the client and networking. In his account of how consultation should be set up, he emphasises the importance of obtaining a clear, detailed account of the problem as presented by the consultee. Only after sufficient information about the nature, context and severity of the problem has been elicited should the consultant attempt to offer solutions. Nicol also states clearly that the main contribution can be for the consultant to reinforce the consultee's own efforts, although obviously it may be appropriate to attempt to address any lack of knowledge or skills that become apparent during the consultation. His views therefore suggest that the process is analogous in some ways to the process of history-taking in medical practice. Nicol also cautions against the consultee inadvertently seeking personal therapy from the process.

Eminson (2001a) makes similar points, emphasising the importance of establishing ground rules before any ongoing consultation arrangements are established. She highlights how it is important to clarify where responsibility lies for decisions arising out of the consultation process. Eminson rightly asserts that the consultant should expend as much time as necessary in finding out about the level of training, skills and managerial arrangements of the consultee before proceeding. The young person's and family's awareness of and consent to the proposed consultation also need to be considered.

Lask (1994) sees five main tasks as being needed in successful liaison: consultation, treatment, support, teaching and research. He cites as being particularly relevant the ideas of Lipowski (1974), who differentiated consultation further into patient-oriented, consultee-oriented and situation-oriented. Lask also cautioned against the child psychiatrist using jargon or pseudo-analytical terminology. Oritz's description is similar to Lask's (Oritz, 1997), and he also asserts that good communication is a prerequisite for effective liaison, suggesting that if this is mainly done through verbal rather than written requests, the outcome will be more satisfactory.

How often is consultation or liaison practised?

Despite consultation and liaison being generally recognised as important components in comprehensive service delivery, there is evidence that current provision in the UK falls some way short of this. The Audit Commission's report *Children in Mind* found that 'only 2% of specialist CAMHS staff time was spent providing consultation to others' (Audit Commission, 1999). Clinical pressures on specialist services are the likely explanation for this gap and the report highlights the importance of commissioners from health, social services and education working across their boundaries in inter-agency groups. Some experts view the consequences of this collaboration not happening as potentially serious. Kraemer (1995), for example, points out that 'breakdown between agencies is common when the problems are severe' (as in the case of inquiries into child deaths).

Paediatric liaison

Paediatrics and child psychiatry have much in common and even more to learn from each other. Although the training received by child psychiatrists is predominantly in adult psychiatry, the day-to-day practice of most clinicians in child mental health has more in common with paediatrics. In particular, some developmental disorders such as autism or attention-deficit hyperactivity disorder (ADHD) can become the specialty of either a child psychiatrist or a paediatrician, depending on local variation and personal interest. Some authors have described wryly how the relationship between consultants in paediatrics and child psychiatry can be considered analogous to a friendship, flirtation or marriage, with Apley (1984) strongly advocating the latter 'if only for the sake of the children'. Garralda (2001) proposes that the Royal College of Paediatrics and Child Health and the Royal College of Psychiatrists need to make a business case about the requirement for 'specialised multi-disciplinary treatment which is not appropriately administered in either a psychiatric or paediatric ward'.

Leaving aside for a moment the shared interest in promoting children's welfare and having an interest in the causes and treatment of their suffering, there are practical reasons why the two disciplines have a need to work closely together:

1. Young people with medical illnesses are at increased risk of psychiatric disorder (Gortmaker *et al*, 1990). This is particularly true of conditions that affect the central nervous system, such as epilepsy (Rutter *et al*, 1970), but also applies to diseases such as asthma, diabetes and eczema. Life-threatening conditions such as cystic fibrosis and cancer are also associated with psychological morbidity, and it is important not to forget the emotional and behavioural concomitants that apply to children with physical or intellectual impairments (Rutter *et al*, 1970; Gillberg *et al*, 1986).

2. In some cases of psychological disorder afflicting children and teenagers, there will be physical concomitants. Hence, cases of self-harm will often need assessment and delivery of treatment on medical wards. Eating disorders have a characteristic pattern of somatic sequelae (whether related to weight loss, self-induced vomiting, purgative misuse or a combination of all three), and the disorders of attention and hyperactivity may present with more than their fair share of accidents, fractures, etc. More recently, the increased usage of alcohol and illicit substances by teenagers makes it more likely that some will be admitted in states of either intoxication or withdrawal.

3. Psychosomatic presentations such as dissociative disorder, somatisation and chronic fatigue are often seen initially by paediatric

services. The CAMHS may be asked to become involved after a search for an organic cause has been unsuccessful.

Some of these issues will now be expanded on.

Young people with chronic medical illness

There are some descriptions in the literature about liaison approaches for children with particular medical conditions, for example renal disease (North & Eminson, 1998), cancer (Jones, 1998) and diabetes (Josse & Challener, 1987), or in settings such as a neonatal intensive care unit (Boris & Abraham, 1999; Colville, 2001) or child development centre (Evered *et al*, 1989).

- **Psychiatric presentations** There are several ways in which the psychological problems associated with long-standing medical conditions in children can manifest. There may be features akin to a bereavement reaction after the diagnosis, particularly if this is a life-threatening condition; if severe, this reaction may require input from mental health professionals. The impact on acceptance of, sometimes painful, physical treatments can be profound, resulting perhaps in oppositional, non-compliant behaviour. A child with diabetes mellitus, for example, may refuse insulin injections. In addition, disorders such as depression or anxiety may be precipitated or a coexisting conduct disorder may make it difficult to engage the young person in the management of their medical condition.

- **Developmental issues** The onset of adolescence can create difficulties in the management of a physical illness. The prospect of maturity and independence presents challenges to many teenagers and their families. Battles for control and autonomy are not uncommon. In a young person who has previously complied passively with treatment, the constraints created by dietary control in diabetes or restriction of alcohol ingestion in epilepsy may provide fertile ground for rebelling against adult authority.

- **Family factors** Parents of children with chronic physical disorders are sometimes liable to become more overprotective and to unwittingly increase the likelihood of separation anxiety. All parents have the unenviable task of balancing their wish to keep their children safe with the requirement to allow them independence and autonomy if they are to fulfil their developmental potential. When a child has a long-standing physical illness, this task is even more difficult. The issue is complicated by the fact that there is inevitably no precise 'cut-off' between childhood and adult life; a young person's social, emotional and physical development do not always progress hand-in-hand. In practice, the aim is for parents to find ways of managing their own anxiety about both their child's illness and their increasing independence. An approach that is either overprotective or too lax can be harmful.

Self-harm

The majority of young people who deliberately take tablets or inflict lacerations to themselves will spend a short time on a paediatric ward as a consequence of these actions. This may be to allow necessary physical treatment to occur, but is likely to happen even when the self-harm is medically trivial so that a full risk assessment can take place. This practice differs from that within adult medicine, where assessments in accident and emergency departments might be more common than on medical wards, and derives from recommendations about the management of school-age children who harm themselves (Royal College of Psychiatrists, 1998). A significant minority will repeatedly self-harm, and become regular 'revolving-door' patients on children's wards. The child and adolescent mental health service has a role not only in making an assessment of the child, but also in supporting its staff. The act of self-harm can be very challenging for health service staff to contend with. Sutton (1986) eloquently describes how medical nurses and doctors may use a range of defences to manage their own uncomfortable feelings about such acts. When a young person is repeatedly taking overdoses or having a prolonged paediatric admission owing to the lack of an appropriate discharge placement, these processes can be magnified. Hence, the patient may unwittingly create splits among the staff, some of whom express sympathy, whereas others voice irritation at what they perceive as a self-inflicted problem. Either emotion can be unhelpful. The CAMHS team members may find themselves the targets of some of these frustrations, and perhaps also may be seen unrealistically as the providers of a magical solution.

Primary psychiatric disorders

A severe case of depressive illness or psychosis can be associated with malnourishment or dehydration due to marked reduction in appetite and self-care. Paediatric input will be indicated if this occurs and frequent liaison will be important in this acute phase. First presentations of adolescent psychosis require a thorough physical evaluation to exclude organic causes, with some authorities recommending investigations such as magnetic resonance imaging (MRI) scans (Clark & Lewis, 1998).

The physical consequences of an eating disorder may be the first presentation to a health professional, in that the young person may be malnourished or at risk because of electrolyte disturbance brought about by purging or vomiting.

Children with behavioural problems associated with conduct disorder or attention deficit are at a theoretically increased risk of accidents and injuries; whether such risk translates to more admissions to paediatric wards is debatable. Higher rates of attendance at accident and emergency departments is perhaps more likely, but nevertheless when such children are admitted, they may present challenges to the ward staff (apart from those cases already benefiting from the expert treatment of CAMHS teams, where the children will naturally be models of good behaviour!).

Substance and alcohol misuse

There is evidence that the use by teenagers in the UK of substances such as alcohol, solvents or illegal drugs is increasing (Glaze, 2001). This growing misuse can be predicted to lead to an increased likelihood of paediatric admission due to the physical complications associated with this behaviour; in addition, it may complicate the management of admissions for other psychological problems such as overdoses, or physical disorders such as diabetes.

Psychosomatic presentations

The ICD–10 (World Health Organization, 1992) diagnostic categories for psychosomatic disorders are listed in Table 20.1. The relevance of these disorders for this chapter is that paediatric services are likely to be involved in the majority of presentations, usually at an early stage.

Somatisation as a *process* (i.e. the manifestation of emotional distress through physical symptoms) is common. Indeed, the interplay between physical and psychological factors in ill health is vast, and it is hard to imagine any condition or presentation where both factors do not play a part. For example, in any medical (somatic) illness, psychological or family factors may be important in exacerbating the condition (e.g. asthma), maintaining it or complicating the management (Lask & Fossan, 1989). Equally, psychiatric disorders such as depression, eating disorders or psychosis can have physical associations, either directly or

Table 20.1 ICD–10 criteria for psychosomatic disorders in young people

Adjustment disorders	States of subjective distress and emotional disturbance, usually occurring within one month of a stressful event. Can present as physical symptoms, e.g. headaches, dizzy spells
Dissociative disorders	Usually present with loss of function without a physical cause, e.g. paralysis, amnesia or convulsions
Somatoform disorders	Repeated presentations of physical symptoms with no basis in disease, and where psychological explanations are rejected by the patient or family. Includes somatisation disorder and hypochondriacal disorder
Neurasthenia	Long-standing exhaustion after minimal effort as well as various physical symptoms (similar to criteria for chronic fatigue syndrome)
Factitious disorders	Intentional production or feigning of symptoms or disabilities

as a result of the treatments used. Sometimes a physical illness such as thyrotoxicosis can present with symptoms similar to anxiety; a young person with bulimia's first sign of ill-health might be dental caries or a referral for 'unexplained vomiting'; some people will have both physical and psychological disorders rather than one or the other, as in a person with epilepsy who develops marked social anxiety. The contribution of the young person and family's beliefs about sickness and its causes is an important factor. Help-seeking behaviour also varies between families, ranging from frequent consultations for trivial symptoms to minimal-isation of quite profound disability.

What is required, therefore, is for health professionals to aim at always considering both physical *and* psychological aspects in *every* case they see. This is more difficult than it sounds and a Cartesian split between mind and body is more common than it should be. Under-standably, this is even more likely when the first presentation of sickness is through an organic symptom; here the likely process will be for parents and then professionals to want to look for a treatable physical cause. For the parents, this quest will be for a 'cure'; for the professional the wish to find something treatable; both will fear missing something sinister or potentially fatal. Mental health professionals will often be invited to contribute once such searches have been unsuccessful and when parents, and maybe paediatricians, are becoming exasperated. Engaging families in such circumstances can be difficult, but is a crucial step in the management of cases of psychosomatic disorder. Eminson (2001*b*) writes about the various ways in which CAMHS can be helpful in these scenarios when acting as liaison professionals to the paediatric team. This is particularly relevant when the family rejects the need for direct referral for psychological assessment and intervention. The three roles that Eminson proposes are: support, containment and prevention of avoidable impairment. She suggests that CAMHS staff can help paediatricians to keep psychosomatic formulations in their minds and thereby avoid unnecessary investigations or treatment.

Models of sickness

In many situations in which children (or indeed adults) present as unwell, it may also be difficult for professionals to arrive at an actual 'diagnosis'. For example, somatisation disorder could be viewed as mental health professionals' way of saying that there is nothing life-threatening about the symptoms but that the suffering, as in an unexplained pain, is real and that psychological factors are paramount. Nevertheless, the danger is that one quest for diagnostic categorisation is replaced with another.

There are many common scenarios that are familiar to child mental health professionals where even a psychiatric diagnosis is somewhat unsatisfactory. For example, a teenage girl who takes an overdose after an unresolved family conflict, who lacks any symptoms or signs of depression or other serious mental illness but who is distressed and unable to give assurances that the act will not be repeated may, if diagnostic criteria are rigidly adhered to, be said to have an adjustment disorder; but what does this tell us about the girl's difficulties or what can be done to help them? A formulation using the five axes from ICD–10 (World Health Organization, 1992) is more helpful, but can also end up being a merely mechanistic exercise unless professionals remember that the person being assessed is an individual. Here, Taylor (1979) has some clear and helpful ideas. In describing the various ways in which people can present as 'sick', he proposes three components: diseases, illnesses and predicaments. Disease infers pathology but need not necessarily be serious; hence the common cold is an infectious disease but is usually trivial. Equally one can have a disease without actually being aware of the fact, as in a person with atheroma who is not yet experiencing symptoms. Illnesses can be thought of as a subjective account of suffering, which might suggest an underlying disease but not necessarily. Disorders like depression may perhaps be thought of as 'illnesses'. Predicaments, on the other hand, are the unique situations in which people find themselves, caused by circumstances in their lives and akin to 'scripts' in the dramas of everyday existence. When a predicament occurs in which no solution seems possible, then intense suffering can occur and may be unconsciously played out through physical symptoms, behaviours or other manifestations of distress. The importance of this model is that it emphasises that the only way to fully understand, and therefore help, many of the children and teenagers who present to us is by taking time to hear and understand their own unique situation. Narrative approaches to healthcare use similar underlying principles and are being increasingly recommended in all aspects of medicine (Greenhalgh, 1999). By being mindful of these points, mental health professionals can more effectively liaise with paediatric doctors and nurses, who, by dint of their training, may adopt a more linear, diagnostic and problem-solving approach to the children they see.

The practice of paediatric liaison and consultation

The actual structure and components of a paediatric liaison service will depend on local resources. Unfortunately, some CAMHS teams, while recognising the value a well-established, systematic liaison service, will be restricted by paucity of staffing to merely offering an emergency assessment response to cases of self-harm. However, even the most richly funded service will fail to provide effective and valued liaison if this is not founded on mutual respect between the professionals. There are some potential pitfalls that can hinder collaborative working relationships: psychiatrists and paediatricians may enter into psychological jousting matches in which each tries, subtly, to score points off the other. In extreme but fortunately rare situations, the psychiatrist will try to impress the paediatrician with his knowledge of disease processes and take great delight in uncovering a hitherto undiagnosed physical problem. The paediatrician, on the other hand, may attempt to demonstrate expertise in the understanding of psychological mechanisms in the child or family and effect a cure in cases that have proved impervious to therapies offered by the CAMHS team. Both parties can end up devoting an inordinate amount of time to areas in which the other has more expertise.

There is a useful account by Black *et al* (1999) of the actual mechanics of setting up a paediatric liaison service in York. Weekly meetings were used as a way of providing mutual consultation and liaison as well as general discussion. In addition, potential referrals were discussed. The authors recommended detailing these discussions in a book designed for the purpose, which also allowed them to audit the process. The results were interesting, in that not only were there benefits in terms of levels of communication, increased respect and closer working relationships, but there was also an impact on referral patterns. Hence, subsequent to the liaison meetings there were increased numbers of eating problems, autism, ADHD and non-organic cases referred, i.e. the sort of cases that most CAMHS teams would view themselves as having expertise in managing. They also found that the case discussions could 'provide new ideas and support for those already involved with families and often averted the need for formal child mental health involvement'.

Whether or not the family is included in the consultation process is another issue. Proctor & Loader (2000) use a case report to describe how the advantage of the family taking part is that their own views and beliefs can be accommodated.

Joint ward rounds

There can be advantages in a member of the CAMHS team being present on the paediatric ward round; this provides opportunities for psychosocial issues to be kept alive in the discussion of children's ill health. This should therefore be advantageous not just to the children and families who are being discussed, but also to any accompanying paediatric trainees or students who, by a process akin to osmosis, will learn that psychological factors are important to consider in children who are physically unwell.

Clinics

In the same way as in joint ward rounds, there can be opportunities for psychiatric team members to attend paediatric clinics. Specialist clinics for children with diabetes or epilepsy are an example. Taylor (1986) describes the benefits of mutual discussion of difficult cases, in writing about his experience of joint clinics at a teaching hospital.

Teaching

Teaching and training can include more formal didactic sessions to junior medical staff or nurses, paediatric trainees sitting in on CAMHS clinical sessions, multidisciplinary case discussions or shared journal clubs. In some centres these ideas have been elaborated to include opportunities for higher trainees in paediatrics to have a long attachment in child and adolescent psychiatry.

Case example 1

A children's ward in a district general hospital had recently had three admissions of teenage girls with anorexia nervosa. Each had presented their own particular management problems: the first had been rather quiet and passive but had steadfastly refused attempts to encourage increased eating; the second was more openly defiant and the nursing staff suspected that she had been secretly vomiting in the toilets; in the third case the girl had spent a short time on the ward after an emergency referral from her general practitioner (who had become alarmed at her weight loss and requested an urgent assessment to exclude physical causes). The CAMHS team had been involved to a greater or lesser extent in each girl's admission, but in none of the cases had the paediatric admission been brought about at the request of the mental health service. A discussion between the paediatric and child psychiatry consultants at their regular monthly meeting proved useful in allowing one of the paediatric consultants to air his anxieties about eating disorders, which were that if patients in cases of anorexia were not admitted, there was a risk that they would deteriorate or fail to get better. It became apparent that he strongly believed that such an admission would 'kick start' a recovery by engendering a sort of 'surrender' by the teenager, who would thus be frightened into eating and gaining weight. Some general information-sharing about the evidence base for treatments in anorexia nervosa helped to modify some of these views.

In addition, it was proposed that the CAMHS team might offer some teaching sessions about eating disorders to both the junior medical and nursing staff. Two members of the mental health team, a family therapist and a specialist registrar offered three support sessions to the staff. This enabled a majority of the staff to attend as it took account of shifts and on-call commitments. The group was run on informal lines and the two team members attempted to identify common assumptions, fears and beliefs about eating disorders. A brief, didactic component was incorporated, as the junior doctors in particular wanted some 'facts' about the condition. The most rewarding aspect of the process was the extent to which the nurses and junior doctors helped each other by ventilating and alternately challenging the assumptions they all had. For example, one of the nurses expressed an opinion in strong terms that teenagers with anorexia were manipulative and 'needed to sort themselves out'. The CAMHS staff had already been aware of this belief, but their own previous attempts to shift this conviction had been fruitless. In allowing each person to express his or her feelings without being criticised, the group format facilitated a subtle shift in the nurse's viewpoint, as some of her own colleagues were able to challenge it in way that had not been possible before (owing to time constraints and other commitments). An excerpt from a book about anorexia written by people who had recovered from this disorder consolidated this step, by conveying the important message that the teenager with an eating disorder is often terrified about weight gain, but also fearful about the consequences of the condition.

Consultation and liaison with other health professionals

A hypothetical model for child and adolescent mental health services was outlined by the NHS Health Advisory Service (1995). This proposes a four-tiered model, with Tier 1 meant to describe the problems and relevant therapeutic approaches delivered within primary care, including schools and other environments (Table 20.2).

There are some drawbacks to this model, particularly as it could imply that, by portraying Tier 3 as specialised services that manage complex problems, Tier 1 is concerned with more mild difficulties. However, it was useful for an attempt to be made to highlight the growing demand on child psychiatry services during the 1990s. Whereas in adult mental health, workers in primary care such as general practitioners were used to manage milder cases of depression or anxiety or were able to invoke the help of trained counsellors within the surgery, there had been comparatively little such progress in child and adolescent mental health. *Together We Stand* (NHS Health Advisory Service, 1995) therefore highlighted the disparity between services at Tier 1 and those at Tiers 2 and 3 and proposed the development of primary mental health workers to

Table 20.2 Tiered model of child and adolescent mental health services

Tier 1	Social workers, general practitioners, voluntary agencies, health visitors, teachers
Tier 2	Psychiatrists, community psychiatric nurses, clinical psychologists, psychotherapists, educational psychologists, etc. (usually working in isolation)
Tier 3	Specialist CAMHS multidisciplinary teams
Tier 4	In-patient CAMHS units, specialised neuropsychiatric services, secure forensic mental health services, very specialised out-patient services for complex or refractory problems

plug this gap. Tier 3 teams are increasingly using consultation with primary care professionals as a way of managing the demand, as a means of providing ongoing learning for these workers and, ideally, as a means of benefiting the young people as well.

Appleton (2000) cites the literature as proposing two main methods of training for primary care. On the one hand, training can be provided for primary care professionals who will be continuing to offer a 'generalist' service; on the other hand it can be aimed at helping those at Tier 1 who wish to spend a specific amount of their time on child mental health-related work. There are some articles published on both the former approach (Bernard *et al*, 1999) and the latter (Davis *et al*, 1997). Appleton emphasises the need to obtain agreement from those at the top of the management and commissioning hierarchy if professionals at the Tier 1 level can be released from other duties to offer this work. Appleton's model for how consultation can operate between Tier 1 and the specialist service is to subdivide this into informal, client-centred, consultee-centred, mediation or consultation about organisational change.

Case example 2

A health visitor made a referral of two children, Jack aged 3 years and Sophie aged 6 years, who had both been passengers in their parents' car when it had been involved in a minor accident. Since then Jack had been fretful at night and had begun to sleep in his parents' bed after formerly being well established in a night-time routine. Sophie generally seemed clingier and had wet the bed on a couple of occasions. The health visitor was requesting that both children be seen and that Sophie perhaps receive play therapy. On receipt of the referral, the child and adolescent mental health team decided to offer a consultation with the health visitor. The team's primary mental health worker met therefore with the referrer who had obtained consent from the children's parents for this to occur.

At the consultation, the CAMHS professional obtained some more information about the children's functioning, drawing on the skills and experience of the health visitor, who had known the family since the birth of Sophie 6 years previously. Her knowledge of normal developmental processes was highlighted, but she expressed a view that she was less certain about when school-age children might need therapy. One of the possible areas for further exploration that emerged was that the children's mother was possibly suffering from anxiety herself. The session was also used to discuss concepts of post-traumatic stress in young children as well as issues relating to normal regressive behaviours following a stressful event. The agreed outcomes were that the health visitor would visit the mother of the children and discuss her own anxiety symptoms further and suggest some potential help she might obtain for them. It was also apparent that Jack's symptoms might then respond to some parental strategies. Finally, with Sophie an intervention based on solution-focused brief therapy was proposed. In essence this would involve the health visitor seeing the parents and Sophie for three or four appointments with the primary mental health worker joining them for the first and fourth appointment. The focus was to reframe Sophie's clinginess and bedwetting as an understandable reaction to an upsetting event, to emphasise the family's strengths and coping strategies that they had already been using and which had helped prevent the symptoms becoming worse.

Both parents found the approach helpful, commenting that, having previously been worried that their daughter was badly affected and in need of 'fixing', they were now able to see that her day-to-day functioning was well within normal limits. Sophie's mother expressed her relief at her realisation that she had not somehow caused her daughter to develop an anxiety disorder, as she herself had felt responsible for the accident and had been nursing unspoken fears of having failed her daughter.

Liaison with social services

Within the UK there has been a philosophical shift away from children being received into care, with a drive towards keeping young people in their families of origin wherever possible. Despite this, the numbers of children in care within the UK has increased slightly (Department of Health, 2001). The main reduction has been in the number of young people accommodated in residential establishments as opposed to foster placements. This parallels the reduction in health service beds for mentally ill adolescents. As a consequence, those children who do end up being accommodated in children's homes are by definition either those who are more out of control or those who have endured more severe abusive or neglectful experiences. Second, some young people within fostering placements will display a greater level of disturbance than perhaps 20 years ago. There is certainly evidence that young people in care, whether in residential or foster placements, have a high level of psychiatric disorder. A study by Williams *et al* (2001), which examined the health needs of 142 children in local authority care, found a high degree of problems, including emotional and behavioural difficulties. McCann *et al* (1996) established that 67% of 13- to 17-year-olds in Oxford who were in the care system had a psychiatric disorder. The figures were strikingly high for those in residential units (96%) and the prevalence of disorder in fostered teenagers (57%) was substantially greater than in their control group (15%). As expected, conduct disorder was the most common actual diagnosis, but rates of mood disorder (23%) and psychosis (8%) were not insignificant. The study by McCann *et al* was with a group of teenagers who had been in the care system for an average of 2.9 years. Another study by Dimigen *et al* (1999) in Glasgow used a questionnaire-based survey to evaluate rates of psychological problems in young people at the point of being taken into care. Their findings were similar, with conduct disorder and depression again being common. The authors commented that 'a considerable proportion of young children have a serious psychiatric disorder at the time they enter local authority care but are not being referred for psychological help' (Dimigen *et al*, 1999).

Social workers are often the first port of call for foster carers or children's home staff who have become concerned about a child in their care. Naturally they may then seek advice from CAMHS teams, who tend to prioritise cases of possible psychosis, depression or self-harm. A young person with a conduct disorder may be given a lower priority. However, the social worker who is involved with such a case is still faced with a young person who may be acting out and creating anxiety for the carers and professionals. In addition to this potential pressure, social services staff have new challenges and demands to meet in response to the expectations that all families seen by their workers will receive a full and comprehensive assessment (Department of Health, 2000). In such a climate, there is considerable potential for relationships between social services and child mental health to become somewhat strained. To prevent such a cooling of interactions, there needs to be much effort expended in increasing mutual understanding of the respective stresses and pressures. Sir William Utting, in his foreword to the useful publication on the mental health needs of looked after children (Richardson & Joughin, 2000), comments that 'professional and organisational separation between child care and mental health has left each with only partial understanding of the other'. Regular liaison forums can help prevent distrust and irritation building up between agencies. Pearce (1999) suggests a number of ways in which greater collaboration between the NHS and social services might occur in the arena of child and adolescent mental health. Commenting that relationships can often be good at either the fieldwork or managerial level, this is not a consistent finding across services. He observes that as health and social services often have differing, conflicting models of understanding clinical and social problems, it is important that these differences are accepted and understood. Pearce also identifies three main factors that can foster or hinder good relationships, namely personalities, power struggles and misconceptions. Once these issues are acknowledged, there is the potential for further development of liaison to occur by closer working, e.g. by secondments or attachments.

The practice of liaison and consultation with social services

Social workers placed in CAMHS

In some services a social worker may be an integral part of the CAMHS team. Links with the local authority will be maintained by external supervision or sessions at the social service office, but the workers will see themselves as full members of the health service's multidisciplinary team. Their clinical work will therefore be supervised within the CAMHS. A secondment or attachment, on the other hand, is slightly different, in that the social worker is temporarily part of the CAMHS, either for personal development or to help foster links between the two agencies. Supervision will be held outside the health service.

Training sessions

Lectures, workshops or group discussions can be provided for common themes such as self-harm, attachment disorder and other concerns.

Regular input to children's homes

Children and young people in residential care homes may present a number of behaviours that cause concern to the staff managing them. Emotional distress may take the form of running away or self-harm, whereas accompanying conduct problems can include aggression or sexualised behaviour. Care staff may therefore value input on the management of some of these concerns either through specific training sessions or by means of ongoing support groups. In addition, the tensions and stresses involved in working in such an environment may be played out in conflicts between staff. The theories underpinning group therapy can be beneficial here and the provision of more psycho-dynamically oriented groups could be appropriate.

Innovations and research into collaborative approaches

In some parts of the UK there have been innovative developments where health and social services (and other agencies) have joined together to develop a particular initiative. One such example is called Sure Start (Hall, 2000). This is funded from central government, and was established towards the end of the 1990s. The aim of this venture is to improve the emotional well-being of future generations of young people by targeting those most at risk in the pre-school years. It is known that a number of factors increase the risk of emotional and behavioural problems in children; poverty and social disadvantage are two such issues. Hence, Sure Start is targeted at families living in areas that suffer higher rates of poverty, unemployment and other variables. The keystones of the approach are to increase resilience and prevent disorder among children under 5 years old. Improving early detection of psychological disorder is another aim. The approach is a good example of true multi-agency work and it is particularly innovative that some of the inter-ventions are available at the pre-birth or even pre-conception stage. Strategies aimed at increasing parental self-esteem and employability, as well as the availability of therapies such as Webster-Stratton groups (a type of intervention known to be effective at treating conduct disorder in children; see Chapter 19), should be helpful not only to the target population and age group, but also in preventing more serious disturbance in later life. Research provides support for the hypothesis that such interventions and innovations will be of value to disadvantaged children and families (White *et al*, 2002).

With regard to collaboration between specialist CAMHS and social services, Cottrell *et al* (2000) have written about their experience in Leeds. Here, the CAMHS team were aware that the needs of social services referrers were not being met and the Tier 3 service felt increasingly under pressure too. Several components of an effective liaison approach were identified, namely social services identifying their high-priority referrals, regular consultation being offered from CAMHS about complex cases, and the organisation of training seminars for field work staff. The authors reported that a greater consensus between health and social workers developed, although the need for more therapeutic services was also highlighted.

Case example 3

A children's home requested some regular consultation sessions from their local child and adolescent mental health service. The CAMHS team felt this request was reasonable, as they had noticed that there had been a spate of referrals from the home. Some of these had merited mental health assessment, whereas others had been considered inappropriate. The CAMHS workers were aware that the different responses to the referrals were creating some confusion, and it was thought that the consultation sessions would allow an information-sharing exercise to occur as well as hopefully developing the confidence and skills of the residential staff. Following a meeting with the officer in charge of the home and the local social services team leader, it was agreed that two CAMHS members would offer to meet with the staff of the home. An introductory meeting ensued, in which a number of issues were generated and written on a flip chart. These included the pressures the staff felt in working with the children, many of whom had been neglected or abused in the past and some of whom were aggressive, sexually disinhibited or prone to absconding; a need for help in understanding what was meant by 'mental disorder'; varying views about the different manifestations of, and risks associated with, self-harm; a somewhat vague awareness of how psychological therapies might or might not help, including in some cases an obvious desire to see the young people have something that could 'cure' them, and also a sense of frustration at the general lack of resources, both in their own establishment and in terms of the CAMHS waiting list.

The outcome of this was that a number of developments occurred. First, regular consultation sessions were set up so that the care staff could book slots with a senior member of the mental health service. These sessions were welcomed as a guaranteed forum for the staff to air their worrying cases, which they had to prioritise to some extent so that only the most difficult or perplexing cases were brought to the consultation.

Second, two focused training sessions were held at the home on the two subjects that had caused most concern, namely self-harm and psychiatric disorder. It was felt that the issue of helping the staff understand the indications for therapy would be addressed through the opportunities for consultation. Third, it was recommended that the social services management look into providing a staff support group with an external facilitator, as it was clear that many of the care home staff had ongoing anxieties, concerns and conflicts, which were having a negative effect not only on themselves but also potentially on the children.

Liaison with education

Schools feature largely in young people's lives. In England, it is a legal requirement for people to receive formal education from about the age of 5 years to 16 years. Some children start school earlier than this (as in the private sector) and many young people stay on until 18 or over. The UK government has stated its commitment to improving the standards in its schools with the development of a national curriculum, an emphasis on improving literacy and numeracy, and promoting the notion of healthy schools (Department for Education and Employment, 1999). Although these targets are not directly concerned with mental health, their achievement would be expected to have positive effects on children's emotional well-being. The important role of schools in recognising emotional and behavioural problems in young people and the strategies they can adopt to ameliorate them has been written about by leading authorities such as Rutter *et al* (1970) and Kolvin *et al* (1981).

In many areas, child and adolescent mental health services will accept referrals from professionals such as teachers, educational welfare officers and educational psychologists. In having experience of seeing children and teenagers for up to 7 hours a day, teachers develop a wealth of experience in seeing at first hand normal child development. The more empathic will also have skills in helping young people who have worries or other difficulties, and the majority should be able to compare a child's level of psychosocial functioning with the norms of other children. However, even in areas where teachers have the means to refer to CAMHS, this is not a common finding (Ford & Nikapota, 2000), and the recognition and understanding by schools of childhood psychological disorders is variable.

There a number of ways in which CAMHS team members can help by offering their expertise to schools. Some of these approaches, such as consultation and liaison, have similar underlying principles to those pertinent to the other agencies described earlier. In addition, there have been efforts to translate clinic-based therapies to the school environment, as in the Help Starts Here project (Kolvin *et al*, 1981). A significant minority of children will receive their schooling not in the mainstream sector, but in a specialised environment. Some comprehensive schools have units attached to cater for young people with problems such as learning disability, visual or hearing impairments, or behavioural disorders. Occasionally, however, children will receive some of their education in a specialised residential establishment. Here, the issues described in the discussion on liaison with social services units apply. When considering the particulars of consultation with schools and their staff, some further discussion is merited. Bostic & Rauch (1999) comment that in the USA schools have been faced with the task of managing greater numbers of pupils with psychiatric illnesses, as a result of a diminution in hospital and residential admissions. The same could be said to be occurring in Britain. They suggest three basic tenets of good consultation, namely to strengthen relationships, foster recognition of dynamic forces (such as resistances and other defences) and facilitate responses in the consultees. Rather neatly, they refer to these as the 'three Rs'.

In England and Wales, the Department for Education and Skills produced a document aimed at helping staff promote children's mental health in schools (Department for Education and Skills, 2001).

Suggestions were also made on how to facilitate this in pre-school settings such as nurseries. General ideas such as schools being advised to promote emotional health through the personal, social and health education (PSHE) curriculum are mentioned; specific multi-agency practices are also outlined, including a number of initiatives as follows:

- peer coping-skills training;
- school nurse screening clinics to detect psychological disorder;
- within-school counselling;
- a multi-agency team (in Rochdale) which intervenes with children under 12 who are at risk of exclusion;
- a child behaviour intervention initiative (in Rutland) aimed at helping schools develop programmes to improve children's psychological health; in addition, children at risk of developing problems are identified, and 'drop-ins' are organised for concerned parents;
- an early-years intervention team (in Camden), offering support and advice to nurseries.

Case example 4

A local CAMHS team received a referral from a mainstream comprehensive school seeking help with a disruptive and oppositional teenage boy. The overt request was for anger management for the young person, but the head of year who made the referral also stated that the boy's mother was not particularly in favour of the need for input from CAMHS. The CAMHS team felt that further clarification was required; it was likely that an appointment sent to the family would not be accepted, but the team were also concerned about comments that the referrer had made about the boy having a low self-esteem and the fact that on one occasion he had threatened self-harm. A plan was agreed whereby one of the team would offer a joint consultation to the teacher but also including the mother. During the meeting it rapidly became apparent that the mother felt that the school were blaming her for her son's difficulties. This belief was explored and, having been able to express this and having her concerns acknowledged, the mother became less angry and for the first time began to describe her own worries about the boy. The teacher was surprised but pleased to hear that, having formerly denied that her son presented any problems at all outside of school, the mother was now admitting that she had always found him hard to manage. Further discussion ensued and the CAMHS professional began to suspect that the boy might have some of the symptoms and behaviours characteristic of attention-deficit hyperactivity disorder. The possibility of this helped both parent and teacher to develop a new and improved relationship as they both recognised that neither of them was the cause of the boy's difficulties.

Liaison approaches with services for young people who commit offences

There is increasing evidence that rates of psychiatric disorder are high in persistent young offenders (Dolan *et al*, 1999). The establishment of youth offending teams (YOTs) by the government in Britain was an attempt to reduce the amount of delinquent behaviour by teenagers. It was also an aim of the new teams to help identify the concomitant psychiatric disorders that many of the young people who commit offences have. Most youth offending teams have a health worker as part of their complement and it is with this professional that the CAMHS may most often relate. The principles of such liaison are as described earlier in other sections, and the youth offending team worker will usually be seeking advice and consultation about disorders such as psychosis, depression or attention-deficit disorder.

The other area in which CAMHS teams may be asked to help is in the provision of reports for the legal system. How teams respond will often be a matter for local agreement. Regular liaison can help clarify what the CAMHS is being asked to provide by way of a report. There is a difference, for example, between a 'professional' report (which is a summary of the input being provided for an ongoing case) and an 'expert' opinion (in which specific questions will be addressed and evaluated independently by the expert).

References

Apley, J. (ed.) (1984) *If a Child Cries*. London: Butterworth.

Appleton, P. (2000) Tier 2 CAMHS and its interface with primary care. *Advances in Psychiatric Treatment*, **6**, 388–396.

Audit Commission (1999) *Children in Mind: Child and Adolescent Mental Health Services*. London: Audit Commission.

Bernard, P., Garralda, M. E., Hughes, T., *et al* (1999) Evaluation of a teaching package in adolescent psychiatry for general practitioner registrars. *Education for General Practitioners*, **10**, 21–28.

Black, J., Wright, B., Williams, C., et al (1999) Paediatric liaison service. Psychiatric Bulletin, **23**, 528–530.

Boris, N. W. & Abraham, J. (1999) Psychiatric consultation to the neo-natal care unit: liaison matters. Journal of the American Academy of Child and Adolescent Psychiatry, **38**, 1310–1312.

Bostic, J. Q. & Rauch, P. K. (1999) The 3Rs of school consultation. Journal of the American Academy of Child and Adolescent Psychiatry, **38**, 339–341.

Clark, A. F. & Lewis, S. W. (1998) Practitioner review: the treatment of schizophrenia in childhood and adolescence. Journal of Child Psychology and Psychiatry, **39**, 1071–1081.

Colville, G. (2001) The role of a psychologist on the paediatric intensive care unit. Child Psychology and Psychiatry Review, **6**, 102–109.

Cottrell, D., Lucey, D., Porter, I., et al (2000) Joint working between child and adolescent mental health services and the department of social services: the Leeds model. Clinical Child Psychology and Psychiatry, **5**, 481–489.

Davis, H., Spurr, P., Cox, A., et al (1997) A description and evaluation of a community child mental health service. Clinical Child Psychology and Psychiatry, **2**, 221–238.

Department for Education and Employment (1999) National Healthy School Standard: Guidance. Annesley, Nottingham: DfEE Publications.

Department for Education and Skills (2001) Promoting Children's Mental Health Within Early Years and School Settings. Nottingham: DfEE Publications.

Department of Health (2000) Framework for the Assessment of Children in Need and Their Families. London: Stationery Office.

Department of Health (2001) Children Looked After in England 2000/2001. London: Department of Health.

Dimigen, G., Del Priore, C., Butler, S., et al (1999) Psychiatric disorder among children at time of entering local authority care: questionnaire survey. BMJ, **319**, 675.

Dolan, M., Holloway, J., Bailey, S., et al (1999) Health status of juvenile offenders. A survey of young offenders appearing before the juvenile courts. Journal of Adolescence, **22**, 137–144.

Eminson, D. M. (2001a) Treatment in non-psychiatric settings. In Adolescent Psychiatry in Clinical Practice (ed. S. G. Gowers), pp. 346–366. London: Arnold.

Eminson, D. M. (2001b) Somatising in children and adolescents: 2. Management and outcomes. Advances in Psychiatric Treatment, **7**, 388–398.

Evered, C. J., Hill, P. D., Hall, D. M., et al (1989) Liaison psychiatry in a child development clinic. Archives of Disease in Childhood, **64**, 754–758.

Ford, T. & Nikapota, A. (2000) Teachers' attitudes towards child mental health services. Psychiatric Bulletin, **24**, 457–461.

Garralda, M. E. (2001) Need for paediatric–psychiatric liaison. British Journal of Psychiatry, **179**, 369.

Gillberg, C., Persson, M., Grufman, M., et al (1986) Psychiatric disorders in mildly and severely mentally retarded urban children and adolescents: epidemiological aspects. British Journal of Psychiatry, **149**, 68–74.

Glaze, R. (2001) Classification and epidemiology. In Adolescent Psychiatry in Clinical Practice (ed. S. G. Gowers), pp. 60–96. London: Arnold.

Gortmaker, S. L., Walker, D. K., Weitzman, M., et al (1990) Chronic conditions, socio-economic risks and behavioral problems in children and adolescents. Pediatrics, **85**, 267–276.

Greenhalgh, T. (1999) Narrative-based medicine in an evidence-based world. BMJ, **318**, 323–325.

Hall, D. M. B. (2000) What is Sure Start? Archives of Disease in Childhood, **82**, 435–437.

Jones, J. (1998) Liaison psychiatry in a paediatric oncology clinic. Bulletin of the Royal College of Psychiatrists, **12**, 213–215.

Josse, J. D. & Challener, J. (1987) Liaison psychotherapy in a hospital paediatric diabetic clinic. Archives of Disease in Childhood, **62**, 518–522.

Kolvin, I., Garside, R. F., Nicol, A. R., *et al* (1981) *Help Starts Here: The Maladjusted Child in the Ordinary School.* London: Tavistock.

Kraemer, S. (1995) The liaison model – a guide to mental health services for children and adolescents. *Psychiatric Bulletin,* **19**, 138–142.

Lask, B. (1994) Paediatric liaison work. In *Child and Adolescent Psychiatry; Modern Approaches* (3rd edn) (eds M. Rutter, E. Taylor & L. Hersov), pp. 996–1005. Oxford: Blackwell Science.

Lask, B. & Fossan, A. (1989) *Childhood Illness: The Psychosomatic Approach.* New York: Wiley.

Lipowski, Z. (1974) Consultation-liaison psychiatry: an overview. *American Journal of Psychiatry,* **131**, 623–630.

McCann, J. B., James, A., Wilson, S., *et al* (1996) Prevalence of psychiatric disorders in young people in the care system, *BMJ,* **313**, 1529–1530.

NHS Health Advisory Service (1995) *Together We Stand: The Commissioning, Role and Management of CAMHS.* London: HMSO.

Nicol, A. R. (1994) Practice in non-medical settings. In *Child and Adolescent Psychiatry, Modern Approaches* (3rd edn) (eds M. Rutter, E. Taylor & L. Hersov), pp. 1040–1054. Oxford: Blackwell Science.

North, C. & Eminson, D. M. (1998) A review of a psychiatry-nephrology liaison service. *European Child and Adolescent Psychiatry,* **7**, 235–245.

Oritz, P. (1997) General principles in child liaison consultation service: a literature review. *European Child and Adolescent Psychiatry,* **6**, 1–6.

Pearce, J. B. (1999) Collaboration between the NHS and social services in the provision of child and adolescent mental health services: a personal view. *Child Pychology and Psychiatry Review,* **4**, 150–152.

Proctor, E. & Loader, P. (2000) Getting it right: a dilemma of multi-disciplinary working in a paediatric liaison team. *Clinical Child Psychology and Psychiatry,* **5**, 491–496.

Richardson, J. & Joughin, C. (2000) *The Mental Health Needs of Looked After Children.* London: Gaskell.

Royal College of Psychiatrists (1998) *Managing Deliberate Self-Harm in Young People* (Council Report CR64). London: Royal College of Psychiatrists.

Rutter, M., Tizard, J. J. & Whitmore, K. (eds) (1970) *Education, Health and Behaviour.* London: Longman.

Sutton, A. (1986) Management of teenagers who take overdoses. *Hospital Update,* 15 July, 144–151.

Taylor, D. C. (1979) The components of sickness: diseases, illnesses and predicaments. *Lancet, ii,* 1008–1010.

Taylor, D. C. (1986) Child psychiatric/ paediatric liaison: a discussion paper. *Journal of the Royal Society of Medicine,* **79**, 726–728.

White, C., Agnew, J. & Verduyn, C. (2002) The Little Hulton project: a pilot child clinical psychology service for pre-school children and their families. *Child and Adolescent Mental Health,* **7**, 10–15.

Williams, J., Jackson, S., Maddocks, A., *et al* (2001) Case-control study of the health of those looked after by local authorities. *Archives of Disease in Childhood,* **85**, 280–285.

World Health Organization (1992) *The ICD-10 Classification of Mental and Behavioural Disorders. Clinical Descriptions and Diagnostic Guidelines.* Geneva: WHO.

CHAPTER 21

Forensic services

Sue Bailey

Young people at the interface of the criminal justice system and mental health services risk double jeopardy for social exclusion, alienation and stigmatisation (Bailey, 1999). The definition of this group varies across and within agencies; their needs are diverse and require a range of mental health services that can only be effective if integrated with the services of other agencies.

Young people account for an estimated 7 million crimes a year. The psychosocial and biological factors placing young people at risk of offending and/or of developing mental health problems are well established (Junger-Tas, 1994; Kazdin, 1995; Rutter & Smith, 1995; Shepherd & Farrington, 1996; Rutter et al, 1998; Rutter, 1999). Despite the available research literature, young offenders with mental health problems often only become the subject of mental health assessments late in their careers. The focus is then on the medico-legal issues in the arena of juvenile court proceedings.

Definitions

Forensic mental health has been defined as an area of specialisation that, in the criminal sphere, involves the assessment and treatment of those who are both mentally disordered and whose behaviour has led or could lead to offending (Mullen, 2000). Defining forensic psychiatry in terms of the assessment and treatment of the mentally abnormal offender delineates an area of concern that could potentially engulf much of mental health. Offending behaviour is common in the whole community and, as Mullen notes, among adolescents it approaches the universal. Criminal convictions are spread widely through society and even more widely among people with mental disorders.

Patients often gravitate to adult forensic services when the nature of their offending or the apprehension created by their behaviour is such as to overwhelm the tolerance or confidence of a professional in the general mental health services. In part these referrals are also driven by the emerging culture of blame, in which professionals fear being held responsible for failing to protect their fellow citizens from the violent behaviour of those who have been in their care. Of particular importance, Mullen stresses, is making mental health expertise address the mental health component of social problems. This should not conflict with traditional medical practice if the aim is to identify and relieve disorder to benefit patients, but also, through their more adequate care and management, to benefit those whom they potentially threaten. Mullen highlights the importance of rigorous risk assessments and management.

There is an association between substance misuse, mental disorder and offending. Nowhere is this more important than in the field of adolescent forensic psychiatry.

Background

In England and Wales since the 1980s there have been major changes in legislation meant to bring about an improvement in services for children. The Children Act 1989 reformed the law, bringing public and private law under one statutory system. More recently, there has been a major review of the legislative framework relating to the involvement of young people in criminal and antisocial activities, in the form of the Crime and Disorder Act 1998. In particular, Section 37 of the Act lays the statutory duty on services including health, education, the police, probation and local authority social services to prevent crime through effective inter-agency practice and appropriate forms of intervention. This focus on youth crime is not surprising, as nearly half of all known offenders are under 21 years old, although most of this offending happens as part of a maturational process, as adolescents test boundaries. However, some of the behaviour becomes entrenched and a small percentage of these youths go on to become persistent offenders.

Surveys of young people at different points in the criminal justice system both in the UK and in the USA show high rates of psychiatric disorder, particularly in persistent offenders (Kazdin, 2000; Lader et al, 2000). In a health needs survey of established young offenders appearing before a large city-centre youth court, 19% had significant medical problems, 42% a history of substance misuse and 7% psychiatric problems requiring treatment and intervention. Over a quarter engaged in a variety of dangerous behaviours, which can be seen partly as the sensation-seeking of a young offender population in general, but also an expression of their emotional instability (Dolan et al, 1999). Despite some positive policy moves (Ashford & Bailey, 2004), a large number of young offenders still end up remanded or sentenced to custody, as illustrated by the rising number of young people and children who now find themselves in the new secure estate provision. This includes over two-and-a-half thousand young people incarcerated, at any one time, in local authority secure care units, young offenders institutions and secure training centres, and the small number in designated adolescent psychiatric medium secure units – commissioned nationally and in the independent sector.

When young people become involved in the criminal justice system, the focus on their offending behaviour often takes precedence over developmental and mental health issues. In Britain the young offender with a mental health problem tends to fall into the gap between the organisational boundaries of different agencies such as social services, youth offending teams, educational provision and child and adolescent mental health services (CAMHS). Of particular concern to probation services are those over 16 years old who are not registered with a general practitioner. The absence of a holistic approach with identified key-workers, as occurs in the adult care programme approach, which could maintain continuity of care for the young person, is starkly apparent. A 1997 review of young prisoners (HM Chief Inspector of Prisons for England and Wales, 1997) found that between the ages of 16 and 24 years, mental and emotional difficulties are major problems for young people in prison. Over 50% of remanded young males and over 30% of sentenced young males have a diagnosable mental disorder. At every level of intervention, from the entry point of prison reception, the excessive delay in transferring the assessed patient from the prison to the National Health Service (NHS), to the fragmented arrangements for care after release, the report chronicles a range of failings. It argues that these failings can only be addressed by the NHS taking over responsibility for the healthcare of young people in custody, so that there is more consistency with provision offered in the community. This becomes more important when the suicide rate for young men, and its rise over recent years, is considered. In 1996 in the UK, 547 men aged 15–24 years took their own lives. The Crime and Disorder Act 1998 proposals, with the establishment of youth offending teams, should aid coordination and cooperation for offenders under 18 years old. However, such cooperation can only be effective if there are resources within CAMHS, and professionals trained and willing to do the job. Real opportunities now present themselves to improve the mental health of young offenders with the new joint running of prison healthcare services by the Department of Health, the Home Office and the prison service, and with the opportunities arising from a Children's National Service Framework.

Young people are often referred to health services as a list of problems that conflate diagnosis and behaviour, a tendency reinforced in research findings. A focus on health need enables professionals working as part of a multidisciplinary health team to consider how interventions can make an impact on career pathways.

Problem profiles

Emerging findings from the long-term follow-up studies of young people in secure care appear to demonstrate five categories of offenders (Bullock & Millam, 1998):

- young people who have been in long-term care;
- young people who have required prolonged special education;
- young people whose behaviour has suddenly deteriorated in adolescence;
- one-off grave offenders;
- serious and persistent offenders.

Broad and overlapping sets of problems associated with offending have been identified and will need to be addressed concurrently. These are illustrated by Rutter *et al* (1998), who stress the heterogeneity of antisocial behaviour, related to the pervasiveness, persistence, severity and pattern of such behaviour. The following offender profiles illustrate the relationship between developmental features, offending behaviour and mental health problems:

- Early onset of antisocial behaviour with aggressive, violent or disruptive acts, coercive sexual activity or arson, with fluctuations in mood state and levels of social interaction.
- Repetitive high-risk behaviours in female adolescents presenting with serious suicide attempts and self-mutilation interspersed with externalising destructive behaviours. Such young people raise grave anxieties within generic service provision, but even here violent behaviour in girls is underestimated, partly due to the non-specific and insensitive diagnostic criteria for conduct disorders in girls (Jasper *et al*, 1998).
- Male offenders with a history of sexual and physical abuse in their childhood who currently show mood disturbance and self-harm (Bailey *et al*, 2005).
- Those in the prodrome of severe mental illness, which may last for 1–7 years before florid psychosis develops. During this time there is marked variation in the degree of non-psychotic behavioural disturbance. The importance of the accurate assessment of young offenders who show multiple high-risk episodes associated with a fluctuating mental state needs to be more fully recognised.
- Young people with particular vulnerability and risk are the homeless and those subject to penal remand detention. Interconnections between homelessness, mental disorders, substance misuse and offending are complex and remain poorly understood.

In addition, these profiles can be compounded by comorbidity in the following areas:

- attention-deficit hyperactivity disorder (Scott, 1998);
- drug use and misuse (which have increased rapidly over the past 10 years);
- learning disability.

Addressing the problem

The challenge of child and adolescent forensic psychiatry is to tease out levels of unmet need, provide a careful assessment of mental state and problem behaviours, bring together collated information to assist in formulating a safe multi-agency care plan, and play a part in its delivery. Scott (1998) has stressed the need for CAMHS to offer an integrated assessment with other agencies. The aim is to work with young children with antisocial behaviour in a family context using parent management training strategies, combined with individual interventions for the child. The full range of psychological therapies should be available to vulnerable adolescents, particularly those leaving care and at risk of custody (Royal College of Psychiatrists, 1999). Multisystemic therapy involving family and community-based interventions can be effective in terms of improved clinical outcomes and cost savings in future life (Henggeler, 1999). These outcomes may include reduction in the risk of development of personality disorder in adulthood.

Interventions

Young offenders require:

1. a strategic approach to commissioning and delivering services for them, which:
   - develops effective and predictable services that meet their current and future needs;
   - builds upon established concepts of service;
   - ensures workforce planning issues are addressed and met by longer-term training;
2. a better understanding of their needs across all involved agencies, which should develop inter-agency strategies at the locality level, such as flexible working in court diversion schemes with innovative partnerships with the voluntary sector (Maziade et al, 1996);
3. access to primary healthcare;
4. speedy access to CAMHS, as their needs are unlikely to be met by adult mental health services;
5. services to overcome a reluctance to treat them that sometimes arises out of a fear of stigmatisation;
6. speedy access to drug and alcohol education and treatment centres (intensive forms of intervention for drug users with complex care

needs should involve specialist residential services and mental health teams closely linked to CAMHS and forensic services;

7. speedy access to HIV testing;

8. for those adolescents who display the criminal behaviours of interpersonal violence, arson and sexual offences, an increased drive to approach the assessment, risk, management and treatment of them as a specific entity; this requires a focus on developmental issues rather than past tendencies to apply adult treatment models to young people (Vizard & Usiskin, 1999);

9. improved inter-agency training of non-health professionals in identifying the indicators of mental vulnerability in young people, thus strengthening the communications with professionals in the mental health services;

10. a recognition that adolescents with learning disability will have a slower pace of developing coping strategies and changing that must always be balanced against their risk to others;

11. social regimes that help to promote the health of young people in prison; girls and young people from ethnic minorities are recognised to be particularly vulnerable to aversive prison regimes, but at present there are no specialised facilities available to young girls in prison in the UK: 16- and 17-year-olds still find themselves in adult female prisons (NHS Executive & HM Prison Service, 1999);

12. an awareness by all agencies of the gaps in the capacity of existing services;

13. the establishment, on a regional basis, of adolescent forensic mental health teams to promote and coordinate:

    • improved outreach services;
    • the development of programmes for young people before they reach the courts and custody, including adolescent in-patient services and access to secure forensic facilities;
    • rehabilitation and support for young offenders on a post-custodial basis;
    • a shared approach to risk assessment and management, together with agreed protocols for better information exchange, between the health service and criminal justice agencies;
    • an awareness of the current growth points in professional practice, service developments and research.

A health perspective

The government strategy for mental health (Department of Health, 1998) put forward, for the first time, a health strategy with risk and public protection as the top priority. Child and adolescent mental health professionals have traditionally been involved at the interface between the law and the welfare of children, but historically this has often been through the need for their professional opinion on children in the child care system rather than in forensic matters. The CAMHS are important in helping professionals in other agencies to recognise developmental and interactional influences on offending behaviour.

Traditionally, CAMHS are generalist, which means they might include forensic work. They must be aware that in addressing such issues, the rights of children have to be seriously considered. The rights of children to be involved in decisions about their own treatment for either physical or mental illness is set in three legal frameworks: common law, the Children Act 1989 and the Mental Health Act 1983, as well as the European Human Rights Act (Bailey & Harbour, 1998).

Solutions

Ways to develop services have been described from assessments of need, commissioning exercises and clinical experience (Kurtz *et al*, 1997; Bailey & Farnworth, 1998; Audit Commission, 1999; Knapp & Henderson, 1999; Bailey & Williams, 2005). The NHS Health Advisory Service review of the adolescent forensic services at Salford (NHS Health Advisory Service *et al*, 1994) concluded that the greatest immediate need was for an increase in secure NHS-funded provision for:

- mentally disordered offenders;
- sex offenders and abusers;
- severely suicidal and self-harming adolescents;
- adolescents with severe mental illnesses;
- adolescents who need to begin psychiatric rehabilitation in secure circumstances;
- brain-injured adolescents and those with severe organic disorder, recognising that some of these services are being developed within the independent sector.

A strategic framework to address such services would be based on a four-tier model in which local generic and regional specialist services allow for the multidimensional problems encountered by these young people to be tackled by local CAMHS in conjunction with other agencies. Other solutions could include:

- Local CAMHS provision for young offenders, while ensuring resources for the rest of the locality CAMHS are not depleted by this work.
- Local CAMHS augmented by advice and training offered by a peripatetic outreach team that is based in and works from a specialised centre of expertise in forensic child and adolescent mental health. This patient group would have high mobility, their

families frequently moving from one local authority to another, and their residential placements often changing. Funding and services must follow the child and not be obstructed by agency and geographical boundaries, to ensure continuity of care. As this is going to be inherently difficult for a locality CAMHS, Tier 3 services may be required.

- Peripatetic specialised forensic services in which the young people are seen directly by members of outreach services from a specialised centre of expertise, sharing responsibility with the local CAMHS.

- Tier 4 centres of specialist forensic expertise, which deliver services directly to patients and their families. These may involve open units, high-dependency units, and intensive assessment and care units with security between medium and high, considerable emphasis being placed on staff training and dissemination of expertise.

Such a strategic framework is ambitious and requires:

- staff wanting to work in this area;
- comprehensive training systems;
- evidence-based interventions;
- a national adolescent forensic mental health research and development network, which has now been established to ensure that what is learnt from research is promptly put into practice.

Working in this field is always challenging for psychiatrists, but can be very rewarding, as sustained mental health input can bring about real change over time.

References

Ashford, M. & Bailey, S. (2004) The Youth Justice System in England and Wales. In *Adolescent Forensic Psychiatry* (eds S. Bailey & M. Dolan), pp. 409–416. London: Hodder Arnold.

Audit Commission (1999) *Children in Mind: Child and Adolescent Mental Health Services*. London: Audit Commission Publications.

Bailey, S. (1999) The interface between Mental Health, Criminal Justice and Forensic Mental Health Services for Children and Adolescents. *Current Opinion in Psychiatry*, **12**, 425–428.

Bailey, S. & Farnworth, P. (1998) Forensic mental health services. *Young Minds Magazine*, **34**, 12–13.

Bailey, S. & Harbour, A. (1998) The law and a child's consent to treatment (England and Wales). *Child Psychiatry Review*, **4**, 1–5.

Bailey, S. & Williams, R. (2005) Forensic mental health services for children and adolescents. In *Child and Adolescent Mental Health Services: Strategy, Planning, Delivery and Evaluation* (eds R. Williams & M. Kerfoot), pp. 271–295. Oxford: Oxford University Press.

Bailey, S., Jasper, A. & Ross, K. (2005) Social diversity. In *Adolescent Forensic Psychiatry* (eds S. Bailey & M. Dolan), pp. 179–181. London: Hodder Arnold.

Bullock, R. & Millam, S. (1998) *Secure Treatment Outcomes: The Care Careers of Very Difficult Adolescents*. Darlington: Ashgate.

Department of Health (1998) *Modernising Mental Health Services*. London: Department of Health.

Dolan, M., Holloway, J., Bailey, S., *et al* (1999) Health status of young offenders appearing before juvenile courts. *Journal of Adolescence*, **22**, 137–144.

Henggeler, S. W. (1999) Multi-systemic therapy: an overview of clinical procedures, outcomes and policy indications. *Child Psychology and Psychiatry Review*, **4**, 2–10.

HM Chief Inspector of Prisons for England and Wales (1997) *Young Prisoners: A Thematic Review*. London: Stationery Office.

Jasper, A., Smith, C. & Bailey, S. (1998) 100 girls in care referred to an adolescent forensic mental health service. *Journal of Adolescence*, **21**, 555–568.

Junger-Tas, J. (1994) *Delinquent Behaviour Among Young People in the Western World*. Amsterdam: Kugler.

Kazdin, A. E. (1995) *Conduct Disorder in Childhood and Adolescence*. London: Sage.

Kazdin, A. E. (2000) Adolescent development, mental disorders and decision making of delinquent youths. In *Youth on Trial. A Developmental Perspective on Juvenile Justice* (2nd edn) (eds T. Grisso & R. G. Schwartz), pp. 33–65. Chicago, IL: Chicago University Press.

Knapp, M. & Henderson, J. (1999) Health economic perspectives and evaluation of child and adolescent mental health services. *Current Opinion in Psychiatry*, **12**, 393–397.

Kurtz, Z., Thorne, R. & Bailey, S. (1997) *Study of the Demands and Needs for Forensic Child and Adolescents Mental Health Services in England and Wales. Report to the Department of Health*. London: Department of Health.

Lader, D., Singleton, N., Meltzer, H. (2000) *Psychiatric Morbidity Among Young Offenders in England and Wales*. London: Office for National Statistics.

Maziade, M., Bouchard, S., Gingras, S., *et al* (1996) Long-term stability of diagnosis and symptom dimensions in a systematic sample of patients with onset of schizophrenia in childhood and early adolescence. II: Positive/negative distinction in childhood predictors of adult outcome. *British Journal of Psychiatry*, **169**, 371–378.

Mullen, P. E. (2000) Forensic mental health. *British Journal of Psychiatry*, **176**, 307–311.

NHS Executive & HM Prison Service (1999) *The Future Organisation of Prison Health Care*. London: Department of Health.

NHS Health Advisory Service, Mental Health Act Commission, Department of Health Social Services Inspectorate (1994) *A Review of the Adolescent Forensic Psychiatry Service Based on the Gardener Unit, Prestwich Hospital, Salford, Manchester*. London: NHS Health Advisory Service.

Royal College of Psychiatrists (1999) *Offenders with Personality Disorder* (Council Report CR71). London: Royal College of Psychiatrists.

Rutter, M. (1999) Psychosocial adversity and child psychopathology. *British Journal of Psychiatry*, **174**, 480–493.

Rutter, M. & Smith, D. J. (1995) *Psychosocial Disorders in Young People: Time Trends and Their Causes*. Chichester: John Wiley.

Rutter, M., Giller, H. & Hagell, A. (1998) *Antisocial Behaviour by Young People*. Cambridge: Cambridge University Press.

Scott, S. (1998) Aggressive behaviour in childhood. *BMJ*, **316**, 202–206.

Shepherd, J. P. & Farrington, B. P. (1996) The prevention of delinquency with particular reference to violent crime. *Medicine, Science and the Law*, **36**, 331–336.

Vizard, E. & Usiskin, J. (1999) Providing individual psychotherapy for young sexual abusers of other children. In *Children and Young People Who Sexually Abuse Others: Challenges and Responses* (eds M. Erooga & H. Massen), pp. 179–210. London: Routledge.

CHAPTER 22

In-patient units

Sean Maskey

In-patient units are part of a continuum of child and adolescent mental health service (CAMHS) provision. There are about 70 adolescent units in the British Isles and around 20 units that admit children. Some units admit both (O'Herlihy & Brook, 2002). A third are in the private sector. In-patient services can be classified in several different ways, such as by age, specialisation or regional distribution (Fig. 1).

In-patient units aim to provide assessment, treatment and education in a highly structured therapeutic environment, which is created and managed by the nursing team and teachers if they are based on the unit. In-patient units deliver a wide range of interventions in parallel, which produce a synergistic effect that it is not usually possible in an out-patient setting. In-patient adolescent psychiatry services are the intensive care services of CAMHS, admitting those few children who need and can benefit from the concentration of intensity that can be provided. Like most high-cost, low-volume services in the National Health Service (NHS), provision has been haphazard and outcome evaluation limited.

By setting clear objectives for admission and discharge, and by reviewing these regularly, services aim to minimise length of stay, and so maximise access to a scarce resource. Admission to, and discharge from, in-patient services necessitates active engagement with the local network of health, education and social services, if the benefits are to be maximised and time away from home minimised. For young people who have left school, the links should be with further education and employment services, and voluntary organisations working with adolescents in these fields. Case management will often be organised under the integrated care programme approach (CPA) (Mind, 2002).

Treatment principles

Any intervention should impose the minimum necessary restrictions on the young person. In-patient admission significantly reduces autonomy

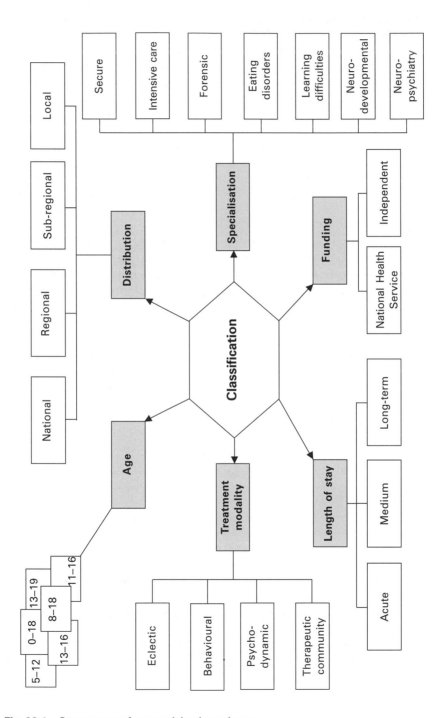

Fig. 22.1 Some ways of categorising in-patients.

and separates adolescents from their families – aspects of life subject to the Human Rights Act 1998 and the UN Convention on the Rights of the Child (http://www.unhchr.ch/html/menu3/b/k2crc.htm). While the in-patient unit ethos, structure and management is designed to minimise harm to the adolescent, it inevitably places young patients at greater physical and psychological risk than if they were living with their family. Young people who are in-patients are more likely than others to have suffered serious adverse life events, abusive experiences and disrupted care, all of which predispose individuals to aggressive, violent and abusive behaviours. Any in-patient may then be the victim of this behaviour, either directly or as a witness to it. Separation from known caregivers and a familiar environment is itself stressful. For an adolescent experiencing the fear and uncertainty of severe mental illness for the first time, admission and the associated experiences can be sufficiently distressing as to cause post-traumatic stress disorder (McGorry *et al*, 1991). Exposure to the raw emotions and associated poorly modulated behaviours of other mentally ill adolescents may also add to the distress of the individual patient. It is a sad fact that staff in residential treatment facilities may also abuse children; awareness of the possibility and effective supervision and management strategies can reduce but not eliminate this risk.

Before any in-patient admission is considered, it is imperative therefore that less restrictive alternatives are considered and – if appropriate – implemented. This is a shared task between the referrer, who will know what treatment resources are available locally, and the patient's capacity to utilise them, and the receiving unit, which will have specialist knowledge of specific interventions, such as alternative medication strategies, that may remove the need for admission. This joint planning should ideally take place prior to admission; in urgent cases, it should be scheduled as soon as possible after intake.

In-patient units are a scarce resource, and unnecessary admission (in the sense that appropriate alternatives are available) or protracted duration prevents the admission of other young people, as well as extending the period of exposure to the risk of harmful experiences. On the other hand, a brief admission reduces the ability of nursing staff to get to know individuals well and adjust their interactions precisely to the particular needs of the young person. In these circumstances, management strategies for non-psychiatric aspects of care, such as aggression, have to be predominantly protocol-driven rather than individualised (American Academy of Child and Adolescent Psychiatry, 2002).

There are factors internal and external to the in-patient unit that determine length of stay, independently of patient characteristics and regardless of the type of unit – short-, medium- or long-term. Delays in assessment, or in the delivery of treatment, usually due to organisational processes or the (relative or absolute) lack of appropriate specialist staff or access to investigations such as electroencephalography (EEG), will result in extended stay in hospital. Sadly, but all too frequently, the appalling domestic circumstances of some young people only become apparent when they are admitted to in-patient units. The additional care needs arising from mental illness overwhelm the already chronically inadequate care provision, be it family, foster care or residential setting. Highlighting the likely long-term needs at the point of referral, and including this in the CPA process, will reduce the risk that the adolescent in-patient unit becomes the place where a young person lives; if patients have no home outside hospital, ending the period of admission becomes impossible as one cannot 'discharge' someone from their home. In-patient units are also understandably reluctant to discharge patients in the absence of appropriate education or day unit facilities at the end of treatment.

Attention to and engagement with the network of people (families and friends) and agencies (health, education, social services, youth justice and voluntary agencies) who surround all young people, and who have specific responsibilities for parts of their lives, focuses in-patient treatment on those who are in greatest need and minimises the length of stay. The integration of an individual's in-patient care with that provided before and after admission will also serve to increase the accountability of the in-patient component, thereby reducing the risk of abuse and neglect in that setting. The admittedly adult-oriented CPA case management can support this process, and the integration of health (CPA) and social services (care management) models should further improve this (Department of Health, 1999). However, education is a significant component that is not directly engaged by this legislation, and attention needs to be paid to the patient's educational needs from the outset.

Admission decisions

Psychiatric in-patient admission in Britain is at one end of a spectrum of treatment options, which can be subdivided into four tiers (Williams & Richardson, 1995) of increasing specialisation, complexity and cost. The American model (American Academy of Child and Adolescent Psychiatry, 2002) is rather more pragmatic and describes the 'continuum of care' in a community, and recognises that not all aspects may be available in all places. Case management is therefore an explicit compromise between the needs of the young person, the local facilities and (in the USA) their insurance provision.

In-patient treatment is indicated when the problems are severe and/or complex (Maskey, 1998) and in the following situations (Box 22.1):

- the patient needs 24-hour psychiatric nursing care, or
- has a rapidly deteriorating condition, or

- appropriate out-patient treatment has been unsuccessful, or
- there is diagnostic uncertainty.

There is no absolute indication for admission. However, most acute in-patient units avoid admitting patients whose primary problem is significant conduct or attachment disorder. Blanz & Schmidt (2000) reviewed research on in-patient psychiatric services for young people and concluded that despite the lack of robust evidence, admission is likely to be helpful if in-patient care is integrated into other forms of treatment, the focus is problem-oriented and there are clear treatment plans.

In the first three examples in Box 22.1, there may be alternative strategies to in-patient admission, and the decision to admit will depend on the accessibility of day-treatment services, intensive home-based treatment and social services support, as well as the social circumstances. For example, if John's mother had access to child-care support, lived in a quiet residential road and regular contact with a community psychiatric nurse was available, he could easily be managed at home. Earl is the most likely to need admission given the diagnostic uncertainty, which includes organic, psychiatric and drug-induced illness, or a combination or these, as well as dangerous behaviour.

Type and choice of unit

The four patients described in Box 22.1, if they came from the same area, could all be referred to their local sub-regional adolescent unit, if beds were available and the unit had an intensive-care area for Earl. However, if the local service is full or (as some services do) restricts admissions because it has specialised in one particular treatment style, does not use medication or cannot admit emergencies, then these young people might go to a variety of different services. On average, referrers contact two units before a place is found, and this figure can be as high as seven (O'Herlihy et al, 2001). Sharon's family and her referrer may argue that a pre-pubertal girl should not be exposed to the psychotic symptoms and aggression that is manifest in a general unit for 13- to 19-year-olds. Graham's referring team may consider their expertise in treating Tourette syndrome superior to that of the local in-patient service and seek a specialist neuropsychiatric unit. Sharon's team, having engaged well in family work, may negotiate with the local unit to continue this while she is an in-patient.

Most National Health Service adolescent units are now closely linked to their local districts. However, there is a shortfall in bed availability of at least 50%. As a result, patients are placed at considerable distance from their homes, either in NHS facilities that happen to have vacancies or in independent sector units. The latter are more likely to be specialised

> **Box 22.1** Admission examples
>
> **'Needs 24-hour psychiatric nursing care'**
>
> John, a 16-year-old boy, has become severely depressed (anhedonic, apathetic and not eating or washing) and is intent on suicide. There is no clear trigger. He lives with his mother and sister (aged 7) on the 12th floor of a tower block. There are no friends or relatives who will help with childcare, and he is likely to be left alone for periods of time during the day. He has contemplated jumping from the balcony. The out-patient team request admission for risk assessment (and management), supervision, and initiation of treatment with selective serotonin reuptake inhibitors and cognitive–behavioural therapy.
>
> **'Has a rapidly deteriorating condition'**
>
> Sharon, a 14-year-old girl, has had anorexia nervosa for 1 year. She has been treated successfully by a specialist out-patient team, but starts to vomit and her weight drops by a kilogram per week shortly after she is told the family are going to America for 3 years because of her father's work. The referrer asks for a short admission to stabilise the patient, while the out-patient team continue to provide individual and family therapy.
>
> **'Appropriate out-patient treatment has been unsuccessful'**
>
> Graham, a 13-year-old boy, has had 2 years of specialist treatment for Tourette syndrome, comorbid with conduct disorder. Medications have been tried systematically, with limited treatment response. He is taking clonidine and risperidone, and the out-patient team are unable to reduce the medication as his symptoms deteriorate to unacceptable levels. Graham and the out-patient team want all medication to be withdrawn, and a diagnostic review to occur before initiating further treatment.
>
> **'There is diagnostic uncertainty'**
>
> Earl, a 17-year-old boy, living at home and working in a fast-food outlet, suddenly refuses to eat or drink anything he has not observed being prepared from fresh ingredients. He has hit his mother several times and threatened a workmate, claiming they were 'tricking' him about the food. He refuses to eat at all at work and as a result of his restricted intake is losing weight rapidly, becoming dehydrated and appearing confused at times. He is known to use 'street drugs', but his friends cannot say what. His only explanation is that the food is 'contaminated'. He has been brought to the emergency clinic by the police under Section 136 of the Mental Health Act 1983. They were called to a disturbance in the street, after he had threatened a passer-by with a broken bottle, accusing her of poisoning him. He is aggressive in the casualty department and does not want any help. The assessment team wants stabilisation of an acutely deteriorating situation by urgent admission under Section 2 of the Mental Health Act 1983, followed by diagnostic assessment, including a neurological review, drug screening and detoxification if necessary.

services, e.g. for young people with eating disorders or those needing secure (locked) facilities (Table 22.1).

Classification of units, and therefore exclusion criteria, by age, IQ or geography, is convenient in planning terms, but unhelpful clinically if criteria are applied too rigidly. The (emotionally and physically) immature

Table 22.1 Number of adolescent in-patient units in England and Wales in 2002

Units	Generic	Specialist	Total
National Health Service	38	11	49
Independent	8	9	17
Total	46	20	66

Data from Royal College of Psychiatrists' Research Unit (2002).

14-year-old girl with anorexia might do very well in an acute unit where the average age is 14 years, and very poorly when the average age is 16.5 years. Conversely, the same girl might be fine in an eating-disorder unit where the majority of patients are over 16 years old. For clinical purposes, considering units in terms of specialisation and patients by psycho-sexual developmental level is more helpful.

Adolescent units can be divided broadly into generic and specialised units. The generic units are usually eclectic in approach, specialise in the treatment of severe and complex psychiatric disorder irrespective of type, and employ a range of therapeutic skills. The more specialist units, by focusing on particular diagnostic groups, are able to limit the range of interventions offered. A further subdivision by length of stay – acute (6–8 weeks), medium-term (up to 26 weeks) and long-stay (6–36 months) – is sometimes helpful in understanding the reluctance of some units to admit (or discharge) particular patients.

For generic adolescent units, the need to design individual treatment programmes and the maintenance of the therapeutic environment (physical and emotional) for a wide range of patients presents a considerable challenge. In general, services planned on a geographic (regional) basis will be generic; the more specialist services, such as eating-disorder, neuropsychiatric or behavioural services, are likely to be supra-regional or national in scope. Unfortunately, lack of coherent planning of in-patient services has led to some regional services becoming highly specialised (e.g. medium- or long-term psycho-therapeutic services) and thus limiting access for diverse groups of young people. Recent changes in the commissioning process have begun to resolve some of these anomalies.

Staffing

There is uncertainty and debate about the optimal staff mix and levels. The relevant factors to consider include case-mix, age and age range, dependency, length of stay, developmental level and developmental delays, comorbid physical illness, physical layout, group size, education provision, and the therapeutic stance of the unit. There are some tasks that can only be done by specific professionals, e.g. the dispensing of medication by trained nursing staff. All staff (including domestic and clerical staff who may meet patients and families) are expected to have a basic understanding of mental health issues, and to respond accordingly. Some staff will have particular therapeutic skills, such as cognitive–behavioural therapy or family therapy, irrespective of their discipline. Figure 22.2 shows the skills mix in units in England and Wales.

A unit requires a critical mass of staff to undertake the various components of the work, clinical and non-clinical, and there is a real danger that by using minimum staff levels for each professional group, the unit is unable to function safely and effectively. Once the profession-specific tasks have been covered, there remains a considerable amount of generic and specific work to be done that is not the de facto responsibility of any particular group. Generic tasks include communication with patients and other staff, observation and report writing, being with young people in unstructured time, and basic child protection work. Some aspects, such as group work, supervision or clinical audit, and non-clinical tasks such as teaching, training, research and general hospital management activities, will be done by individuals with specific skills, not necessarily because of their professional training (Fig. 22.3).

Guidance on UK in-patient unit staffing comes primarily from two documents, both published by the Royal College of Psychiatrists. *Guidance on Staffing for Child and Adolescent In-patient Psychiatry Units* (Royal College of Psychiatrists, 1999) uses a dependency model to

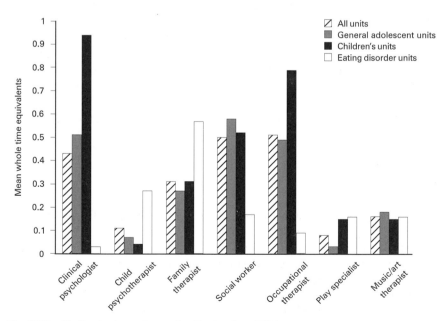

Fig. 22.2 Staff mix: in-patient units, England and Wales.

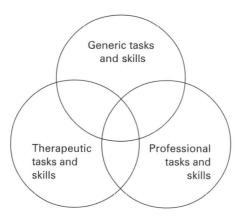

Fig. 22.3 A model of skill and task interaction.

calculate minimum professional staffing numbers, and does not allow for generic or individual specific tasks. *Not Just Bricks and Mortar* (Royal College of Psychiatrists, 1998), which is a more comprehensive report on the requirements of adult units, discusses the options for calculating staffing levels based on professional opinion, dependency and an activity-scheduling model that is essentially a time-and-motion exercise. It concludes that numerical models alone are inadequate, as is unsupported 'judgement'. However, the scenario envisaged to determine staffing levels, using the economies of scale produced by multiple adjacent wards providing flexible cross-cover, does not often arise in adolescent services, which are often deliberately placed away from other (adult) mental health wards. This report does emphasise the need to avoid 'minimum staffing' levels being the norm for the unit, as they are not sustainable in the long term. They lead to a culture of containment rather than therapy, with low morale and minimal development (as the team is focused on 'getting through the next 24 hours'), and high rates of staff turnover and sickness.

Nurses, teachers and doctors form the core of all in-patient services. The extended multidisciplinary team will be drawn from professionals including psychologists, individual and family therapists, occupational, speech and language therapists, physiotherapists, social workers and other staff (such as paediatricians), depending on the specific needs and historic arrangements of the service.

The therapeutic approach also affects team size. In a service that works exclusively with one client group, using a limited range of assessment and treatment tools, many of the staff, regardless of discipline, will be able to deliver most of the treatment programme. Case allocation then becomes a matter of allocating the first person with a gap in their workload. In a general unit, with a broad case mix, scheduling is

> **Box 22.2** Project management for in-patient care
>
> Projects have four phases: conception and definition; planning and scheduling; execution; and closure.
>
> *Conception and definition*
> Clarify ideas
> Identify the stakeholders (patient, family and clinical network)
> Agree the outcomes with them, allocate tasks (to the in-patient and other services) and manage expectations
>
> *Planning and scheduling*
> Resource (beds and staff) availability
> Sort expected time scales (admission, review and discharge dates)
> Allocate staff – key nurse, other therapists, etc.
> Identify and manage risks
>
> *Execution*
> Commence the (clinical) work
> Monitor progress and bridge internal and external systems (ward rounds, update letters and review meetings)
> Manage dissension – there are often multiple possible solutions, but one has to be followed
>
> *Closure and handover*
> Stakeholder agreement that the end-point has been reached
> Planning handover of responsibilities and ongoing work
> Closing meeting
> Closing summary
> Evaluation and project appraisal (outcome and audit)

more complex. The available specialist clinical time can quickly be exceeded if a few similar cases are referred (for example, treatment-resistant obsessive–compulsive disorder needing sophisticated cognitive–behavioural therapy). The options then are to defer admission, defer the provision of expert treatment or offer a less able therapist. All of these options will prolong the distress for the young person and the carers, and require careful judgement and open discussion in agreeing the treatment plan.

The in-patient process and CPA

For all too many people with severe and enduring mental health problems, the revolving door of admission is a continuous process with little (second-order) change. In contrast, the goal of most adolescent admissions is to effect a fundamental change in the psychosocial developmental trajectory of the young person. In order to do this, the admission will consider the whole of the adolescent's context and not just focus on symptoms. Resolution of the person's predicament there-fore requires coordinated input from a number of agencies and services.

Units vary in the extent to which they build the treatment package around individual patients. Some will deliver treatment according to a more or less fixed protocol of assessment, treatment and discharge plans. Others will design their interventions around the assessed needs of each young person and the family. If integrated treatment with out-patient services is to be achieved, there needs to be a clear agreement about the purpose and goals of the admission between the out-patient referrer, the patient and their carers, and the in-patient team. In some circumstances, this is implicit. In the case of Earl, the psychiatrist assessing in accident and emergency wants a safe and secure environ-ment in which Earl could be nursed, fully assessed and have treatment instigated; an acute adolescent unit will expect this type of referral, and the referrer will expect this service. Sharon could be referred to a general psychiatric unit that might be very pleased to have an offer of ongoing family therapy as part of the treatment plan. On the other hand, she might be referred to a specialist eating-disorder service that offers packages of treatment in which the family therapy programme dovetails into individual therapy, group work and the re-feeding programme. In the latter case, the different treatment styles could be experienced as contradictory and confusing. Explicit discussion about the tasks and roles of different members of the treating teams is then essential if misunderstanding and, potentially, mistreatment is to be avoided.

The care programme approach, which was introduced in part to encourage planning and integration between disparate agencies and services and to bridge hospital and community care, requires joint planning and reviews of progress by all the relevant parties for all mental health patients. It makes explicit the areas of need for the young person, and identifies the individuals and agencies responsible for addressing those needs. Any patient referred for tertiary care in an in-patient unit should be on a CPA programme prior to referral. Many, if not most, should have enhanced CPA, given that several professionals will be involved (Centre for Evidence Based Mental Health, 2001). It can be helpful to regard CPA (or indeed any in-patient admission) as a specialised form of project management (Box 22.2). Some specific principles are known that are key to successful projects (Young, 1998), and although the CPA model describes what is to be done, in terms of areas to be addressed it is not informative about how it should be managed.

The ward

The in-patient setting will vary to some extent, depending on the nature and purpose of the service; for example, a secure unit will have an external locked perimeter, whereas a general hospital-based unit might have some hospital-type beds and accommodation to manage young people who are also physically ill. There is a range of standards that apply to the design and layout of adolescent wards, which address safety, comfort, privacy, recreational facilities, therapy rooms and classrooms (Royal College of Psychiatrists' Research Unit, 2002).

The ward accommodation needs to provide a variety of areas for different activities at different levels of intensity, from quiet study and reflection to communal eating and living space, as well as outdoor areas for boisterous play and exercise. Some flexibility of use is helpful, particularly being able to open or close areas of the ward, dependent on gender mix, dependency levels and overall occupancy. A 'low-stimulus' area is invaluable for nursing highly aroused patients with active psychotic symptoms. By creating a calm, contained and emotionally containing space within the ward area, the need for 'as required' medication will be reduced. This should not be confused with seclusion

---

Box 22.3 The ward milieu

This intangible quality of all wards supports young people's sometimes precarious engagement with treatment and their self-regulation of emotion and behaviour. A strong, positive milieu allows groups to work with lower levels of direct supervision and support than does a poorer milieu. As the ward milieu deteriorates, higher levels of one-to-one nursing and 'as required' medication are needed and antisocial behaviour increases.

The milieu is created directly by the nursing team, with the support of the extended multidisciplinary team and the hospital management. Positive staff behaviours include: the systematic attention to the detailed content of each person's treatment plan and respect for scheduled activities; active identification of individual strengths and weaknesses and appropriate management; explicit awareness of interpersonal tensions and support to resolve them; a comprehensive weekly timetable, providing structure to the day, outside as well as within school; active support for the families of patients and their engagement in therapeutic work; a balance of task-focused and reflective groups; the active involvement of the patient group with staff in planning the daily and weekly programme; access to advocacy; clear boundaries on confidentiality; transparent and robust child protection and complaint procedures, and respect for the fabric of the ward.

The fabric of the unit should be regarded as a therapeutic tool and not simply as the box in which 'the treatment' can take place. Damage to the building should be repaired quickly. Soiled or broken furniture and equipment should be removed and replaced, immediately or after an appropriate interval, depending on circumstances. Hard surfaces are easy to clean, but attract graffiti and reflect sound. Dining rooms in particular can be very hard environments, where the noise level rises exponentially as people struggle to be heard. Patients and staff are stressed, and emotional and consequent behavioural disturbance rises.

(enforced isolation) or 'time out' (from positive reinforcement), as part of a behaviour-modification programme.

Smoking is an issue in all adolescent settings and many of the young people will have a long-standing habit. At the minimum, smoking should be confined to set times and areas; better is the provision of a smoking cessation programme available to all patients. Illicit drug use will be an exclusion criterion for some units. However, services for dual-diagnosis adolescents are rare and so there may be real barriers to treatment for this group. Cooperation with, and support from, local substance-misuse teams will reduce the anxiety associated with these patients. A contract of regular screening can be used to good effect.

Assessment

In-patient units provide a unique opportunity for trained and experienced staff to observe patients over the 24-hour period. Reticent patients may reveal their mental state through the observations of the staff. The young person's behaviour should be considered in its own right, and in relation to their family, other young people and staff, in both structured and 'free' time, and across the day and night.

All patients require a full physical evaluation, which may include EEG, electrocardiography, blood tests, drug screens and scans. The exact protocol will depend on the history, presentation and differential diagnoses. If possible, an extended medication-free period will allow differentiation of contextual distress from psychiatric symptoms.

It is essential to pay attention to the family context, and the strengths and difficulties therein should be understood. A reported lack of educational difficulties should not be taken to exclude specific or generalised learning difficulties and formal evaluation should occur, at the minimum through the educational provision on the unit. All patients should have a documented risk assessment; this is routine in secure and forensic settings, but variable in other units. A risk matrix considers frequency (probability) and severity (dangerousness) independently. A high probability of very dangerous behaviour being displayed on the unit should prompt consideration of the appropriateness of the patient for the particular type of unit.

Treatment

Treatment begins with the engagement of the young person and the family at the point of first contact. As the results of assessments become clear, and this is an iterative process, specific interventions will be introduced. The ward milieu is not only the framework within which treatment happens, it is a therapeutic intervention in its own right (Box

22.3). Graham, our patient with Tourette syndrome and conduct disorder, will have been used to chronic rejection from other children and staff at school, and quite possibly at home. His family are probably exasperated and dejected. The recognition and praise for positive attributes and behaviours, coupled with firm, consistent and sympathetic challenging of his conduct problems by nursing and teaching staff who are in continuous contact with him, is likely to be a novel, and ultimately very positive, experience.

The integration of different aspects of treatment is the task of the whole multidisciplinary team. The objective is to find the right intensity of work so that the admission goals are reached as quickly as possible, without overwhelming the young person and the family with too many tasks, activities and ideas. Time is needed for medication to take effect, as well as to practise new skills and consolidate new thinking and behaviours. Medication is usually titrated step-wise to an effective level, pausing at each step, to allow therapeutic effects to become manifest.

All patients should have a copy of their written treatment plan. Changes or problems should be discussed with them. Most adolescents will be able to consent to treatment, but it should be remembered that a greater cognitive maturity is needed, prior to the age of majority, to decline recommended treatment. Parental refusal to consent to treatment for their child who is not able to give consent him- or herself should be considered first within the child protection framework of the Children Act 1989, before thinking of applying the Mental Health Act 1983. The reasoning for this is that if the young person is living with, or dependent upon, parents who do not consent to their treatment, there is a risk that they do not recognise, and therefore will not be able to meet, the immediate and future health needs of their son or daughter.

Discharge

Clinicians working closely with young people will always find justification for more clinical work, and are often anxious that not enough has been done to permit safe discharge. Budget holders, in contrast, may press for premature discharge, or in some cases simply run out of money. Once again, having prior agreement about the goals can minimise these problems, which can be unsettling, if not distressing, for young people and their families, caught up in what can otherwise be a seemingly arbitrary decision-making process.

All patients, regardless of their length of stay, should have a discharge planning meeting under the rubric of the CPA. This should review treatment, identifying the aspects of the in-patient treatment that seemed to contribute to a positive outcome, and also highlighting and recording those interventions that were unhelpful or adverse. An up-to-date risk assessment should be available to the network receiving the patient, and relapse predictors, intrinsic and extrinsic to the young person, listed if they are known or postulated. Ongoing treatment needs should be apparent by this stage, and the purpose of the meeting is to confirm the out-patient arrangements, not to identify needs for the first time. The same applies to educational provision and living arrangements.

Sometimes, although the needs have been clarified, no provision is available. Discharge into inadequate ongoing care raises the risk of re-emergence of problems, relapse and readmission. Unfortunately, an indefinite stay in hospital 'until a place is available' also leads to a loss of purpose and direction for the patient, the family and the staff of the unit, resulting in degradation of the ward milieu, and deterioration in quality of care for all patients. In addition, the 'blocked bed' prevents the admission of other young people. A compromise when satisfactory discharge arrangements are not in place, which is often appropriate clinically and acceptable to the network, is to offer a brief extension to the admission, subject to urgent identification of suitable after-care arrangements. The team can then work on transition into the new placement, or graduated discharge. Setting clear dates for decisions can aid in focusing the attention of external planning groups and in preventing procrastination.

Patients who have been detained 'for treatment' under the provisions of the Mental Health Act 1983 are subject to Section 117 of the Act, and a Section 117 meeting to address after-care and living arrangements, i.e. health and social need, is required. The Act stipulates joint planning and provision between agencies, and this is usually organised within the care programme approach framework. The responsibility to provide care and treatment under Section 117 does not end until there is a joint agreement between the health and social services agencies that it is no longer necessary.

Conclusion

In-patient units are scarce resources in the UK, and their use is rightly limited, for ethical and economic reasons, to young people with the most severe and complex of disorders. Although firm evidence of the clinical value of these units is lacking, there are strong indications that clarity of clinical purpose and well-planned and organised assessment and treatment are important factors in determining outcome. The low-volume, high-cost nature of available services and the lack of coherent commissioning have resulted in a serious decline in the availability of in-patient beds in the UK since the 1980s. Recent government attention to in-patient provision and a focus on child and adolescent mental health should reverse this trend.

References

American Academy of Child and Adolescent Psychiatry (2002) Practice parameter for the prevention and management of aggressive behavior in child and adolescent psychiatric institutions, with special reference to seclusion and restraint. *Journal of the American Academy of Child and Adolescent Psychiatry*, **41** (suppl. 2), 4S–25S.

Blanz, B. & Schmidt, M. H. (2000) Preconditions and outcome of inpatient treatment in child and adolescent psychiatry. *Journal of Child Psychology and Psychiatry*, **41**, 703–712.

Centre for Evidence Based Mental Health (2001) *What is the Care Programme Approach?* Oxford: Centre for Evidence Based Mental Health. http://cebmh.warne.ox.ac.uk/cebmh/elmh/nelmh/schizophrenia/guides/social/page5.html

Department of Health (1999) *Still Building Bridges. The Report of a National Inspection of Arrangements for the Integration of Care Programme Approach with Care Management*. London: Department of Health. http://www.dh.gov.uk/PublicationsAndStatistics/Publications/PublicationsInspectionReports/PublicationsInspectionReportsArticle/fs/en?CONTENT_ID=4006041&chk=Eozlvv

Maskey, S. (1998) Admission. In *Inpatient Child Psychiatry* (eds J. Green & B. Jacobs). London: Routledge.

McGorry, P. D., Chanen, A., McCarthy, E., et al (1991) Posttraumatic stress disorder following recent-onset psychosis. An unrecognized postpsychotic syndrome. *Journal of Nervous and Mental Disease*, **179**, 253–258.

Mind (2002) http://www.mind.org.uk/Information/Factsheets/Community+care/Community+Care+2+-+The+Care+Programme+Approach.htm

O'Herlihy, A. & Brook, H. (2002) *Child and Adolescent In-patient Units in England and Wales – Unit Directory*. London: Royal College of Psychiatrists' Research Unit.

O'Herlihy, A., Worrall, A., Banerjee, S., et al (2001) *National In-Patient Child and Adolescent Psychiatry Study (NICAPS)*. Final Report to the Department of Health. London: Royal College of Psychiatrists' Research Unit.

Royal College of Psychiatrists (1998) *Not Just Bricks and Mortar: Report of the Royal College of Psychiatrists' Working Party on the Size, Staffing, Structure, Siting and Security of New Acute Adult Psychiatric In-Patient Units* (Council Report CR62). London: Royal College of Psychiatrists.

Royal College of Psychiatrists (1999) *Guidance on Staffing for Child and Adolescent In-patient Psychiatry Units* (Council Report CR76). London: Royal College of Psychiatrists.

Royal College of Psychiatrists' Research Unit (2002) *Quality Network for In-patient CAMHS. Service Standards*. London: Royal College of Psychiatrists. http://www.rcpsych.ac.uk/cru/QNICStdsYr2.pdf

Williams, R. & Richardson, G. (eds) (1995) *Child and Adolescent Mental Health Services: Together We Stand*. London: HMSO.

Young, T. (1998) *The Handbook of Project Management: A Practical Guide to Effective Policies and Procedures*. London: Kogan Page.

Index

Complied by Caroline Sheard